# HANDBOOK
## OF
## DIET
## THERAPY

# HANDBOOK
# OF
# DIET
# THERAPY

DOROTHEA TURNER

THE UNIVERSITY OF CHICAGO PRESS
CHICAGO & LONDON

Written and compiled for
the American Dietetic Association


*Library of Congress Catalog Card Number: 65-24984*

THE UNIVERSITY OF CHICAGO PRESS, CHICAGO & LONDON
The University of Toronto Press, Toronto 5, Canada

# FOREWORD

It is with some understanding of the decision-making problems which need to be met in planning diets that I greet with pleasure this, the fourth edition of the *Handbook of Diet Therapy*. For this book to continue to be of timely value, it had to be rewritten with a re-evaluation of the literature in mind; but the vision and clarity of organization of the preceding editions has been retained. While continuing its emphasis on the need "of a state of nutritive sufficiency" for each of us, the book presents a commendable integration of therapeutic nutrition in terms of the individual and his individual needs.

The field of diet therapy has been flooded with a variety of diets presenting controversial ideas. The handbook, by describing dietary modifications in a commonsensical, logical manner, should eliminate the confusion that has plagued dietitians, nutritionists, and physicians. By condensing, editing, and reviewing current knowledge and practice in therapeutic nutrition, this book serves as a valuable resource.

Frequently, we receive requests from hospitals, particularly those not associated with medical centers and those which do not have a dietary teaching program, for assistance in the preparation of a hospital diet manual. It has always seemed to me that the *Handbook of Diet Therapy* should and can take care of these requests. In fact, our reply to such letters usually takes the form of a suggestion that the individual hospital manual be based on this handbook.

This latest revision offers not only an up-dating of previously included dietetic reference material, but much that is new. For example, I am pleased to see that modifications of the diet relating to phenylalanine, fat, and protein incorporate recent scientific findings. Of particular interest is the new chapter by Mildred Kaufman, "Expanding Opportunities in the Practice of Diet Therapy," in which she emphasizes the role of the dietitian and nutritionist in leading the way for the medical health team in developing the proper plan for the dietetic care of the individual. This should serve as a stimulus and a challenge to all concerned with not only the therapeutic needs of a patient, but also with the educational needs of the professional people concerned with the care of the patient.

FREDRICK J. STARE

Chairman, Department of Nutrition
Harvard School of Public Health
Boston, Massachusetts

# PREFACE

The purpose of the *Handbook of Diet Therapy* continues to be to aid in naming, defining, and describing therapeutic diets in terms of current dietetic principles. Up-to-date definitions of dietetic terminology have been included in the Revised Glossary of Dietetic Terms (1965) which appears in toto in this edition.

Since the aim of a normal dietary regimen is to maintain or to bring the patient to a state of nutritive sufficiency, it is to be expected that a therapeutic regimen should meet or exceed this goal. If a certain nutrient (sodium, for example) should be decreased for therapeutic purposes, other nutrients should remain at a level required for nutritive sufficiency. With this principle in mind, the therapeutic diet has again been regarded as a modification of the normal diet.

Therapeutic variants are largely quantitative in nature. For this reason, the normal diet and all therapeutic diets have been reassessed in quantitative terms, which will permit simple and relatively accurate modifications as well as a quick reappraisal of the over-all nutrient content. As in previous editions, a nutrient evaluation of each therapeutic diet appears as well as a sample menu pattern, and a description of the food groups and sample meals.

The changing content and bibliographies record the phenomenal growth of basic information on food composition and the use of food in therapy. New attention has been given to the 1964 revision of the *Recommended Dietary Allowances* and the greatly expanded compilations of data on many new food items. Current figures on fatty acid composition of foods, cholesterol, sodium and potassium analyses, and magnesium content of foods have been incorporated. As a result, chapters on fat modifications, protein modification, phenylalanine restriction, sodium restriction, and diabetes have been largely rewritten.

Since many important therapeutic diets require long-range changes in food habits, special attention has again been given to the patient's ability to make these changes. The chapter by Margaret Mead on "Interviewing the Patient" serves as an excellent introduction to this matter. New and relevant references have been added at the end of this chapter.

Greatly expanding facilities for health care in the nursing homes and home-care programs have brought about a vast need for improvements in the continuum of good patient care. Mildred Kaufman, in a new chapter entitled "Expanding Opportunities in the Practice of Diet Therapy," discusses the need for an informative diet history, individualized diets, frequent assessment of food intake in the hospital, education of the patient, and improvements in communications between the physicians, the patients, and all community agencies and supporting workers in the community.

The intent of the *Handbook* has been to bring together new information heretofore scattered in various sources. In so doing, it is hoped that both professional workers and students will have a convenient reference and guide for use in dietetic practice.

# CONTENTS

SECTION **III**

## INTERVIEWING THE PATIENT

SECTION **IV**

## EXPANDING OPPORTUNITIES
## IN THE PRACTICE OF DIET THERAPY

### GLOSSARY OF DIETETIC TERMS, REVISED, 1965

### INDEX

# LIST OF TABLES

# SECTION I | NORMAL DIET

Since the aim of a dietary regimen is to maintain or bring the patient to a state of nutritive sufficiency, it is logical to assume that a therapeutic diet will be planned to meet or exceed the dietary allowances for a normal individual. On the other hand, there are instances in planning a therapeutic diet in which less than the normal requirement may be indicated, as in caloric or sodium restrictions. Other nutrients, in these instances, should remain at or above the levels of the normal diet. With this principle in mind, it follows that the therapeutic diet will be planned as a modification of the normal diet.

In the organization of a plan for practical use, the first step will be to outline and appraise a basic plan of food intake for the normal dietary regimen. Since most modifications for therapeutic purposes will be of a quantitative nature, in terms of calories, protein, or other nutrients, the basic plan of normal diet will be appraised in these terms to make possible quick and easily assessed adjustments.

To achieve this goal as concisely as possible, space will not be given to itemizing and calculating individual items in a diet. Instead, a basic pattern of diet will be outlined simply in terms of commonly used food groups. With this plan, foods may be combined into groups that are comparable enough in nutrient content to permit substitution within a group. This plan has the advantage of permitting variety in choice, minimizing dietary calculations, and insuring a good nutrient content.

Four food groups have been used in amounts required to meet the protein, mineral, and vitamin recommendations for the healthy

3

individual. These four groups include the milk group, the vegetable and fruit group, the meat group, and the bread-cereal-potato-legume group. A fifth group—fats and sweets—has been considered separately, since this group adds comparatively little in protein, minerals, and vitamins but may instead be a major source of calories.

In the dietary patterns which follow, these groups have been out-lined in the amounts necessary to meet the needs of the individual during childhood, adolescence, adult life, pregnancy and lactation, and after age fifty-five. In each case a nutrient evaluation has been made of the basic diet; each food group has been described; and a sample menu pattern and sample meals have been outlined as illus-trations of the food plan.

In appraising the nutrient content of any dietary pattern, a question arises concerning the selection of figures on food composi-tion for this purpose. In the past, nutritional accounting has been based on various tables of food composition. Widdowson and McCance (1)* have pointed out that there are two extreme schools of thought concerning food tables: "One tends to regard the figures in them as having the accuracy of atomic weight determinations; the other dismisses them as valueless on the ground that a foodstuff may be so modified by the soil, the season, or its rate of growth that no figure can be a reliable guide to its composition. The truth, of course, lies somewhere between these points of view."

To meet the need for representative values suitable for use in dietary calculations, the Food and Nutrition Board, National Re-search Council, and the Bureau of Human Nutrition and Home Eco-nomics, United States Department of Agriculture, in 1945 published *Tables of Food Composition in Terms of Eleven Nutrients* (2). Subse-quent publications have now been superseded by *Composition of Foods—Raw, Processed, Prepared* (U.S. Department of Agriculture, Agriculture Handbook No. 8 [December, 1963]). Numerous foods not listed in the previous tables and different forms of food—especially frozen and cooked foods—as well as a number of foods of tropical or semitropical origin have brought the total items to nearly 2,500. In this publication, data are presented on energy,

---

* Numbers in parentheses refer to works cited in the References at the end of each chapter.

vitamins, and the minerals, calcium, phosphorus, and iron, per 100 gm. and per pound of product. New values for sodium and potassium have been incorporated together with data on selected fatty acids, cholesterol, and magnesium.

A condensed source of this information, relating to the 500 most commonly used foods in the United States, appears in the 1964 publication (3) entitled *Nutritive Value of Foods* (U.S. Department of Agriculture, Home and Garden Bulletin No. 72). In this publication items are described in common household measures and weights. For convenience these data are reproduced in Table 36.

TABLE 1

FOODS AVAILABLE FOR CONSUMPTION PER
PERSON PER WEEK (6)

Vegetables and fruit................................ 9.7 lb.
    Dark-green and deep-yellow vegetables...... 0.6 lb.
    Citrus fruit............................ 1.2 lb.
Milk, cream, cheese................................ 4.4 qt.
Eggs.......................................... 0.6 doz.
Meat, poultry, fish................................ 4.2 lb.
Separated fats and oils............................ 0.9 lb.
Sugars.......................................... 1.4 lb.
Flour, cereals, baked goods........................ 2.8 lb.

Although figures taken from these tables serve a valuable function in making values on individual food items available, it would still be a laborious task to make detailed computations of menus over a prolonged number of days, unless use were made of a shortened method of dietary calculation. One such method has been developed jointly by The American Dietetic Association, the American Diabetes Association, and the U.S. Public Health Service (4). Foods have been combined into groups roughly equivalent in nutrient content. These groups have been called Exchanges and assigned the values shown in Table 20. Since the Exchanges have come into common use in making gross assessments of carbohydrate, protein, fat, and calories, these values have been used in the tables on normal diet which follow. The mineral and vitamin contents of the food groups have been grossly estimated from appraisal of the most commonly used foods in each group.

A *menu pattern* and *sample meals* have been outlined to illustrate

## TABLE 2—EVALUATION OF A BASIC PLAN OF NORMAL DIET FOR AN ADULT (1,415–2,415 Calories; 70 Gm. Protein)

| DAILY FOOD INTAKE | QUANTITY | | CALO-RIES* | FOODSTUFFS | | | MINERALS | | | VITAMINS | | | |
| | Weight (Gm.) | Approximate Measure | | Protein* (Gm.) | Fat* (Gm.) | Carbo-hydrate* (Gm.) | Ca (Mg.) | Fe (Mg.) | A (I.U.) | Ascorbic Acid (Mg.) | Thia-mine (Mg.) | Ribo-flavin (Mg.) | Niacin (Mg.) |
|---|---|---|---|---|---|---|---|---|---|---|---|---|---|
| Milk, whole | 488 | 1 pint | 340 | 16 | 20 | 24 | 576 | 0.2 | 700 | 4 | 0.16 | 0.84 | 0.2 |
| Egg | 50 | 1 medium | 75 | 7 | 5 | ...... | 27 | 1.1 | 590 | ...... | 0.05 | 0.15 | Tr. |
| Meat, poultry, fish, cooked† | 120 | 4 oz. E.P.§ | 300 | 28 | 20 | ...... | 16 | 3.4 | 35 | ...... | 0.40 | 0.25 | 5.9 |
| Bread, whole-grain or enriched white‡ | 180 | 6 slices | 420 | 12 | ...... | 90 | 123 | 4.6 | Tr. | ...... | 0.46 | 0.31 | 4.0 |
| Cereal, whole-grain or enriched | 20 | ½ cup, cooked | 70 | 2 | ...... | 15 | 21 | 0.7 | Tr. | ...... | 0.07 | 0.05 | 0.7 |
| Potato, cooked | 100 | 1 small | 70 | 2 | ...... | 15 | 5 | 0.5 | Tr. | 16 | 0.09 | 0.03 | 1.1 |
| Vegetable (A)‖ | 150 } | 2 servings | 20 | 1 | ...... | 4 | 43 | 1.2 | 2,180 | 32 | 0.10 | 0.10 | 0.9 |
| (B)# | 50 } | | | | | | 12 | 0.5 | 1,660 | 5 | 0.03 | 0.03 | 0.4 |
| Including deep green and yellow | | | | | | | | | | | | | |
| Fruit, citrus** | 100 | 1 serving | 40 | | | 10 | 18 | 0.1 | 140 | 40 | 0.05 | 0.01 | 0.1 |
| Other fruit†† | ...... | 2 servings | 80 | | | 20 | 14 | 0.8 | 945 | 9 | 0.04 | 0.06 | 0.8 |
| Subtotal | ...... | ...... | 1,415 | 68 | 45 | 178 | 855 | 13.1 | 6,250 | 106 | 1.45 | 1.83 | 14.1 |
| Fats and oils§§ | ...... | ...... | 1,000 | | | | | | 660 | | | | |
| Sugar and sweets§§ | ...... | ...... | | | | | | | | | | | |
| Total‡‡ | ...... | ...... | 2,415‖‖ | 68 | ...... | ...... | 855 | 13.1‡‡ | 6,910 | 106 | 1.45 | 1.83 | 14.1 |

* Values for calories, carbohydrate, protein, and fat from the Food Exchange Lists Table 20, p. 000 have been used to evaluate foods and food groups.

† Weighting was adapted from *Meat Consumption Trends and Patterns* (U.S. Department of Agriculture, Agriculture Handbooks, No. 187 [Washington, D.C., July, 1960]). Weekly consumption estimated as 350 gm. beef, 280 gm. pork, 140 gm. poultry, and 70 gm. fish.

‡ 30 gm. (1 oz.) has been the weight assigned to one slice of bread in the exchange lists. It is recognized that variation is common. Adjustments should be made where usage varies.

§ Edible portion.

‖ Commonly used vegetables selected from the vegetable A group of the exchange lists were tomatoes, snap beans, spinach, asparagus, broccoli, cabbage, lettuce, and cucumber. It was estimated that these vegetables might be used 10 times weekly, averaging 150 gm. daily. Weighting was adapted from Agriculture Handbook No. 215, *Consumption, Trends, and Patterns for Vegetables* (U.S. Department of Agriculture, Economic and Statistical Analysis Division, Economic Research Service [July, 1961]).

# It was assumed that the most commonly used vegetables from the vegetable B group of the exchange lists were peas, carrots, beets, and squash. It was estimated that these vegetables might be used 4 times weekly averaging 50 gm. daily. Weighting was adapted from Agriculture Hand-book No. 215, *Consumption Trends and Patterns for Vegetables* (U.S. Department of Agriculture, Economic and Statistical Analysis Division, Economic Research Service [July, 1961]).

** Fresh orange, fresh grapefruit, canned orange juice, blended grapefruit and orange and frozen citrus juice were considered to be commonly used citrus fruits or juice. Weighting was adapted from *Consumption of Food in the United States*, Supplement for 1962 to Agriculture Handbook No. 62 (U.S. Department of Agriculture, Agricultural Marketing Service [October, 1963]).

†† Apple, banana, canned peaches, pineapple, pear, apricot, and plum were considered commonly used. Weighting was adapted from *Consumption of Food in the United States*, Supplement for 1962 to Agriculture Handbook No. 62 (U.S. Department of Agriculture, Agricultural Marketing Service [October, 1963]).

‡‡ Meets Recommended Dietary Allowances (Table 3) for an adult in good health except for iron level for women.

§§ Per capita consumption of fats and sweets has been estimated as 2 oz. separated fat or oil and 3 oz. sugar daily. *National Food Situation, NFS-108* (U.S. Department of Agriculture, Economic Research Service [May, 1964]).

‖‖ Caloric needs should be adjusted to individual requirements. For variations in need, see Table 3.

## TABLE 2A

### DESCRIPTION OF THE DAILY FOOD PLAN OF NORMAL DIET
(70 Gm. Protein, 1,415–2,415 Calories; Derived from Table 2)

| Daily Food Plan | Description |
|---|---|
| **MILK GROUP** | |
| 1 pint* | *One pint whole milk* contains 340 calories, 16 gm. protein, calcium, phosphorus, and the B complex in important amounts. One pint buttermilk made from whole milk or ½ pint evaporated milk are similar. |
| | *One pint skim milk* contains 180 calories, 18 gm. protein, and important amounts of calcium, phosphorus, and the B complex. If completely skimmed, no fat will be present, accounting for the 50 per cent decrease in calories. One pint of buttermilk made from skim milk or ½–⅔ cup (depending on brand) of non-fat milk solids is similar. |
| **MEAT GROUP†** | |
| 5 meat equivalents | *One meat equivalent* is approximately equal to 1 oz. (edible portion—weighed after cooking) beef, veal, lamb, pork, poultry, fish, cheese, or 1 egg. The five equivalents may be distributed throughout the day as desired. Liver and other variety meats are exceptional sources of vitamin A, iron, and the B complex. Four ounces of cooked meat may contain about 28 gm. protein and 300 calories. |
| **VEGETABLE AND FRUIT GROUP** | |
| 5 servings | *A dark-green or deep-yellow vegetable* is important each day for its vitamin A value. Asparagus, green beans, broccoli, carrots, green pepper, winter squash, pumpkin, and other greens make up this group. Carrots, winter squash, and pumpkin may contain about 35 calories per serving. The others will be negligible. |
| | *Other vegetables*, as beets, cabbage, cauliflower, celery, cucumber, eggplant, lettuce, mushrooms, onions, peas, tomatoes, or turnips contribute varied amounts of all nutrients. Beets, onions, peas, or turnips may contribute about 35 calories per ½ cup serving. Others will be negligible. |
| | *Citrus fruit or other fruit rich in vitamin C* is important each day. One orange or ½ cup juice, or ½ grapefruit or ½ cup juice, or 1 cup tomato juice or 1 cup strawberries or 1 cup red raspberries or ¼ cantaloupe or 1 large tangerine contains about 40 calories per serving and important amounts of vitamin C. |

\* 1 qt. of milk during last trimester of pregnancy; 1½ qts. of milk during lactation.

† If more meat is desired, 1 additional meat equivalent (edible portion—1 oz. cooked meat) may be substituted for 1 serving of the bread group without a significant change in calories. Other rearrangements or omissions should be assessed by reference to Tables 2 and 36.

| Daily Food Plan | Description |
|---|---|

**VEGETABLE AND FRUIT GROUP—*Continued***

5 servings—

*Other fruits*, such as 1 apple or 1 peach or 1 pear or 2 prunes or 4 halves apricots or 12 grapes or ½ banana, contribute varied amounts of all nutrients and contain about 40 calories per serving. For other fruits see Table 26, page 000. If sugar or syrup is added, additional calories must be calculated.

**BREAD-CEREAL-POTATO-LEGUME GROUP**

8 servings

*One serving provides approximately 70 calories*, important amounts of the B complex, and iron. One serving is equal to 1 slice enriched or whole-wheat bread, ½ cup white potato, ¼ cup sweet potato, ⅓ cup corn, ½ cup cooked macaroni, noodles, spaghetti, rice, cornmeal, or ½ cup cooked dried beans or peas, ½ cup cooked cereal, or ¾ cup flake-type cereal or 2 graham crackers. For other equivalents see Table 27, page 000.

**FATS AND SWEETS**

*Without this group* the calories for the day approximate 1,245–1,415 (depending on whether skim milk is used). The 2 oz. separated fats and oils and 3 oz. sugar available per capita in the United States would add approximately 1,000 calories. Adjustments to fit individual needs may be made as follows:

*If one level teaspoon fat or oil* is used on bread, in vegetables, or in cooking, about 45 calories may be added. One thin slice crisp bacon, 2 tablespoons light cream or 1 tablespoon heavy cream, 1 teaspoon mayonnaise or oil, 1 tablespoon cream cheese or French dressing, or 5 small olives or 6 small nuts, also contain 45 calories each.

*One level teaspoon sugar, jelly, or honey* in cooking, on cereal, in fruit, or in coffee adds 20 calories. One-half cup ice cream, pudding, or gelatin dessert may add between 150 and 300 calories, and one serving cake or pie between 300 and 700 calories (see Table 36, p. 154, for additional caloric values).

**IODIZED SALT**

Iodized salt should be used in regions where iodine is lacking. Iodized salt is especially important in adolescence and pregnancy.

MENU PATTERN AND SAMPLE MEALS—NORMAL DIET FOR AN ADULT
(70 Gm. Protein; 1,415–2,415 Calories; derived from Tables 2 and 2A)

| DAILY FOOD PLAN* | SAMPLE MENU PATTERN* | SAMPLE MEALS* |
|---|---|---|
| | **A.M.** | |
| **MILK GROUP**<br>1 pint† | ½ cup citrus fruit or juice<br>1 egg<br>1 cup cooked enriched or whole-grain cereal<br>or<br>1½ cups flake-type cereal with milk and sugar§<br>1 slice enriched or whole-grain toast with spread§<br>Coffee or tea, if desired, with sugar§ and milk | Orange juice<br>1 egg<br>1 cup farina with milk and sugar§<br>1 slice toast with spread§<br>Coffee or tea if desired |
| **MEAT GROUP**<br>5 meat equivalents‡<br>One equivalent equals 1 oz. meat (edible portion) weighed after cooking | | |
| | **Noon** | |
| **VEGETABLE AND FRUIT GROUP**<br>5 servings or more<br><br>**BREAD-CEREAL-POTATO-LEGUME GROUP**<br>8 servings‡<br><br>**FATS AND SWEETS§**<br>(Without this group the calories are approximately 1,415) | 2 oz. meat, poultry, fish, cheese, or 2 eggs‡<br>½ cup potato or substitute<br>Dark-green or deep-yellow vegetable<br>Other vegetable<br>Fruit<br>2 slices enriched or whole-grain bread or alternate* with spread§<br>Milk | Broiled chicken breast<br>Baked potato<br>Broccoli<br>Tomato and lettuce salad<br>Baked apple<br>2 small hot rolls<br>Milk |
| | **P.M.** | |
| | 2 oz. meat‡ or substitute, as at noon<br>Vegetable<br>Fruit<br>Milk<br>Enriched or whole-grain bread 2 slices or alternate* with spread§<br>Dessert§ | Vegetable soup<br>Sandwich—cheese and ham<br>Sliced fresh peaches with ice cream§<br>Milk |

* See Table 2A for alternates.

† The use of 1 pt. skim milk instead of 1 pt. whole milk will reduce the calories by 160. One quart of milk should be used daily during last trimester of pregnancy and 1½ qt. during lactation.

‡ If 1 additional meat equivalent (1 oz. E.P.) is desired, 1 serving of the bread group may be omitted with no important change in the calories. Other rearrangements or omissions should be reassessed by reference to Table 2.

§ Without sweets and fats, the diet contains about 1,415 calories. Per capita separated fats and sugar in United States average 1,000 calories. One teaspoon sugar, jelly, or honey adds 20 calories; 1 teaspoon fat or oil, 45 calories. A dessert like gelatin, ice cream, or pudding may add 150 to 300 calories. A dessert like cake or pie may add between 300 and 700 calories (see Table 36 in Appendix).

the "daily food plan" and some of the choices within each of the four food groups in the normal diet. Obviously, there is no "one" normal diet which must be consumed to insure a dietary sufficiency. Many foods may be combined in amounts which will meet individual needs. In selecting a basic plan, then, it would seem most suitable to combine commonly used foods in amounts which are the most generally acceptable.

Gross guides to the per capita consumption of food are available in the *National Food Situation* published quarterly by the Economic Research Service, U.S. Department of Agriculture, and in special reports from the Household Food Consumption Surveys, U.S. Department of Agriculture (5).

The kind and average quantity of foods available for consumption per person per week are summarized in Table 1, page 5. The nutrient evaluation by Stiebeling (6) indicated that these foods met or exceeded the Recommended Dietary Allowances (7). As such, then, they serve to suggest a framework for the basic plan.

In the basic plan of normal diet which follows (Table 2), the amounts of the milk group, the meat group, and the fruit and vegetable group closely approximate the "average diet" given in Table 1. Fats and sweets have been considered separately to permit modifications in calories, fat, and carbohydrate for various therapeutic purposes. A nutrient evaluation of the basic plan of normal diet appears in Table 2 and a menu pattern and sample meals in Tables 2A and 2B.

In setting up this framework for normal diet it is intended only that this pattern of eating be regarded as a flexible guide from which basic foods may be selected in proper amounts and with a wide variety of choice. It is not to be inferred that all individuals must use this exact allotment of foods. Modifications should be made for individuals as appropriate. A quick reassessment of nutrient content can then be made by a comparison with the basic plan in Table 2.

## REFERENCES

1. WIDDOWSON, E. M., and McCANCE, R. A. Food tables, Lancet, 1:230–32, 1943.
2. BUREAU OF HUMAN NUTRITION AND HOME ECONOMICS in cooperation with the NATIONAL RESEARCH COUNCIL. Tables of food composition in terms of eleven nutrients. (U.S. Department of Agriculture, Miscellaneous Publications, No. 572.) 1945.

3. CONSUMER AND FOOD ECONOMICS RESEARCH DIVISION. Nutritive Value of Foods. (U.S. Department of Agriculture, Agricultural Research Service Home and Garden Bulletin No. 72.) 1964.

4. CASO, E. K. Calculation of diabetic diets, J. Am. Dietet. A., **26**: 575–83, 1950.

5. Household Food Consumption Survey, 1955. (U.S. Department of Agriculture, Agricultural Research Service Reports, Nos. 1–10.) 1957.

6. STIEBELING, H. K. Food and nutrient consumption trends and consumer problems: talk at American Institute of Nutrition, Chicago. (U.S. Department of Agriculture, Agricultural Research Service. Mimeo.) 1957.

7. FOOD AND NUTRITION BOARD, NATIONAL RESEARCH COUNCIL. Recommended dietary allowances, revised, 1958. ("NAS-NRC Publications," No. 589.)

Chapter 2 | *Correlation of Basic Diet with*

| *Recommended Dietary Allowances*

 

The next step will be to compare the plan of diet with nutrient needs. Two guides to nutrient sufficiency are desirable: one for the needs in good health and one for the requirements in disease states. At the present time, only an accepted guide to the former has been established.

In 1943, the Food and Nutrition Board of the National Research Council prepared the first established guide to the needs of healthy individuals covering recommended allowances from infancy to old age (3). Subsequent revisions appeared in 1945 (4), 1948 (5), 1953 (6), 1958 (2), and again in 1964 (1). An adaptation of recently revised recommendations appears in Table 3. The following notes and excerpts accompanying this table have been taken from the National Academy of Sciences, National Research Council, Publication No. 1164 (1964).

### RECOMMENDED DIETARY ALLOWANCES
(Revised 1964)

#### PURPOSES AND INTENDED USES

The title, "Recommended Dietary Allowances," was selected in order to make it clear that the levels of nutrient intake recommended were judgments which were not to be considered final and which should be revaluated periodically as new information became available. Moreover, the use of this term was meant to avoid the misinterpretation of the allowances as representing either minimal or optimal requirements.

The allowances are designed to afford a margin of sufficiency above average physiological requirements to cover variations among essentially all individuals in the general population. They provide a buffer against the increased needs during common stresses and permit full realization of growth and productive

## TABLE 3

### RECOMMENDED DAILY DIETARY ALLOWANCES*

Designed for the maintenance of good nutrition of practically all healthy persons in the U.S.A.

(Allowances are intended for persons normally active in a temperate climate)

| Persons | Age§ (Yr.) From | up to | Wt. (Lb.) | Ht. (In.) | Food Energy† (Calories) | Protein (Gm.) | Calcium (Gm.) | Iron (Mg.) | Vitamin A (I.U.) | Thiamine (Mg.) | Riboflavin (Mg.) | Niacin Equivalent‡ (Mg.) | Ascorbic Acid (Mg.) | Vitamin D (I.U.) |
|---|---|---|---|---|---|---|---|---|---|---|---|---|---|---|
| Men | 18 | 35 | 154 | 69 | 2,900 | 70 | 0.8 | 10 | 5,000 | 1.2 | 1.7 | 19 | 70 | .... |
|  | 35 | 55 | 154 | 69 | 2,600 | 70 | .8 | 10 | 5,000 | 1.0 | 1.6 | 17 | 70 | .... |
|  | 55 | 75 | 154 | 69 | 2,200 | 70 | .8 | 10 | 5,000 | .9 | 1.3 | 15 | 70 | .... |
| Women | 18 | 35 | 128 | 64 | 2,100 | 58 | .8 | 15 | 5,000 | .8 | 1.3 | 14 | 70 | .... |
|  | 35 | 55 | 128 | 64 | 1,900 | 58 | .8 | 15 | 5,000 | .8 | 1.2 | 13 | 70 | .... |
|  | 55 | 75 | 128 | 64 | 1,600 | 58 | .8 | 10 | 5,000 | .8 | 1.2 | 13 | 70 | .... |
| Pregnant (second and third trimester) | .... | .... | .... | .... | +200 | +20 | +.5 | +5 | +1,000 | +.2 | +.3 | +3 | +30 | 400 |
| Lactating | .... | .... | .... | .... | +1,000 | +40 | +.5 | +5 | +3,000 | +.4 | +.6 | +7 | +30 | 400 |
| Infants‖ | 0 | 1 | 18 | .... | lb.×52±7 | lb.×1.1±0.2 |  | lb.×0.45 | 1,500 | .4 | .6 | .... | 30 | 400 |
| Children | 1 | 3 | 29 | 34 | 1,300 | 32 | .7 | 8 | 2,000 | .5 | .8 | 9 | 40 | 400 |
|  | 3 | 6 | 40 | 42 | 1,600 | 40 | .8 | 10 | 2,500 | .6 | .8 | 11 | 50 | 400 |
|  | 6 | 9 | 53 | 49 | 2,100 | 52 | .8 | 12 | 3,500 | .8 | 1.0 | 14 | 60 | 400 |
| Boys | 9 | 12 | 72 | 55 | 2,400 | 60 | 1.1 | 15 | 4,500 | 1.0 | 1.3 | 16 | 70 | 400 |
|  | 12 | 15 | 98 | 61 | 3,000 | 75 | 1.4 | 15 | 5,000 | 1.2 | 1.4 | 20 | 80 | 400 |
|  | 15 | 18 | 134 | 68 | 3,400 | 85 | 1.4 | 15 | 5,000 | 1.4 | 1.8 | 22 | 80 | 400 |
| Girls | 9 | 12 | 72 | 55 | 2,200 | 55 | 1.1 | 15 | 4,500 | .9 | 1.3 | 15 | 80 | 400 |
|  | 12 | 15 | 103 | 62 | 2,500 | 62 | 1.3 | 15 | 5,000 | 1.0 | 1.5 | 17 | 80 | 400 |
|  | 15 | 18 | 117 | 64 | 2,300 | 58 | 1.3 | 15 | 5,000 | .9 | 1.3 | 15 | 70 | 400 |

* Source: Adapted from Recommended Dietary Allowances, Publication 1146, 59 pp., revised 1964. Published by National Academy of Sciences—National Research Council, Washington, D.C., 20418. Price $1.00. Also available in libraries. The allowance levels are intended to cover individual variations among most normal persons as they live in the United States under usual environmental stresses (3).

† Tables 4 and 5 and figures 1 and 2 show calorie adjustments for weight and age.

‡ Niacin equivalents include dietary sources of the preformed vitamin and the precursor, tryptophan. 60 milligrams tryptophan represent 1 milligram niacin.

§ Entries on lines for age range 18 to 35 years represent the 25-year age period. All other entries represent allowances for the midpoint of the specified age periods, i.e., line for children 1 to 3 is for age 2 years (24 months); 3 to 6 is for age 4½ years (54 months), etc.

‖ The calcium and protein allowances per pound for infants are considered to decrease progressively from birth. Allowances for calcium, thiamine, riboflavin, and niacin increase proportionately with calories to the maximum values shown.

NOTE.—The Recommended Daily Dietary Allowances should not be confused with Minimum Daily Requirements. The Recommended Dietary Allowances are amounts of nutrients recommended by the Food and Nutrition Board of National Research Council, and are considered adequate for maintenance of good nutrition in healthy persons in the United States. The allowances are revised from time to time in accordance with newer knowledge of nutritional needs.

The Minimum Daily Requirements are the amounts of various nutrients that have been established by the Food and Drug Administration as standards for labeling purposes of foods and pharmaceutical preparations for special dietary uses. These are the amounts regarded as necessary in the diet for the prevention of deficiency diseases and generally are less than the Recommended Dietary Allowances. The Minimum Daily Requirements are set forth in the Federal Register (Nov. 22, 1941), beginning on p. 5921, and amended as stated in the Federal Register (June 1, 1957), 22, No. 106, p. 3841.
See Table 46.

potential: *but they are not to be considered adequate to meet additional requirements of persons depleted by disease or traumatic stresses.*

Actual nutritional status of groups of people or individuals must be judged on the basis of physical, biochemical, and clinical observations on food and nutrient intakes. If the recommended allowances are used as reference standards for interpreting records of food consumption, it should not be assumed that malnutrition exists because the recommendations are not completely met.

The margin of sufficiency above normal physiological requirements is different for each nutrient because of differences in the body storage capacity, in the range of individual requirements, in the precision of assessing requirements, and in the possible hazard of excessive intake of certain nutrients.

The scientific bases for the revised Recommended Dietary Allowances appear in the text of the original report as well as a discussion of essential nutrients not tabulated. In addition, dietary allowances and standards for adults developed by other countries, by the Food and Agriculture Organization, and jointly by the Food and Agriculture Organization and the World Health Organization have been tabulated, including the differences in objectives.

TABLE 4*

DESIRABLE WEIGHTS FOR HEIGHT

| Height† (Inches) | Weight† in Pounds | |
| --- | --- | --- |
| | Men | Women |
| 60. | . . . . . . . . . . . . | 109 ± 9 |
| 62. | . . . . . . . . . . . . | 115 ± 9 |
| 64. | 133 ± 11 | 122 ± 10 |
| 66. | 142 ± 12 | 129 ± 10 |
| 68. | 151 ± 14 | 136 ± 10 |
| 70. | 159 ± 14 | 144 ± 11 |
| 72. | 167 ± 15 | 152 ± 12 |
| 74. | 175 ± 15 | . . . . . . . . . . . . |

* Modified from Table 80, Hathaway and Ford, 1960, *Height and Weight of Adults in the U.S.* (Home Economics Research Report, No. 10, ARS, USDA.)

† Heights and weights are "without shoes and other clothing." To convert inches to centimeters, multiply by 2.54. To convert pounds to kilograms, multiply by 0.454.

## SCIENTIFIC BASES FOR THE RECOMMENDED
## ALLOWANCES OF CALORIES

The present revision continues to utilize the device of the "reference" man or woman. As in the 1958 revision, the "reference" man is 25 years old and weighs 70 kg. The "reference" woman is 25 years of age and weighs 58 kg. Both the man and woman are presumed to live in an environment with a mean temperature of 20° C. They are considered to be "moderately" active physically, with occupations that could be described neither as sedentary nor as hard physical labor. The allowance for the "reference" man is 2,900 calories and the woman, 2,100 calories.

Adjustments must be made when individuals or population averages differ from the "reference" in characteristics of age, body size, or activity. Procedures for these adjustments are described below.

*Age.*—Energy requirements decline progressively after the years of early adulthood because of a decrease in basal metabolic rate as well as lessened physical activity. It is proposed that caloric allowances be reduced by 5 per cent per decade between ages 35 and 55, and by 8 per cent per decade from ages 55 up to 75. A further decrement of 10 per cent is recommended for age 75 and the years beyond.

*Body Size.*—In adapting allowances for differences in size, weight may be used as a basis provided the subjects are not overweight or underweight.

TABLE 5

ADJUSTMENT OF CALORIE ALLOWANCES FOR ADULT INDI-
VIDUALS OF VARIOUS BODY WEIGHTS AND AGES*

| DESIRABLE WEIGHT | | CALORIE ALLOWANCE† | | |
|---|---|---|---|---|
| Kilograms | Pounds | 25 Years | 45 Years | 65 Years |
| | | Men | | |
| | | (1) | (2) | (3) |
| 50.......... | 110 | 2,300 | 2,050 | 1,750 |
| 55.......... | 121 | 2,450 | 2,200 | 1,850 |
| 60.......... | 132 | 2,600 | 2,350 | 1,950 |
| 65.......... | 143 | 2,750 | 2,500 | 2,100 |
| 70.......... | 154 | 2,900 | 2,600 | 2,200 |
| 75.......... | 165 | 3,050 | 2,750 | 2,300 |
| 80.......... | 176 | 3,200 | 2,900 | 2,450 |
| 85.......... | 187 | 3,350 | 3,050 | 2,550 |
| | | Women | | |
| | | (4) | (5) | (6) |
| 40.......... | 88 | 1,600 | 1,450 | 1,200 |
| 45.......... | 99 | 1,750 | 1,600 | 1,300 |
| 50.......... | 110 | 1,900 | 1,700 | 1,450 |
| 55.......... | 121 | 2,000 | 1,800 | 1,550 |
| 58.......... | 128 | 2,100 | 1,900 | 1,600 |
| 60.......... | 132 | 2,150 | 1,950 | 1,650 |
| 65.......... | 143 | 2,300 | 2,050 | 1,750 |
| 70.......... | 154 | 2,400 | 2,200 | 1,850 |

Formulas

(1) $725+31W$  (2) $650+28W$  (3) $550+23.5W$
(4) $525+27W$  (5) $475+24.5W$  (6) $400+20.5W$
$W$ = weight in kg.

* At a mean environmental temperature of 20° C (68° F) assuming average physical activity.

† Values have been rounded to nearest 50 calories. To convert formulas for weight in pounds, divide factor by 2.2.

Actuarial statistics and other data indicate that the most favorable health expectation is associated with conditions under which weight as normally achieved by age 25 is maintained throughout life. Table 4 may be used as a guide for this adjustment. Heights and weights as recorded are without shoes and clothing. Adjustment of caloric allowances for individuals whose weight and height are different from those of the reference man and woman is illustrated in Table 5. Figures 1 and 2 are designed to be helpful in calorie adjustment for *children* of varying size and age.

*Pregnancy and Lactation.*—Additional calories are needed to meet the energy costs of pregnancy. It is proposed that daily allowances be increased by 200 calories during the second and third trimesters. Some women, however, may so reduce physical activity during the third trimester that the extra demands for calories may be largely compensated without the addition of food calories. The suitability of the allowance for the individual woman should be evaluated at frequent intervals by a physician, nurse, or nutritionist.

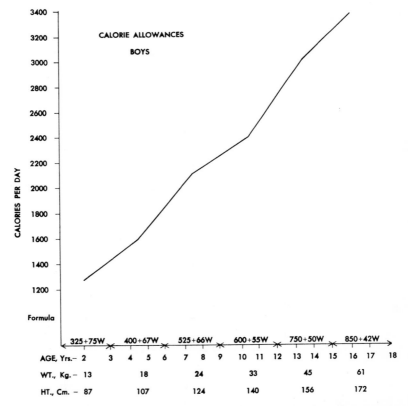

FIG. 1.—Calorie allowances for boys by age and formulas for adjustment by weight. *W* in formulas is weight in kilograms. To convert formulas for weight in pounds, divide factor by 2.2.

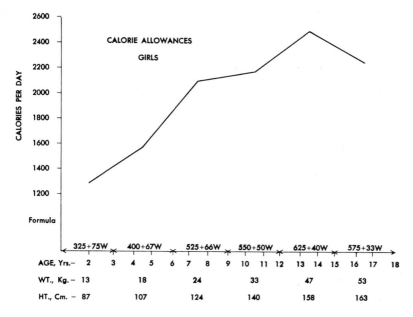

FIG. 2.—Calorie allowances for girls by age, and formulas for adjustment by weight. $W$ in formulas is weight in kilograms. To convert formulas for weight in pounds, divide factor by 2.2.

TABLE 6

ARBITRARY EXAMPLES OF ENERGY EXPENDITURE
BY REFERENCE MAN AND WOMAN

| ACTIVITY | TIME (HRS.) | MAN | | WOMAN | |
|---|---|---|---|---|---|
| | | Rate (Cals/Min) | Total | Rate (Cals/Min) | Total |
| Sleeping* and lying... | 8 | 1.1 | 540 | 1.0 | 480 |
| Sitting† | 6 | 1.5 | 540 | 1.1 | 420 |
| Standing‡ | 6 | 2.5 | 900 | 1.5 | 540 |
| Walking§ | 2 | 3.0 | 360 | 2.5 | 300 |
| Other‖ | 2 | 4.5 | 540 | 3.0 | 360 |
| | | | 2,880 | | 2,100 |

* Essentially basal metabolic rate plus some allowance for turning over or getting up or down.

† Includes normal activity carried on while sitting, e.g., reading, driving automobile, eating, playing cards, and desk or bench work.

‡ Includes normal indoor activities while standing and walking spasmodically in limited area, e.g., personal toilet, moving from one room to another, etc.

§ Includes purposeful walking, largely outdoors, e.g., home to commuting station to work site, and other comparable activities.

‖ Includes spasmodic activities in occasional sports, exercises, limited stair climbing or occupational activities involving light physical work. This category may include week-end swimming, golf, tennis, or picnics using 5–20 cals. per min. for limited time.

The increased requirements of lactation are proportional to the quantity of milk produced. Approximately 120 calories for each 100 ml. of milk produced is suggested. Assuming an average milk yield of 650 ml. per day for between one and four months, it is proposed that an additional allowance of 1000 calories per day be afforded. If in the post-partum period the mother increases her activity through the care of the infant and the return to household duties, an additional caloric allowance will be necessary, whether breast feeding takes place or not.

*Infants, Children, and Adolescents.*—During the first year of life caloric allowances are reduced in suitable steps from a level of 130 calories per kg. at birth to 100 calories per kg. at the end of the year. There are wide individual variation in physical activity in infants and children. Allowances in Figures 1 and 2 and in the tabulated recommendations pertain to children of average activity in the United States. More appropriate allowances for individual children may be derived by observation of growth, appetite, activity, and body fatness.

*Activity.*—Although physical activity is the major variable affecting caloric requirements, no simple procedure has been derived for estimating caloric allowances in relation to energy expenditure. Arbitrary examples of energy expenditure by the reference man and reference woman are given in Table 6. Persons engaged in heavy labor will have increased requirements; but will probably need no more than 25 per cent above the standard allowance. In the United States it is more common to encounter persons with reduced requirements because of a relatively sedentary existence. There is evidence that inactive persons tend to consume more calories than they need to remain in energy balance. Proper caloric balance for an individual is that which will maintain body weight and health at a level most conducive to his well-being.

*Protein, Minerals, and Vitamins.*—The bases for the selection in these categories have been discussed in some detail in the original publication. (See National Academy of Sciences, National Research Council, Publication No. 1146 [1964]).

## REFERENCES

1. FOOD AND NUTRITION BOARD, NATIONAL RESEARCH COUNCIL. Recommended dietary allowances, revised, 1964. ("NAS-NRC Publications," No. 1146.)

2. ———. Recommended dietary allowances, revised, 1958. ("NAS-NRC Publications," No. 589.)

3. NATIONAL RESEARCH COUNCIL. Recommended dietary allowances. ("National Research Council Reprint and Circular Series," No. 115.) 1943.

4. ———. Recommended dietary allowances, revised, 1945. ("National Research Council Reprint and Circular Series," No. 122.)

5. ———. Recommended dietary allowances, revised, 1948. ("National Research Council Reprint and Circular Series," No. 129.)

6. ———. Recommended dietary allowances, revised, 1953. ("National Research Council Reprint and Circular Series," No. 302.)

Chapter 3 | *Modification of Basic Diet at*

*Various Phases of Life*

DIET DURING PREGNANCY AND LACTATION

There is an increased need above the normal maintenance allowances for protein, minerals, vitamins, and calories during pregnancy and lactation. (See Table 3 from *Recommended Dietary Allowances*, 6th Revised Edition, 1964 [1].)

*During pregnancy increased energy needs* arise due to the building of new tissue in placenta and fetus, the increased work load associated with the movement of the mother, and the increase in basal metabolic rate in the second and third trimesters. It is suggested in the Recommended Dietary Allowances that 200 calories per day be added to meet this need. The suitability of this allowance should be evaluated at frequent intervals by a physician, nurse, or nutritionist.

*During lactation, the increase in energy requirements* is proportional to the quantity of milk produced. Since this varies widely for each individual, adjustment may be made by approximating 120 calories for each 100 ml. of milk produced. Assuming an average milk yield of 850 ml. per day for between one and four months, it is proposed that an allowance of 1,000 calories per day be afforded during the period of lactation.

In the post-partum period the mother may increase her activities by the care of the infant and return to household duties. If such an increase occurs, additional calories should be provided whether breast feeding takes place or not.

*Increases in protein need* come about as a result of the growth of the fetus and accessory tissues. Although evidence for a high protein diet is limited, the Food and Nutrition Board recommends an addi-

19

## TABLE 7

### NUTRIENT CONTENT OF DIET FOR USE DURING PREGNANCY AND LACTATION‡‡
#### (Protein 82 Gm.; Calories 1,645–2,645)

| DAILY FOOD INTAKE | QUANTITY Weight (Gm.) | Approximate Measure# | CALORIES** | FOODSTUFFS Protein (Gm.)‖ | Fat (Gm.)‖ | Carbohydrate (Gm.)‖ | MINERALS Ca (Mg.) | Fe (Mg.) | VITAMINS A (I.U.) | Ascorbic Acid (Mg.) | Thiamine (Mg.) | Riboflavin (Mg.) | Niacin (Mg.) |
|---|---|---|---|---|---|---|---|---|---|---|---|---|---|
| Milk, whole† | 976 | 1 quart | 680 | 32 | 40 | 48 | 1,152 | 0.4 | 1,400 | 8 | 0.32 | 1.68 | 0.4 |
| Egg | 50 | 1 medium | 75 | 7 | 5 | ...... | 27 | 1.1 | 590 | ...... | 0.05 | 0.15 | Tr. |
| Meat, poultry, or fish, cooked* | 120 | 4 oz. edible portion | 300 | 28 | 20 | ...... | 16 | 3.4 | 35 | ...... | 0.40 | 0.25 | 5.9 |
| Bread, whole-grain or enriched white† | 150 | 5 slices | 350 | 10 | ...... | 75 | 103 | 3.7 | Tr. | ...... | 0.37 | 0.25 | 3.2 |
| Cereal, whole-grain or enriched white | 20 | ½ cup | 70 | 2 | ...... | 15 | 21 | 0.7 | Tr. | ...... | 0.07 | 0.05 | 0.7 |
| Potato, cooked | 100 | 1 small | 70 | 2 | ...... | 15 | 5 | 0.5 | Tr. | ...... | 0.09 | 0.03 | 1.1 |
| Vegetable (A)‡ | 150 } | 2 servings | 20 | 1 | ...... | 4 | 43 | 1.2 | 2,180 | 16 | 0.10 | 0.10 | 0.9 |
|     (B)§ | 50 } | | ...... | ...... | ...... | ...... | 12 | 0.5 | 1,660 | 5 | 0.03 | 0.03 | 0.4 |
| Including green and yellow | | | | | | | | | | | | | |
| Fruit, citrus | 100 | 1 serving | 40 | ...... | ...... | 10 | 18 | 0.1 | 140 | 40 | 0.05 | 0.01 | 0.1 |
| Fruit, other‖ | ...... | 1 serving | 40 | ...... | ...... | 10 | 7 | 0.4 | 473 | 5 | 0.02 | 0.03 | 0.4 |
| Subtotal | ...... | ...... | 1,645 | 82 | 65 | 177 | 1,494 | 12.0 | 6,478 | 106 | 1.50 | 2.58 | 13.1 |
| Vitamin D concentrate‡‡ | ...... | ...... | ...... | ...... | ...... | ...... | ...... | ...... | ...... | ...... | ...... | ...... | ...... |
| Separated fats and sweets† | ...... | ...... | 1,000 | ...... | ...... | ...... | ...... | ...... | 660 | ...... | ...... | ...... | ...... |
| Total§§ | ...... | ...... | 2,645 | 82 | 65 | 177 | 1,404 | 12.0§§ | 7,138 | 106 | 1.50 | 2.58 | 13.1 |

* Estimate based on weekly consumption of 350 gm. beef, 280 gm. pork, 70 gm. fish, and 140 gm. poultry. *Meat Consumption Trends and Patterns* (U.S. Department of Agriculture, Agricultural Marketing Service, Agricultural Economics Division, Agriculture Handbook, No. 187 [Washington, D.C., July, 1960]).

† Each slice of bread has been considered to weigh 30 gm. (1 oz.) as in the values assigned to the exchange lists. It is recognized, however, that sliced bread may range between 20 and 30 gm. in weight. Adjustments should be made where usage varies.

‡ In making this estimate, it was considered that the commonly used vegetables A, tomatoes, snap beans, spinach, asparagus, broccoli, cabbage, lettuce, and cucumber, might be used 10 times weekly. Weighting was adapted from Agriculture Handbook, No. 215, *Consumption Trends and Patterns for Vegetables* (U.S. Department of Agriculture, Economic and Statistical Analysis Division, Economic Research Service [July, 1961]).

§ It was assumed that the most commonly used vegetables were peas, carrots, beets, and squash. It was estimated that these vegetables might be used 4 times weekly averaging 50 gm. daily. Weighting was adapted from Agriculture Handbook, No. 215, *Consumption Trends and Patterns for Vegetables* (U.S. Department of Agriculture, Economic and Statistical Analysis Division, Economic Research Service [July, 1961]).

‖ Apples, bananas, canned peaches, pineapples, pears, apricots, and plums were considered commonly used. Weighting was adapted from *Consumption of Food in the United States*, Supplement for 1962 to Agriculture Handbook, No. 62 (U.S. Department of Agriculture, Agricultural Marketing Service [October, 1961]).

# Weights and measures assigned to the Exchanges are indicated in Tables 21–29.

** Calories are rounded off to the nearest 5.

†† Per capita consumption of fats and sweets has been estimated as 2 oz. separated fat or oil and 3 oz. sugar daily. *National Food Situation, NFS-108* (U.S. Department of Agriculture, Economic Research Service [May, 1964]).

‡‡ 400–800 I.U. vitamin D may be obtained from fortified milk or a concentrate. During lactation 1½ quarts of milk should be used to provide extra protein and other nutrient levels proposed in the Recommended Dietary Allowances (Table 3). The use of skim milk would reduce the calories in 1 quart by approximately 340.

§§ The total minerals, vitamins, and protein will approximate the recommended dietary allowances (Table 3), with the exception of iron. Liver and other iron-rich foods may be used to augment this level. Caloric needs should be adjusted to the individual.

‖ Values for calories, carbohydrate, protein, and fat from the Food Exchange Lists, Table 20, p. 000, have been used to evaluate foods and food groups.

MENU PATTERN AND SAMPLE MEALS DURING PREGNANCY AND LACTATION†
(82 Gm. Protein and 1,645–2,645 Calories; Derived from Table 7)

| DAILY FOOD PLAN‡ | SAMPLE MENU PATTERN‡ | SAMPLE MEALS‡ |
|---|---|---|
| | **A.M.** | |
| **MILK GROUP** | | |
| 1 qt. whole milk# | 1 citrus fruit or ½ cup juice | ½ grapefruit |
| | ½ cup cooked cereal or ¾ cup flake-type with milk and sugar§ | ¾ cup flakes with milk and sugar§ |
| **MEAT GROUP** | 1 slice enriched or whole-grain toast with spread§ | 1 slice toast with spread§ |
| | Milk—1 glass | Milk—1 glass |
| 5 ounces or equivalent‖ Cooked beef, pork, veal, lamb, poultry or fish | | |
| | **Noon** | |
| **VEGETABLE AND FRUIT GROUP** | 2 oz. meat, poultry, fish, cheese or 2 eggs‖ | Sandwich: |
| 4 servings or more | Vegetable | 2 slices meat |
| A dark-green or deep-yellow vegetable daily for vitamin A value | 2 slices enriched or whole-grain bread or substitute | 2 slices bread Sliced tomatoes and |
| A citrus fruit or other fruit rich in vitamin C daily | Milk—1 glass | lettuce Milk—1 glass |
| | **P.M.** | |
| **BREAD-CEREAL-POTATO-LEGUME GROUP** | | |
| 7 servings | 3 oz. meat,‖ poultry, fish or substitute | Meat loaf Baked potato |
| | ½ cup potato or substitute | Asparagus tips |
| | Dark-green or deep-yellow vegetable | Cabbage slaw Fresh strawberries |
| **FATS AND SWEETS** | Other vegetable | 2 hot rolls with |
| (Without this group the diet contains 1,645 calories) | Fruit 2 slices enriched or whole-grain bread with spread§ or substitute | spread§ Milk—1 glass |
| 10 teaspoons fat or oil contain 450 calories | Milk—1 glass | |
| 10 teaspoons sugar, jelly, or honey contain 200 calories | **Between** | |
| **Vitamin D#** | Milk—1 glass | Milk—1 glass |

\* The Recommended Dietary Allowances (Table 3) during pregnancy may be met by this pattern, with the exception of iron. Liver and other iron rich foods may be used to augment this level.

† During lactation 1½ quarts of milk per day would provide the extra protein and other nutrients required to meet the Recommended Dietary Allowances.

‡ For alternates within each food group see Tables 21–29.

§ 1 teaspoon sugar adds 20 calories; 1 teaspoon fat or oil adds 45 calories. Desserts like ice cream, pudding, and gelatin may add 150–300 calories. For additional caloric values see Table 36. Adjustments in this group should be made to suit caloric needs of the individual patient.

‖ If additional meat is desired, one serving of the bread group (as 1 slice bread) may be omitted for each 1 oz. meat added, without changing the caloric value or reducing nutrient content. Other rearrangements or omissions should be assessed by reference to the values in Table 7.

# The use of skim milk would reduce calories in 1 quart of milk by 360.
If 400 I.U. of vitamin D is not contained in 1 quart of milk a concentrate should be prescribed.

tional allowance of 20 gm. protein per day above the normal requirement. It is noted, however, that normal gestation seems to occur with less than this added amount.

The protein requirement for lactation may be estimated from the fact that a liter of breast milk contains approximately 12 gm. protein. If the efficiency of conversion of dietary protein to milk protein approaches 50 per cent, an additional requirement of 25 gm. might be projected. Since milk production may actually exceed a liter per day, the Recommended Dietary Allowances indicate an additional 40 gm. protein during lactation. It is recognized that lower protein intakes are common in other parts of the world and that acceptable growth occurs during the first six months of life. Whether continuous low levels of protein intake are detrimental to the mother is not clear.

These recommendations for increased protein and other nutrients may be met, with the exception of iron, by adding to the basic dietary plan for the normal diet 1 pint of milk during pregnancy and 1 quart of milk during lactation. Without the fats and sweets, the basic dietary pattern indicated in Table 7 will approximate 1,645 calories and 82 grams of protein. A further reduction of 340 calories may be attained with the use of skim milk. If the milk is not fortified with 400 International Units vitamin D per quart, an additional supplement should be prescribed. An example of a menu pattern together with sample meals is indicated in Table 7A. Any modifications in the kind and amount of foods or food groups in a resultant diet may be reassessed by reference to Table 7.

#### DIETS DURING INFANCY, CHILDHOOD, AND ADOLESCENCE

Relatively more calories, protein, minerals, and vitamins are recommended per unit of weight during the growth period of an individual. A wide range of normality exists in the development pattern. Data on heights and weights of children and youth in the United States have been compiled by Hathaway (2). The compilation includes general tables giving height-weight data from research studies on children and youth from thirty-four states and the District of Columbia; height-weight standards used in appraisal of growth and nutritional status; special tables relating height-weight-age data to some factors affecting growth patterns; and an annotated list of references, which furnishes pertinent details of methodology and supplementary information concerning the studies from which data have been quoted. Mean figures indicating height and weight appear in Table 3.

*Allowances for energy needs of infants* during the first year range from 130 calories per kg. at birth to 100 calories per kg. by the end of the year. There are wide individual variations in physical activity in both infants and children. Inactive children may become obese with less than these allowances; very active children may require more. For this reason much caution should be used in selecting a value for any one individual.

Major differences in growth rates between boys and girls after age nine also contribute to wide individual differences. Appropriate allowances for individual children must be derived from observation of growth, appetite, activity, and body fatness. Figures 1 and 2, pages 16 and 17, may be used as a general guide to caloric adjustments for body size.

*Protein need* during growth must be relatively higher than that of the adult to provide for the formation of new tissues. The evidence from studies of young children indicates that their protein metabolism is similar to that of the adult except for the larger amount required for growth.

The protein allowances proposed for children after infancy provide approximately 10 per cent of the caloric intake as protein. The dietary protein ordinarily comes from a variety of sources including 25 to 50 per cent of the total from animal sources or other high quality protein. This can be expected to provide approximately twice the minimal need for the average child and allow a reasonable margin for growth. The bases for the Recommended Dietary Allowances for minerals and vitamins, fats and carbohydrates are discussed in the text of Publication 1146, *A Report of the Food and Nutrition Board*, 6th revised edition, 1964 (National Academy of Sciences, National Research Council).

Although the relative amounts of each food consumed will vary during the child's developmental period, the selection of food is derived ordinarily from the commonly consumed foods and food groups indicated in the basic dietary patterns. For example, the Recommended Daily Allowances for protein indicate a variation in

## TABLE 8

### Nutrient Content of Diet for Child Between Four and Six Years of Age

(64 Gm. Protein; 1,355–1,700 Calories)

| Daily Food Intake | Quantity — Weight (Gm.) | Quantity — Approximate Measure# | Calories** | Foodstuffs — Protein (Gm.)‖‖ | Foodstuffs — Fat (Gm.)‖‖ | Foodstuffs — Carbohydrate (Gm.)‖‖ | Minerals — Ca (Mg.) | Minerals — Fe (Mg.) | Vitamins — A (I.U.) | Vitamins — Ascorbic Acid (Mg.) | Vitamins — Thiamine (Mg.) | Vitamins — Riboflavin (Mg.) | Vitamins — Niacin (Mg.) |
|---|---|---|---|---|---|---|---|---|---|---|---|---|---|
| Milk, whole | 976 | 1 quart | 680 | 32 | 40 | 48 | 1,152 | 0.4 | 1,400 | 8 | 0.32 | 1.68 | 0.4 |
| Egg | 50 | 1 medium | 75 | 7 | 5 | … | 27 | 1.1 | 590 | … | 0.05 | 0.15 | Tr. |
| Meat, poultry, or fish, cooked* | 60 | 2 oz. edible portion | 150 | 14 | 10 | … | 8 | 1.7 | 18 | … | 0.20 | 0.13 | 3.0 |
| Bread, whole-grain or enriched white† | 90 | 3 slices | 210 | 6 | … | 45 | 62 | 2.3 | Tr. | … | 0.23 | 0.16 | 2.0 |
| Cereal, whole-grain or enriched | | | | | | | | | | | | | |
| Potato, cooked | 20 | ½ cup | 70 | 2 | … | 15 | 21 | 0.7 | Tr. | … | 0.07 | 0.05 | 0.7 |
| Vegetable (A)‡ | 100 | 1 small | 70 | 2 | … | 15 | 5 | 0.5 | Tr. | 16 | 0.09 | 0.03 | 1.1 |
| Vegetable (B)§ | 150 | 2 servings | 20 | 1 | … | 4 | 43 | 1.2 | 2,180 | 32 | 0.10 | 0.10 | 0.9 |
| Including green and yellow | 50 | | | | | | 12 | 0.5 | 1,660 | 5 | 0.03 | 0.03 | 0.4 |
| Fruit, citrus | 100 | 1 serving | 40 | … | … | 10 | 18 | 0.1 | 140 | 40 | 0.05 | 0.01 | 0.1 |
| Fruit, other‖ | 100 | 1 serving | 40 | … | … | 10 | 7 | 0.4 | 473 | 5 | 0.02 | 0.03 | 0.4 |
| Vitamin D concentrate§§ | | | | | | | | | | | | | |
| Separated fats and sweets†† | | | | | | | | | | | | | |
| Total‡‡ | | | 1,355 | 64 | 55 | 147 | 1,355 | 8.9‡‡ | 6,461 | 106 | 1.16 | 2.37 | 9.0 |

* Estimate based on weekly consumption of 175 gm. beef, 140 gm. pork, 35 gm. fish, and 70 gm. poultry. *Meat Consumption Trends and Patterns* (U.S. Department of Agriculture, Agricultural Marketing Service, Agricultural Economics Division, Agriculture Handbook, No. 187 [Washington, D.C., July 1960]).

† Each slice of bread has been considered to weigh 30 gm. (1 oz.) as in the values assigned to the exchange lists. Sliced bread, however, may range between 20 and 30 gm. in weight. Adjustments should be made where usage varies.

‡ In making this estimate, it was considered that the commonly used vegetables A, tomatoes, snap beans, spinach, asparagus, broccoli, cabbage, lettuce, and cucumber, might be used 10 times weekly. Weighting was adapted from Agriculture Handbook, No. 215, *Consumption Trends and Patterns for Vegetables* (U.S. Department of Agriculture, Economic and Statistical Analysis Division, Economic Research Service [July, 1961]).

§ It was assumed that the most commonly used vegetables from the vegetable B group of the exchange lists were peas, carrots, beets, and squash. It was estimated that these vegetables might be used 4 times weekly averaging 50 gm. daily. Weighting was adapted from Agriculture Hand-

book, No. 215, *Consumption Trends and Patterns for Vegetables* (U.S. Department of Agriculture, Economic and Statistical Analysis Division, Economic Research Service [July, 1961]).

‖ Apples, bananas, canned peaches, pineapples, pears, apricots, and plums were considered commonly used. Weighting was adapted from *Consumption of Food in the United States*, Supplement for 1962 to Agriculture Handbook No. 62, U.S. Department of Agriculture (Agricultural Marketing Service [October, 1963]).

# Weights and measures assigned to the Exchanges are indicated in Tables 21–29.

** Calories are rounded off to the nearest 5.

†† 1 teaspoon sugar adds 20 calories; 1 teaspoon fat or oil adds 45 calories. Such desserts as ice cream, pudding, and gelatin may add 150–300 calories. For additional caloric values see Table 36.

‡‡ Meets Recommended Dietary Allowances (Table 3) for child in good health except for iron.

§§ 400–800 I.U. vitamin D may be obtained from fortified milk or a concentrate.

‖‖ Values for calories, carbohydrate, protein, and fat from the Food Exchange Lists, Table 20,

# TABLE 8A

## MENU PATTERN AND SAMPLE MEALS FOR CHILD BETWEEN FOUR AND SIX YEARS OF AGE

(64 Gm. Protein; 1,355–1,700 Calories; Derived from Table 8)

| DAILY FOOD PLAN* | SAMPLE MENU PATTERN* | SAMPLE MEALS* |
|---|---|---|
| | **A.M.** | |
| MILK GROUP | | |
| 1 qt. milk | 1 citrus fruit or ½ cup juice<br>½ cup cereal with sugar‡<br>1 slice toast with spread‡<br>1 glass milk | Orange juice<br>Enriched farina with sugar‡<br>Toast with spread‡<br>1 glass milk |
| MEAT GROUP | | |
| 3 equivalents† | | |
| (One equivalent is equal to 1 oz. cooked beef, veal, pork, lamb, liver, poultry, fish, cheese or one egg) | **Noon** | |
| | 2 oz. meat, poultry, fish, cheese or 2 eggs<br>½ cup potato or substitute<br>Dark-green or deep-yellow vegetable<br>Dessert‡<br>1 slice enriched or whole-grain bread with spread‡<br>Milk—1 glass | Broiled ground beef<br>Baked potato<br>Carrot rings<br>Ice cream<br>Bread with spread‡<br>Milk—1 glass |
| VEGETABLE AND FRUIT GROUP | | |
| 4 servings<br>A dark-green or deep-yellow vegetable is important for vitamin A<br>A citrus fruit or other fruit rich in vitamin C is important daily | **P.M.** | |
| BREAD-CEREAL-POTATO-LEGUME GROUP | 1 egg or 1 oz. cheese, meat, poultry, or fish<br>Vegetables, raw or cooked<br>Fruit<br>1 slice enriched or whole-grain bread with spread‡<br>Milk—1 glass | Liver in tomato sauce<br>Shredded lettuce<br>Baked apple<br>Bread with spread‡<br>Milk—1 glass |
| 5 servings | | |
| FATS AND SWEETS | | |
| (Without this group the diet contains 1,355 calories) | **Between** | |
| 5 teaspoons fat or oil add 225 calories | | |
| 4 teaspoons sugar, jelly or honey add 80 calories | Milk—1 glass | Milk—1 glass |

* For alternates within each food group see Tables 21–29.

† If additional meat is desired, one serving of bread group (as 1 slice bread) may be omitted for each 1 oz. meat added, without changing the caloric value or reducing nutrient content. Other rearrangements or omissions should be assessed by reference to the values in Table 8.

‡ 1 teaspoon sugar adds 20 calories; 1 teaspoon fat or oil adds 45 calories. Such desserts as ice cream, pudding, and gelatin may add 150–300 calories. For additional caloric values see Table 36.

25

## TABLE 9

### NUTRIENT CONTENT OF DIET FOR AN ADOLESCENT BETWEEN TWELVE AND FIFTEEN YEARS OF AGE

(Protein 82 Gm.; Calories 1,645–2,645)

| DAILY FOOD INTAKE | QUANTITY | | CALORIES** | FOODSTUFFS | | | MINERALS | | VITAMINS | | | | |
|---|---|---|---|---|---|---|---|---|---|---|---|---|---|
| | Weight (Gm.) | Approximate Measure# | | Protein (Gm.)‖‖ | Fat (Gm.)‖‖ | Carbohydrate (Gm.)‖‖ | Ca (Mg.) | Fe (Mg.) | A (I.U.) | Ascorbic Acid (Mg.) | Thiamine (Mg.) | Riboflavin (Mg.) | Niacin (Mg.) |
| Milk, whole | 976 | 1 quart | 680 | 32 | 40 | 48 | 1,152 | 0.4 | 1,400 | 8 | 0.32 | 1.68 | 0.4 |
| Egg | 50 | 1 medium | 75 | 7 | 5 | | 27 | 1.1 | 590 | | 0.05 | 0.15 | Tr. |
| Meat, poultry, or fish, cooked* | 120 | 4 oz. edible portion | 300 | 28 | 20 | | 16 | 3.4 | 35 | | 0.40 | 0.25 | 5.9 |
| Bread, whole-grain or enriched white† | 150 | 5 slices | 350 | 10 | | 75 | 103 | 3.7 | Tr. | | 0.37 | 0.25 | 3.2 |
| Cereal, whole-grain or enriched white | 20 | ¼ cup | 70 | 2 | | 15 | 21 | 0.7 | Tr. | | 0.07 | 0.05 | 0.7 |
| Potato, cooked | 100 | 1 small | 70 | 2 | | 15 | 5 | 0.5 | Tr. | 16 | 0.09 | 0.03 | 1.1 |
| Vegetable (A)‡ | 150 | 2 servings | | 1 | | | 43 | 1.2 | 2,180 | 32 | 0.10 | 0.10 | 0.9 |
| (B)§ Including green and yellow | 50 | | 20 | | | 4 | 12 | 0.5 | 1,660 | 5 | 0.03 | 0.03 | 0.4 |
| Fruit, citrus | 100 | 1 serving | 40 | | | 10 | 18 | 0.1 | 140 | 40 | 0.05 | 0.01 | 0.1 |
| Fruit, other‖ | | 1 serving | 40 | | | 10 | 7 | 0.4 | 473 | 5 | 0.02 | 0.03 | 0.4 |
| Subtotal | | | 1,645 | 82 | 65 | 177 | 1,404 | 12.0 | 6,478 | 106 | 1.50 | 2.58 | 13.1 |
| Vitamin D concentrate‡‡ | | | | | | | | | | | | | |
| Separated fats and sweets†† | | | 1,000 | | | | | | 660 | | | | |
| Total§§ | | | 2,645 | | | | 1,404 | 12.0§§ | 7,138 | 106 | 1.50 | 2.58 | 13.1 |

* Estimate based on weekly consumption of 350 gm. beef, 280 gm. pork, 70 gm. fish, and 140 gm. poultry. *Meat Consumption Trends and Patterns* (U.S. Department of Agriculture, Agricultural Marketing Service, Agricultural Economics Division, Agriculture Handbook, No. 187 [Washington, D.C., July, 1960]).

† Each slice of bread has been considered to weigh 30 gm. (1 oz.) as in the values assigned to the exchange lists. It is recognized, however, that sliced bread may range between 20 and 30 gm. in weight. Adjustments should be made where usage varies.

‡ In making this estimate, it was considered that the commonly used vegetables A, tomatoes, snap beans, spinach, asparagus, broccoli, cabbage, lettuce, and cucumber, might be used 10 times weekly. Weighting was adapted from Agriculture Handbook, No. 215, *Consumption Trends and Patterns for Vegetables*, (U.S. Department of Agriculture, Economic and Statistical Analysis Division, Economic Research Service [July, 1961]).

§ It was assumed that the most commonly used vegetables from the vegetable B group of the exchange lists were peas, carrots, beets, and squash. It was estimated that these vegetables might be used 4 times weekly averaging 50 gm. daily. Weighting was adapted from Agriculture Handbook, No. 215, *Consumption Trends and Patterns for*

*Vegetables* (U.S. Department of Agriculture, Economic and Statistical Analysis Division, Economic Research [July, 1961]).

‖ Apples, bananas, canned peaches, pineapples, pears, apricots, and plums were considered commonly used. Weighting was adapted from *Consumption of Food in the United States*, Supplement for 1962 to Agriculture Handbook, No. 62 (U.S. Department of Agriculture, Agricultural Marketing Service [October, 1963]).

# Weights and measures assigned to the Exchanges are indicated in Tables 21–29.

** Calories are rounded off to the nearest 5.

†† Per capita consumption of fats and sweets have been estimated as 2 oz. separated fat or oil and 3 oz. sugar daily. *National Food Situation, NFS-108* (U.S. Department of Agriculture, Economic Research Service [May, 1964]).

‡‡ 400–800 I.U. vitamin D may be obtained from fortified milk or a concentrate.

§§ Meets Recommended Dietary Allowances (Table 3) for adolescents in good health except for iron level for girls.

‖‖ Values for calories, carbohydrate, protein, and fat from the Food Exchange Lists, Table 20, have been used to evaluate foods and food groups.

MENU PATTERN AND SAMPLE MEALS FOR AN ADOLESCENT
BETWEEN TWELVE AND FIFTEEN YEARS OF AGE
(82 Gm. Protein and 1,645–2,645 Calories; Derived from Table 9)

| DAILY FOOD PLAN‡ | SAMPLE MENU PATTERN‡ | SAMPLE MEALS‡ |
|---|---|---|
| MILK GROUP | A.M. | |
| 1 qt. whole milk# | 1 citrus fruit or ½ cup juice<br>½ cup cooked cereal or ¾ cup flake-type with milk and sugar†<br>1 slice enriched or whole-grain toast with spread†<br>Milk—1 glass | ½ grapefruit<br>¾ cup flakes with milk and sugar†<br>1 slice toast with spread†<br>Milk—1 glass |
| MEAT GROUP<br><br>5 ounces or equivalent§<br>Cooked beef, pork, veal, lamb, poultry or fish | | |
| VEGETABLE AND FRUIT GROUP | Noon | |
| 4 servings or more<br>A dark-green or deep-yellow vegetable daily for vitamin A value<br>A citrus fruit or other fruit rich in vitamin C daily | 2 oz. meat, poultry, fish, cheese or 2 eggs§<br>Vegetable<br>2 slices enriched or whole-grain bread or substitute<br>Milk—1 glass | Sandwich:<br>2 slices meat<br>2 slices bread<br>Sliced tomatoes<br>Milk—1 glass |
| BREAD-CEREAL-POTATO-LEGUME GROUP§ | P.M. | |
| 7 servings<br><br>FATS AND SWEETS†<br><br>(Without this group the diet contains 1,645 calories)<br>10 teaspoons fat or oil contain 450 calories<br>10 teaspoons sugar, jelly, or honey contain 200 calories | 3 oz. meat, poultry, fish or substitute§<br>½ cup potato or substitute<br>Dark-green or deep-yellow vegetable<br>Other vegetable<br>Fruit<br>2 slices enriched or whole-grain bread with spread† or substitute<br>Milk—1 glass | Meat loaf<br>Baked potato<br>Asparagus tips<br>Cabbage slaw<br>Fresh strawberries<br>2 hot rolls with spread†<br>Milk—1 glass |
| | Between | |
| Vitamin D** | Milk—1 glass | Milk–1 glass |

* The Recommended Dietary Allowances (Table 3) during adolescence may be met by this pattern, with the exception of iron. Liver and other iron rich foods may be used to augment this level.

† 1 teaspoon sugar adds 20 calories; 1 teaspoon fat or oil adds 45 calories. Desserts like ice cream, pudding, and gelatin may add 150–300 calories. For additional caloric values see Table 36. Adjustments in this group should be made to suit caloric needs of the individual patient.

‡ For alternates within each food group see Tables 21–29.

§ If additional meat is desired, one serving of the bread group (as 1 slice bread) may be omitted for each 1 oz. meat added, without changing the caloric value or reducing nutrient content. Other rearrangements or omissions should be assessed by reference to the values in Table 9.

# The use of skim milk would reduce calories by 360.

** 400 I.U. vitamin D should be used as a concentrate if not contained in milk.

protein need between 40 and 100 gm., depending upon the age and size of the child. In younger children the 32 gm. protein provided in 1 quart of milk will insure a surplus of animal protein. With 1 egg and 1 oz. meat in addition, it would be possible to provide two-thirds of the protein as animal protein in a diet including 65 gm. protein daily.

A combination of foods given a child between four and six years of age might approximate that given in Table 8. A daily food pattern and sample meals have been illustrated in Table 8A. The nutrient evaluation of the plan in Table 8 meets or exceeds the Recommended Dietary Allowances, 1964 (Table 3).

It is not intended or expected that all children will conform to any one exact pattern of eating. However, if any omissions or gross changes in the basic pattern of eating are made, it is desirable to reassess the resultant nutrient content of the diet by reference to appropriate tables.

A menu pattern and sample meals for an adolescent between twelve and fifteen years of age are outlined in Table 9A. If omissions or gross changes are made in this basic plan, a reassessment of the resultant diet should be made by reference to Table 9.

### DIETS AFTER FIFTY-FIVE YEARS OF AGE

*Energy requirements* decline progressively after the years of early adulthood in part because of a decrease in basal metabolic rate and in part because of a reduction in physical activity. It has been proposed in the Recommended Dietary Allowances (Table 3) that caloric allowances be reduced by 5 per cent per decade between ages 35 and 55 and by 8 per cent per decade from ages 55 to 75. A further decrease of 10 per cent is recommended for age 75 and beyond. However, it is most difficult to estimate precisely the degree of reduction in physical activity in any one individual. For this reason, the Allowances should serve only as a reference, with deviations being determined by the individual's total health status.

With advancing age, the total food consumption will fall markedly in line with the decrease in caloric needs. The total body protein (or "active metabolic mass") also falls with age. The extent to which this is a natural accompaniment of aging, of a change in food habits, or of decreased activity is not certain. The efficiency of protein utilization may decrease, with age. In view of the lack of clear evidence the protein allowance in the Recommended Dietary Allowances has been made 1 gm. per kg. per day for adults of all ages. Other nutrient needs for minerals and vitamins also remain at the level of the young adult.

A reduction in caloric needs will point primarily to a need for reduction in such food groups as the bread and cereal, and fats and sweets if the greatest advantage is to be taken of foods high in good quality protein and other nutrients. For this purpose the basic plan of diet indicated for the young adult in Table 2 will be appropriate with the curtailment of fats and sweets. The basic plan provides approximately 1,415 calories and 70 gm. protein. Modifications in this plan should be made to accommodate the size and health status of the older individual. Any gross omission or change in the resultant plan should be reassessed by reference to Table 2.

A description of the basic dietary pattern containing 1,415 calories may be obtained from Table 2. Sample menu pattern and sample meals are outlined in Table 10. Appropriate modification should be made in fats and sweets to achieve the goal for any one individual.

The following publications for popular use are available from The American Dietetic Association, 620 North Michigan Avenue, Chicago, Illinois, 60611:

*Give Yourself a Break* contains questions and answers on food for teen-agers with hints for weight control. A single copy is available for 3 cents; or fifty copies for $1.25.

*Eating is Fun—For Older People Too* is a 28-page booklet directed to the administrator or manager of a residential home for older people or a nursing home. It contains ideas for planning menus, sample lunches and suppers, comments on modified diets, and tips on saving money. The cost is 50 cents per copy; or $17.50 for fifty copies.

*Forget Birthdays and Enjoy Good Eating* is a folder for the older person who wants sound advice on food selection for healthful living. A single copy is 3 cents; fifty copies, $1.25.

*Food Facts Talk Back* is a booklet designed to combat food misinformation. Questions and answers cover common misconceptions. Single copies are available at 50 cents each; 50 copies may be obtained for $17.50.

TABLE 10

MENU PATTERN AND SAMPLE MEALS FOR INDIVIDUAL
FIFTY-FIVE YEARS OR OVER
(70 Gm. Protein; 1,415–1,615 Calories; Derived from Table 2)‡

| DAILY FOOD PLAN | SAMPLE MENU PATTERN | SAMPLE MEALS |
|---|---|---|
| | A.M. | |
| MILK GROUP† | | |
| 1 pint milk | 1 citrus fruit or ½ cup juice | ½ cup orange juice |
| | ½ cup cooked cereal or ¾ cup flake-type cereal with milk and sugar* | ¾ cup flake-type cereal with milk and sugar* |
| MEAT GROUP† | 1 slice enriched or whole-grain toast with spread* | Toast with spread* |
| 5 equivalents | Coffee or tea if desired* | Coffee or tea if desired* |
| (One equivalent equals 1 oz. edible portion of cooked beef, veal, lamb, poultry, fish, cheese or 1 egg) | | |
| | Noon | |
| VEGETABLE AND FRUIT GROUP† | Meat, poultry, fish or cheese (3 oz. edible portion) | Browned meat pattie |
| | ½ cup potato or substitute† | Baked potato |
| 5 servings or more | Dark-green or deep-yellow vegetable | Broccoli |
| A dark-green or deep-yellow vegetable is important for vitamin A value | Fruit | Tossed lettuce and tomato salad* |
| | 1 slice enriched or whole-grain bread with spread* | Applesauce |
| A citrus fruit or other fruit rich in vitamin C is important daily | Milk | Bread with spread* |
| | | Milk |
| | P.M. | |
| BREAD-CEREAL-POTATO-LEGUME GROUP† | 2 oz. edible portion of meat, poultry, fish, cheese or 2 eggs | Vegetable soup with crackers† |
| | ½ cup potato, or rice, or substitute† | Tuna casserole† |
| 8 servings | Vegetables | Mixed salad greens* |
| | Fruit | Peach custard* |
| FATS AND SWEETS | 2 slices enriched or whole-grain bread or substitute† | 1 slice bread with spread* |
| (Without this group the diet contains 1,415 calories) | Milk | Milk |
| 3 teaspoons fat or oil add 135 calories | Between | Bedtime |
| 3 teaspoons sugar, jelly, or honey add 60 calories | Milk | Milk |
| | 2 Graham crackers† | 2 Graham crackers† |

* 1 teaspoon sugar adds 20 calories; 1 teaspoon fat or oil adds 45 calories. Desserts like ice cream, pudding, or gelatin may add 150–300 calories. Cake or pie may add 300–700 calories. For additional caloric values see Table 36.

† See Tables 21–29 for other alternates within each food group. Five soda crackers (2 inches square) or 2 Graham crackers may be used as an alternate for 1 slice bread.

‡ The nutrient content of the above plan corresponds to the Recommended Dietary Allowances for the older individual.

*The Best of Health to You* includes normal nutrition for the adult. Meals, menus, and modifications for weight control are designed for the adult. Single copy is 5 cents; fifty copies, $1.75.

### REFERENCES

1. FOOD AND NUTRITION BOARD, NATIONAL RESEARCH COUNCIL. Recommended dietary allowances. 6th revised edition, 1964. ("NAS-NRC Publications," No. 1164.)
2. HATHAWAY, M. L. Heights and weights of children and youth in the United States. ("U.S. Department of Agriculture Home Economics Research Reports," No. 2.) 1957.

# SECTION II | MODIFICATIONS OF THE NORMAL DIET

As stated previously, the aim of the normal dietary regimen is to maintain, or bring the patient to, a state of nutritive sufficiency. If, in illness, deterioration has occurred in the digestive or metabolic processes or in the utilization of nutrients, nutritional needs may increase. On the other hand, there are instances in which a decrease is indicated, as in sodium or calories. In such instances, all other nutrients should remain at or above the needs for nutritive sufficiency. From this it is logical to assume that a therapeutic diet may be regarded as a modification of the normal diet. With this principle in mind, two basic guides will be called for, from which appropriate adaptations may be made: first, a guide to the recommended nutrient allowances for healthy individuals and, second, a plan of eating which will meet these needs. Appropriate adaptations may then be made from this to suit the special purposes of therapeutic diets.

Recently a revision of a guide to the nutrient needs of healthy individuals has been prepared by the Food and Nutrition Board of the National Research Council, covering the needs of individuals from infancy to old age. This guide, called *Recommended Dietary Allowances,* 6th Revised Edition, 1964, has been reproduced and discussed on pages 12–18 in the text.

The next step will be to develop a flexible plan of eating which will approximate this level of nutrient content. To achieve this goal as concisely as possible, a basic daily pattern of diet has been outlined simply, in terms of commonly used and available food groups. For this purpose, foods have been divided into the four food groups

33

which supply the major portion of the day's needs for protein, minerals, and vitamins. These four groups include the milk group, the meat group, the bread-cereal-potato-legume group, and the vegetable and fruit group. A fifth group, fats and sweets, has been noted separately because this group contributes a major source of calories but comparatively small amounts of protein, mineral, and vitamins. In this manner it will be possible to think in terms of a small number of food groups with approximately similar nutrient characteristics rather than many individual food items. This plan has the advantage of requiring a minimum of effort on the part of the dietitian, nurse, or physician in suggesting appropriate variety on a modified diet or in re-totaling the nutrient content of a diet if certain omissions or additions are made to the basic plan for therapeutic purposes.

The selection and definition of the therapeutic diets which follow have been made in terms of dietetic principles rather than in terms of diseases or names of physicians in order that more accurate, flexible, and nutritionally appropriate dietary programs may be prescribed for the therapeutic goals established by the physician. The definitions of diets are taken from the *Revised Glossary of Dietetic Terms* prepared by committees of the Diet Therapy Section of The American Dietetic Association. In bringing this material up to date, some changes in definitions have been made as a result of special study and review by member-contributors.

In each therapeutic diet which follows, a definition has been stated; a basic plan of daily food intake has been evaluated for nutrient content; deviations from the Recommended Dietary Allowances for normal diet have been noted; a description of the daily food plan has been presented in terms of food groups; a menu pattern and sample meals have been derived from this, and, where appropriate, foods to restrict have been noted. It is not intended, however, that these patterns should be used without appropriate adaptations for individual needs. It is hoped only that the description of each diet has been made sufficiently concise and flexible that it will be possible easily to formulate diets suitable for individual needs and with full awareness of the nutrient content.

## LIQUID DIETS

Liquid diets are of two kinds—the full liquid and the clear liquid. The full liquid diet consists of a variety of foods that are liquid or that liquefy at body temperature. Milk, plain frozen desserts, pasteurized eggs, fruit juice, vegetable juice, cereal gruels, and broth may be used. Finely homogenized meat or liver may be added to the broth or tomato juice to advantage. If this is not done, dried brewer's yeast will serve to improve the iron, protein, and B complex of this diet. Such a diet becomes a modification of a normal diet as far as physical consistency is concerned. The criterion is that it pour.

The foods enumerated in Table 11 will supply 80 gm. protein, 1,780 calories, and minerals and vitamins which approximate or exceed the Recommended Allowances for normal diet with the exception of iron and thiamine. If more or less of any nutrient is desired for a particular purpose, changes may easily be made by reference to the values given in Table 11 for each of the food groups. A reassessment of the resultant diet may then be made by re-totaling the nutrient content.

Description of the daily plan of food intake has been made in Table 11A, followed by a sample menu pattern and sample meals in Table 11B. Innumerable combinations may be made of these foods. The outlines should be considered examples only.

The clear liquid diet has been defined in the Glossary of Dietetic Terms as one that supplies clear fluids but is of little nutritional benefit. Only fat-free broth, tea, and coffee with sugar but without milk

35

## TABLE 11

### NUTRIENT CONTENT OF FULL LIQUID DIET
#### (80 Gm. Protein; 1,780 Calories)

| DAILY FOOD INTAKE | QUANTITY | | CALORIES | FOODSTUFFS | | | MINERALS | | VITAMINS | | | | |
| --- | --- | --- | --- | --- | --- | --- | --- | --- | --- | --- | --- | --- | --- |
| | Weight (Gm.) | Approximate Measure | | Protein (Gm.) | Fat (Gm.) | Carbohydrate (Gm.) | Ca (Mg.) | Fe (Mg.) | A (I.U.) | Ascorbic Acid (Mg.) | Thiamine (Mg.) | Riboflavin (Mg.) | Niacin (Mg.) |
| Milk‖ | 1,464 | 1½ qt. | 1,020 | 48 | 60 | 72 | 1,728 | 0.6 | 2,100 | 12 | 0.48 | 2.52 | 0.6 |
| Egg | 100 | 2 medium | 150 | 14 | 10 | .... | 54 | 2.3 | 1,180 | .... | 0.10 | 0.30 | Tr. |
| Cereal, refined enriched | 40 | (dry weight) 4 level tablespoons | 140 | 4 | .... | 30 | 42 | 1.4 | Tr. | .... | 0.14 | 0.10 | 1.4 |
| Fruit juice, citrus | 100 | ½ cup | 40 | .... | .... | 10 | 18 | 0.1 | 140 | 40 | 0.05 | 0.01 | 0.1 |
| Tomato juice | 200 | 1 cup | 40 | 2 | Tr. | 8 | 14 | 1.8 | 1,600 | 32 | 0.10 | 0.06 | 1.6 |
| Cocoa, dry | 10 | 4 level teaspoons | 30 | 2 | 2 | 5 | 13 | 1.0 | Tr. | .... | 0.01 | 0.05 | 0.2 |
| Sugar | 15 | 1 level tablespoon | 60 | .... | .... | 15 | | | | | | | |
| Plain gelatin | 3 | 1 level teaspoon | 12 | 3 | Tr. | .... | | | | | | | |
| Bouillon cube | 4 | 1 cube | 5 | 1 | Tr. | Tr. | | | | | | | |
| Fats or oils | 25 | 5 level teaspoons | 225 | .... | 25 | .... | | | 220* | | | | |
| Subtotal† | .... | | 1,722 | 74 | 97 | 140 | 1,869 | 7.2 | 5,240 | 84 | 0.88 | 3.04 | 3.9 |
| Finely strained liver‡ | 60 | 2 oz. | 60 | 8 | 2 | 1 | 4 | 3.4 | 14,400 | 6 | 0.03 | 1.20 | 4.6 |
| Total§ | .... | | 1,782 | 82 | 99 | 141 | 1,873 | 10.6§ | 19,640 | 90 | 0.91 | 4.24 | 8.5 |

\* If 5 gm. butter or fortified margarine is included.

† Does not meet levels of iron, vitamin A, or thiamine in Recommended Dietary Allowances (Table 3) for adult in good health.

‡ Strained liver or other strained meat for baby foods serves conveniently for combination with broth.

§ Approaches Recommended Dietary Allowances (Table 3) for adults in good health except for iron and thiamine.

‖ If a high protein drink is desired, 1-1½ cups non-fat, dry milk solids (100 gm.) may be added to each 1 qt. of fluid milk, thereby adding approximately 34 mg. protein and 330 calories to each quart.

DESCRIPTION OF THE DAILY FOOD PLAN FOR THE FULL LIQUID DIET*
(80 Gm. Protein; 1,780 Calories; Derived from Table 11)

| Daily Food Plan | Description |
|---|---|
| **MILK GROUP** 1½ qt. fluid whole milk† | *One and ½ qt. fluid whole milk* contain approximately 50 gm. protein and 1,000 calories. Three-fourths quart of evaporated milk or 1½ cups whole milk solids may be used as a substitute.‡ |
| **MEAT AND EGG GROUP** 2 oz. finely homogenized meat or 2 eggs or variations | *Two eggs* contain 14 gm. protein and 150 calories. Two ounces finely homogenized meat will contain approximately 14 gm. protein and 60 calories. Liver is of exceptional value in iron, vitamin A, and the B complex. However, other finely homogenized meats may be combined with bouillon or broth and served in soup. Meat and eggs may be interchanged. |
| **VEGETABLE AND FRUIT GROUP** | *The puree or juice* from spinach, asparagus, carrots, tomatoes, string beans, or celery may be used. Mild-flavored vegetables are commonly served in soups. Other vegetable purees or juices may be used if tolerated by the patient. Calories from this source are negligible. *Citrus or tomato juice* daily provides an important source of vitamin C. A half-cup of citrus juice or 1 cup tomato juice provides approximately 40 calories. |
| **CEREAL-POTATO GROUP** 1 or more servings | *One cup strained, cooked cereal* or 1 cup strained potato contains approximately 140 calories as well as a source of iron and the B complex. Combinations may be made with milk in gruels or soups. |
| **FATS AND SWEETS** | *Three teaspoons sugar* contribute approximately 60 calories and serve as flavoring for cocoa or gruel. Five teaspoons fat or oil provide approximately 225 calories and serve as flavoring for gruels or soup. |
| **MEAT SUPPLEMENT** | *Two ounces* finely homogenized calf liver supplies 8 gm. protein, 60 calories, and an important source of iron and the B complex. It may be added to bouillon or tomato juice. If this is not used, additional meat and eggs will supply iron, protein, and the B complex. |

* If any omissions or changes are made in this food plan, it should be reassessed for nutrient content.
† If 1–1½ cups (depending on the brand) non-fat milk solids are added to the 1½ quarts fluid milk, approximately 34 gm. protein and 330 calories will be added to the value of this group.
‡ This fluid whole milk containing non-fat milk solids may be used in beverages, strained cereal gruels, strained soups, ice cream, and desserts such as soft custard and rennet desserts, where high protein drinks or desserts are needed.

or cream are allowed. Occasionally small amounts of ginger ale, clear fruit, or vegetable juice, and gelatin may be added. This diet would be used for very brief periods of time when it is necessary to minimize the amount of fecal material in the colon.

*Tube feedings* may be prepared from a mixture of foods modified in consistency to the point at which the mixture may be passed through a tube. Such feedings may vary from a finely homogenized mixture of foods selected from the "regular or house diet" to food combinations carefully designed to serve particular therapeutic purposes. Barron *et al.* (15 and 16) demonstrated the successful use of

TABLE 11B

MENU PATTERN AND SAMPLE MEALS FOR A FULL LIQUID DIET*
(80 Gm. Protein;‡ 1,780 Calories;‡ Derived from Table 11 and 11A)

| SAMPLE MENU PATTERN† | SAMPLE MEALS† |
|---|---|
| | A.M. |
| ½ cup citrus juice | Citrus juice |
| Cereal gruel (made from 2 tablespoons dry cereal) and milk containing non-fat milk solids with sugar, butter, or margarine | Cream of wheat gruel |
| | Sugar and butter or margarine |
| | Coffee with milk and sugar |
| Coffee or tea if desired | |
| | Noon |
| Broth with finely homogenized liver or other meat‡ | Broth with finely homogenized liver‡ |
| | Soft custard |
| Ice cream, rennet dessert, gelatin dessert, or soft custard | Milk |
| Milk containing non-fat milk solids | |
| | P.M. |
| Strained milk soup or cereal gruel‡ | Strained potato soup‡ |
| Ice cream, or dessert as at noon | Ice cream |
| Milk containing non-fat milk solids | Cocoa |

Between

Midmorning, midafternoon, and bedtime: tomato juice or soup with finely homogenized liver, or additional eggs in desserts. Milk beverage, ice cream, and soft desserts serve as between-meal nourishments. One glass of whole milk to which ⅓ cup instant non-fat dry milk, sugar, and flavoring is added may serve as a "high protein drink."

* If any omissions or changes are made in this food plan, it should be reassessed for nutrient content, by reference to Table 11.

† Foods to restrict: Obviously, anything that has not been finely homogenized or will not pour has been omitted. Although meat, poultry, fish, vegetables, and fruits have been greatly reduced in amount, it would be possible to use more, provided that the food is finely homogenized and diluted to the extent of pouring. Pepper, cloves, mustard, and nutmeg are the spices commonly avoided.

‡ See Table 11A for alternates and for total amounts of foods to be used daily in order to include 80 gm. protein and 1,780 calories.

a small mechanical pump to pass well-blenderized, liquefied natural foods through small plastic tubing at a slow, constant rate. A highly nutritious combination of foods which may be used for this purpose may be derived from the foods outlined in the Full Liquid Diet, Table 11. Commercial products derived from natural foods and supplemented with various nutrients are also available.

## SOFT AND LOW-FIBER DIETS

The soft and low-fiber diets follow the normal diet pattern, with modifications in consistency, that is, including liquid foods and those solid foods which contain a restricted amount of indigestible carbohydrate and no tough connective tissue. If the only modification required is that a diet be made mechanically soft. this may be accomplished by cooking, mashing, pureeing, or homogenizing the foods used in a normal diet. If consideration must also be given to indigestible carbohydrate, connective tissue, or flavor, the following modifications may be made.

*Indigestible carbohydrates.*—These carbohydrates are substances that make up the cell-wall structure of plants, consisting of varying amounts of cellulose, hemicellulose, lignin, pectic substances, gums, and mucin. A number of foods have been analyzed for their cellulose, hemicellulose, and lignin content by Williams and Olmsted (1), by Olmsted and Williams (2), and by Hummel, Shepherd, and Macy (3). Figures for total fiber have been included in the compilation by Chatfield and Adams (4) and in *Composition of Foods—Raw, Processed, Prepared* (U.S. Department of Agriculture, Agriculture Handbook No. 8 [1963]). Information on hemicelluloses, celluloses, and lignins, as well as pectins, gums, and related substances, have been compiled by Hardinge, Swarner, and Crooks (18).

A reduction of the indigestible carbohydrate content of the diet may be effected by the use of refined breads and cereals, immature vegetables, and fruits from which the skins and seeds have been eliminated. During cooking, both the pectic substances and the cellulose are disintegrated (5). For this reason, cooked vegetables and fruits are sometimes used instead of the raw. In extreme instances, still greater reduction in indigestible carbohydrates may be effected by the use of pureed vegetables and fruits or the juice only of the vegetable or fruit.

## TABLE 12

### NUTRIENT CONTENT OF SOFT AND LOW-FIBER DIET
(90 Gm. Protein; 2,075 Calories)

| DAILY FOOD INTAKE | QUANTITY | | CALORIES‖ | FOODSTUFFS | | | MINERALS | | A (I.U.) | VITAMINS | | | |
|---|---|---|---|---|---|---|---|---|---|---|---|---|---|
| | Weight (Gm.) | Approximate Measure | | Protein# (Gm.) | Fat# (Gm.) | Carbo-hydrat# (Gm.) | Ca (Mg.) | Fe (Mg.) | | Ascorbic Acid (Mg.) | Thia-mine (Mg.) | Ribo-flavin (Mg.) | Niacin (Mg.) |
| Milk, whole | 976 | 1 quart | 680 | 32 | 40 | 48 | 1,152 | 0.4 | 1,400 | 8 | 0.32 | 1.68 | 0.4 |
| Egg | 50 | 1 medium | 75 | 7 | 5 | ...... | 27 | 1.1 | 590 | ...... | 0.05 | 0.15 | Tr. |
| Meat, poultry, fish, cooked† | 150 | 5 oz. E.P. | 375 | 35 | 25 | ...... | 20 | 4.3 | 44 | ...... | 0.50 | 0.31 | 7.4 |
| Bread, white, enriched | 150 | 5 slices | 350 | 10 | ...... | 75 | 103 | 3.7 | Tr. | ...... | 0.37 | 0.25 | 3.2 |
| Cereal, refined, enriched | 20 | ½ cup | 70 | 2 | ...... | 15 | 21 | 0.7 | Tr. | ...... | 0.07 | 0.05 | 0.7 |
| Potato, cooked | 100 | 1 small | 70 | 2 | ...... | 15 | 5 | 0.5 | Tr. | 16 | 0.09 | 0.03 | 1.1 |
| Vegetable cooked: | | | | | | | | | | | | | |
| A‡ | 100 | one serving | ...... | ...... | ...... | ...... | 31 | 1.1 | 1,310 | 19 | 0.09 | 0.10 | 0.6 |
| B§ | 100 | one serving | 35 | 2 | ...... | 7 | 24 | 1.0 | 3,320 | 10 | 0.06 | 0.06 | 0.8 |
| Fruit juice, citrus | 100 | ½ cup | 40 | ...... | ...... | 10 | 18 | 0.1 | 140 | 40 | 0.05 | 0.01 | 0.1 |
| Fruit, other, cooked** | ...... | 2 servings | 80 | ...... | ...... | 20 | 14 | 0.8 | 945 | 9 | 0.04 | 0.06 | 0.8 |
| Subtotal | ...... | ...... | 1,775 | 90 | 70 | 190 | 1,415 | 13.7 | 7,749 | 102 | 1.64 | 2.70 | 15.1 |
| Separated fats and oil | 20 | 4 level teaspoons | 180 | ...... | 20 | ...... | ...... | ...... | 220 | ...... | ...... | ...... | ...... |
| Sugar | 30 | 6 level teaspoons | 120 | ...... | ...... | 30 | ...... | ...... | ...... | ...... | ...... | ...... | ...... |
| Total* | ...... | ...... | 2,075 | 90 | 90 | 220 | 1,415 | 13.7 | 7,969 | 102 | 1.64 | 2.70 | 15.1 |

* The mineral, vitamin, and protein content of this basic plan will meet or exceed the Recommended Dietary Allowances (Table 3) for a man in normal good health (70 kg.) or a woman (58 kg.) with the exception of iron. If necessary iron-rich foods could be used more frequently to bring about an increase to meet individual caloric needs. Adjustments should be made as appropriate.

† Weighting was adapted from *Meat Consumption Trends and Patterns* (U.S. Department of Agriculture, Agricultural Marketing Service, Agricultural Economics Division, Agriculture Handbook No. 187 [Washington, D.C., July, 1960]).

‡ An average of snap beans, spinach, asparagus, and tomato juice.

§ An average of cooked carrots, beets, peas, and squash.

‖ Calories rounded off to nearest 5.

# Values for carbohydrate, protein, and fat from exchange lists.

** Apple sauce, pear, peach, apricot, plum.

# TABLE 12A

## Description of the Daily Food Plan for the Soft and Low-Fiber Diet*

(90 Gm. Protein; 2,075 Calories; Derived from Table 12)

| Daily Food Plan† | Description |
|---|---|
| **MILK GROUP** | |
| 1 qt. fluid whole milk | *One quart of fluid whole milk* contains 680 calories and 32 gm. protein. One pint evaporated milk or 1 cup whole milk solids may be substituted for 1 qt. fluid whole milk. |
| **MEAT AND EGG GROUP** | |
| 6 meat equivalents | *One meat equivalent* is approximately equal to 1 oz. cooked (edible portion) beef, veal, pork, lamb, poultry, fish, cheese, or 1 egg. Each equivalent contributes approximately 7 gm. protein and 75 calories. Liver and other glandular meats are exceptional sources of iron, vitamin A, and the B complex. |
| **VEGETABLE AND FRUIT GROUP** | |
| 4 servings | *A dark-green or yellow vegetable* daily is important for vitamin A value. Asparagus, carrots, green beans, yellow squash, pumpkin, spinach, and other greens are in this group. Additional vegetables commonly used include beets, peas, summer squash, and tomato juice or tomato puree. Other vegetables may be used as tolerated by the patient. Yellow squash, pumpkin, carrots, beets, and peas contain approximately 35 calories per serving. The others are negligible in calories. |
| | One-half cup citrus juice or 1 cup tomato juice daily will contribute an important part of the vitamin C needed daily. Approximately 40 calories per serving come from this source. |
| | *Other fruits* without skins or small seeds may be used. One serving of sweetened fruit may contain between 75 and 100 calories. |
| **CEREAL-BREAD-POTATO GROUP** | |
| 7 servings | *One serving provides* approximately 70 calories and is equal to 1 slice enriched bread, ½ cup potato, ½ cup cooked macaroni, noodles, spaghetti, rice, cornmeal or ½ cup cooked cereal or ¾ cup refined flake-type cereal. For other equivalents in calories see Table 27. Other substitutes may be added as tolerated by the individual. |
| **FATS AND SWEETS** | |
| | *Without this group* the diet contains approximately 1,800–2,100 calories. Six teaspoons sugar, jelly, or honey add about 120 calories. Four teaspoons fat or oil add about 180 calories. For additional calories in desserts see Table 36. |

* If any omissions or changes are made in this food plan, it should be reassesssed for total nutrient content by reference to Table 12.

† *Foods to restrict:* This diet has become increasingly liberalized and individualized to the extent that restrictions which would apply to all patients would be difficult to name (14). However, foods highly flavored with pepper, cloves, mustard, and possibly nutmeg are commonly omitted. Foods which are "overfried" or overcooked to the extent of becoming potential mechanical irritants are also commonly omitted. Foods such as bran, corn, dried beans, nuts, raisins, and fruits with small seeds and skins are also commonly avoided in view of the relatively high fiber content.

The trend, however, has been a more liberal one, due in large part to the observation (6) that vegetable purees are notoriously unpopular and that many patients refuse to eat them. The use of immature vegetables such as frozen or canned young vegetables resulted in a more palatable diet and happier patients, who benefited from eating vegetables that had been refused in their pureed state.

There has also been a trend to the use of a wider variety of fruits

TABLE 12B

Menu Pattern and Sample Meals for Soft and Low-Fiber Diet
(90 Gm. Protein; 2,075 Calories; Derived from Tables 12 and 12A)

| Sample Menu Pattern* | Sample Meals* |
|---|---|
| **A.M.** | |
| ½ cup citrus juice or 1 cup tomato juice | Tomato juice |
| 1 egg | 1 egg |
| ½ cup cooked refined cereal or ¾ cup flake-type with milk and sugar† | Cream of wheat with milk and sugar† |
| 1 slice enriched toast with spread† | Toast with spread† |
| Coffee or tea if desired | Coffee |
| **Noon** | |
| 3 oz. tender meat, poultry, fish, or cheese | Roast beef |
| ½ cup potato or alternate | Mashed potato |
| Cooked vegetables such as asparagus, carrots, spinach, yellow squash, pumpkin, or other greens; other vegetables may be used as tolerated | Asparagus tips |
| | Sliced peaches |
| Fruit (no skin or seeds) | Enriched bread with spread† |
| 1 slice enriched bread with spread† | 1 glass milk |
| 1 glass milk | Plain cake† |
| Dessert† | |
| **P.M.** | |
| Cream soup | Cream soup |
| 2 oz. (edible portion) cooked meat, poultry, fish, cheese, or 2 eggs | Tuna with rice casserole |
| | Peas |
| 1 cup rice, spaghetti, noodles, potato, or alternate* | 1 glass milk |
| Cooked vegetables (as at noon) | 1 slice enriched bread or alternate* |
| 1 glass milk | Ice cream† |
| 1 slice enriched bread with spread† or alternate* | |
| Dessert† | |
| **Between** | |
| Milk beverage | Milk shake |

\* See Table 12A for alternates and total amounts to use daily.

† Six teaspoons sugar (120 calories) and 4 teaspoons fat (180 calories) may be used during the day, or, if a substitution is desired for the 300 calories calculated in sugar and fat, ½ cup ice cream, plain pudding, custard, or gelatin dessert may add 150–300 calories. One serving plain cake may add 200–300 calories (see Table 36 for additional caloric values).

and vegetables, including some raw fruits. Removal of skins and
seeds is usually specified, however. Peeled apples, pears, peaches,
apricots, and bananas are frequently recommended.

*Connective tissue.*—Whether meat is tender or less tender is due
chiefly to the relative quantity of connective tissue present. Connective tissue in meat consists of white or collagenous fibers and yellow
elastic fibers called elastin. The total amount of connective tissue depends not only on the extent to which the muscle has been exercised
but somewhat on the age. In general, older animals have denser,
tougher connective tissue than do younger ones, although the tough-
ness may be lessened in an older animal that has been confined and
fattened.

This quantitative difference in the amount of connective tissue
present forms the basis for an appropriate cookery process. Tender-
ness of meat may be increased by cooking with moist heat to convert
the collagen in the connective tissue to gelatin and also by the use of
low-temperature cookery to reduce or lessen the toughening or hard-
ening of soluble proteins. The total effect of these two reactions depends on the composition of the meat, its acidity, the temperature,
and the rate at which it is cooked (7).

*Flavor.*—Muscle tissue contains such non-protein nitrogenous
products as creatine, creatinine, purines, and other products which
are thought to stimulate the flow of gastric juices. The most important non-nitrogenous extractive from a quantitative viewpoint is
lactic acid (8). In the usual mixed diet, the effect of this factor is
minimized, and this consideration becomes of less importance;
however, if it is desirable to limit the extractives, poultry as well as
meat, meat broths, consommé, and gravy will have to be restricted.
In this case adequate compensation for protein and other nutrients
provided by meat may be made by the proportional increase in
other protein-containing foods.

In recent years the trend in the use of a wide variety of meats has
been a liberal one. Beef, veal, pork, lamb, liver, poultry, and fish are
all commonly used. Exceptions are generally in terms of the special
needs of an individual patient.

Strongly flavored vegetables, such as onions, leeks, radishes,
dried beans, and vegetables of the cabbage family—Brussels sprouts,
cauliflower, broccoli, and turnips—have commonly been omitted.

Here again it has been found (6) that many patients can and do eat some of the strongly flavored or "gas-forming vegetables" without particular discomfort if the vegetables are properly prepared. To prevent the decomposition of sinigrin and any other substances yielding disagreeable products that may be present, such vegetables should be heated quickly, to destroy enzymes that catalyze decomposition; the kettle kept uncovered, to prevent the water from becoming acid; the cooking period made as short as possible; and the vegetable drained and served immediately when it is done. Vegetables contain both volatile and non-volatile acids, and these acids are released largely in the first few minutes of cooking. A closed kettle retains not only the volatile sulfur compounds which mar odor and flavor but also volatile vegetable acids, which favor decomposition of the sulfur compounds present (9). With proper cooking, it may be desirable, therefore, to eliminate only those vegetables that the individual patient cannot tolerate rather than to eliminate all strongly flavored vegetables.

It is now less common to restrict all spices. Schneider, DeLuca, and Gray (10) have studied the effect of spice ingestion upon the mucosa of fifty patients with active duodenal or gastric ulcer craters. In periods of up to 180 days, it was found that cinnamon, allspice, mace, thyme, sage, paprika, and caraway seed administered with food did not exert a harmful effect upon the stomach as judged by the rate of ulcer healing and clinical symptomatology, the gastroscopic appearance of the stomach before and after the ingestion of spices, and the effect on gastric secretion of pepsin. Black pepper, chili pepper, cloves, mustard seed, and possibly nutmeg were considered gastric irritants.

*Beverages.*—Coffee contains caffeine, fat, coffalic acid, and chlorogenic acid, which, on oxidation, yields caffeic acid. The chlorogenic acid differs from tannins in that it does not precipitate proteins and is therefore not astringent. The percentage of caffeine varies from $\frac{2}{3}$–$2\frac{1}{2}$ per cent, with an average of $1\frac{1}{4}$ per cent (11). The main change during roasting consists in the production of aromatic, brown, and oily substances. This oil consists of 50 per cent furfurol alcohol, small quantities of valerianic acid, phenol, pyridine, and a nitrogenous aromatic substance. A cup of strong coffee contains about 0.1–0.15 gm. of caffeine. A cup of coffee has also been found to contain about 1 mg. of niacin, as well as small amounts of thiamine and riboflavin.

Tea contains caffeine (1.4–3.5 per cent), tannins (1–30 per cent), and traces of theobromine, theophylline, xanthine, and volatile oils. A cup of strong tea prepared from 1 teaspoon of dried leaves contains about 0.1 gm. of caffeine. A quick infusion extracts practically all the caffeine but only part of the tannins. The customary brief infusion is therefore recommended. Tea also contains traces of riboflavin and niacin.

Cocoa contains $1\frac{1}{2}$–$4\frac{1}{2}$ per cent theobromine, a trace of caffeine, 31 per cent carbohydrate, 9 per cent protein, and approximately 10 per cent fat.

*Nutrient content.*—In the past it was common practice to put more emphasis on "foods to avoid" and less on "foods to eat," with the result that this group of diets has been singled out by Duncan (12) and Pollack *et al.* (13) as one of the hazards of hospitalization, resulting in nutritional deficiency and delayed convalescence. Any such deficiency is unnecessary and can be avoided if care is given to the proper selection and amount of food used.

Milk, eggs, meat, poultry or fish, vegetables, and fruit may be used in amounts sufficient to meet or exceed the Recommended Dietary Allowances. This is particularly important for those individuals who have been ill for some time and who may have had undue dietary restrictions, resulting in an inadequate intake of nutrients. In addition, changes due to the disease itself may impose further nutritional demands to hasten healing of tissue or to compensate for poor absorption. Such extra requirements would justify an increase in all the food groups, above the level recommended for the normal diet. For example, when this diet is used for reduction of gastric acidity, the number of meals and distribution may be given in 6 or more small feedings per day. Since protein-containing foods are effective in buffering the acidity of the stomach, it would be advantageous to fortify fluid milk with sufficient non-fat milk solids at least to double the natural protein content of milk, thus making the total approximately 65 gm. protein per quart. In this instance, it is well to add sufficient eggs, citrus juice, and other foods to exceed the Recommended Dietary Allowances (Table 3) for the normal individual. Special adaptations to suit the needs of any one individual may be made with a full awareness of the total nutrient content by referring to Table 12.

The nutrient content of the soft and low-fiber diet is indicated in Table 12, which shows approximately 90 gm. protein and 2,075 calories. With the exception of iron, minerals and vitamins exceed the levels indicated in the Recommended Dietary Allowances (Table 3) for the normal individual. A description of the daily food plan and a sample menu pattern and sample meals appear in Tables 12A and 12B. It is intended that appropriate adaptations of this plan be made in food selection or in calories and other nutrients to suit individual needs. However, if changes or omissions are made in any of the food groups, a reassessment of the nutrient content should be made by reference to Table 12.

The validity of correlations between food and gastrointestinal symptomatology has been critically reviewed in a report of the Joint Committee on Diet as Related to Gastrointestinal Function of The American Dietetic Association and the American Medical Association (17). Consideration is given to the chemical and physical composition of a food before its ingestion, the effect of that food in altering the gastrointestinal contents, the effect of the food or its products on the digestive tube itself, and the clinical significance of such an effect. The evidence available, the gaps in our knowledge, and the need for further research are pointed out.

## REFERENCES

1. WILLIAMS, R. D., and OLMSTED, W. H. The effect of cellulose, hemicellulose, and lignin on the weight of the stool: a contribution to the study of laxation in man, Nutrition, 11:433–49, 1936.
2. OLMSTED, W. H., and WILLIAMS, R. D. Carbohydrates of certain vegetables and fruits, Proc. Soc. Exper. Biol. & Med., 40:586, 1939.
3. HUMMEL, F. C., SHEPHERD, M. L., and MACY, I. G. Effect of changes in food intakes upon the lignin, cellulose, and hemicellulose content of diets, J. Am. Dietet. A., 16:199–207, 1940.
4. CHATFIELD. C., and ADAMS, G. Proximate composition of American food materials. (U.S. Department of Agriculture Circular No. 549.) 1940.
5. SIMPSON, J. I., and HALLIDAY, E. G. Chemical and histological studies of the disintegration of cell-membrane materials in vegetables during cooking, Food Research, 6:189–206, 1941.
6. KRAUSE, M. V. Some modern concepts concerning hospital diets, J. Am. Dietet. A., 20:610–12, 1944.

7. COMMITTEE ON PREPARATION FACTORS, NATIONAL COOPERATIVE MEAT INVESTIGATIONS. Meat and meat cookery. Chicago: National Live Stock and Meat Board, 1942, p. 76.

8. *Ibid.*, p. 32.

9. HALLIDAY, E. G., and NOBLE, I. T. Food chemistry and cookery. Chicago: University of Chicago Press, 1943, p. 35.

10. SCHNEIDER, M. A., DELUCA, V., JR., and GRAY, S. J. The effect of spice ingestion upon the stomach, Am. J. Gastroenterol., 26:722–32, 1956.

11. SOLLMANN, T. A. A manual of pharmacology. Philadelphia and London: W. B. Saunders Co., 1942, pp. 265–67.

12. DUNCAN, G. C. Some nutritional hazards of the hospitalized patient, J. Am. Dietet. A., 25:330–38, 1949.

13. POLLACK, H., and HALPERN, S. L., with the collaboration of the COMMITTEE ON THERAPEUTIC NUTRITION, FOOD AND NUTRITION BOARD, NATIONAL RESEARCH COUNCIL. Therapeutic nutrition. (Publication No. 234.) 1952.

14. Is there a rationale for the bland diet? J. Am. Dietet. A., 33:608–9, 1957.

15. BARRON, J., and FALLIS, L. S. Tube feeding with natural foods in elderly patients, J. Am. Geriatrics Soc., 4:400–404, 1956.

16. BARRON, J., PRENDERGAST, J. J., and JOCZ, M. W. Food pump: new approach to tube feeding, J.A.M.A., 161:621–22, 1956.

17. REPORT OF THE JOINT COMMITTEE ON DIET AS RELATED TO GASTROINTESTINAL FUNCTION OF THE AMERICAN DIETETIC ASSOCIATION AND THE AMERICAN MEDICAL ASSOCIATION. Diet as related to gastrointestinal function, J. Am. Dietet., A. 38:425–32, 1961.

18. HARDINGE, M. G., SWARNER, J. B., and CROOKS, H. Carbohydrate in foods, J. Am. Dietet. A., 46:197–204, 1965.

## CALORIE-RESTRICTED DIETS

The low-calorie diet is a modification of the normal diet pattern in that the prescribed allowance has a caloric value below the total maintenance energy requirement for the day, thus providing for a depletion of body fat. Protein, minerals, and vitamins remain at or above those given in *Recommended Dietary Allowances*, 6th Revised Edition, 1964 (Table 3).

*Caloric allowance.*—Since weight may be lost on any level of calories below the number required to maintain the actual weight of an individual, it becomes a matter of arriving at an allowance below maintenance that is tolerable to the patient and that permits a rate of weight loss satisfactory to both the physician and the patient. In making an accurate estimate of caloric needs for maintenance of the actual body weight, a reliable record of activity during a 24-hour period and of the food intake would be helpful. In lieu of this, a gross estimate of caloric need may be made by using 12–15 calories per pound as an approximation of the needs of a sedentary adult. Thus a woman weighing 150 pounds might need between 1,800 and 2,250 calories to maintain her actual weight. A more reliable estimate of caloric expenditure may be made by reference to the values compiled by Passmore and Durnin from direct observations of energy expenditure under various conditions of work, recreation, and rest (see Table 44).

In estimating the rate of weight loss which might be expected, a deficit of 500 calories per day under maintenance needs may be used as a gross guide. Such a deficit may be expected to bring about a loss in body weight in the range of 1 pound per week. The exact loss on the scale, however, will be influenced by factors affecting water balance, heat loss, metabolism, activity, and the presence of disease. Most women lose weight satisfactorily on diets between 1,000 and 1,500 calories and most men on diets between 1,500 and 2,000.

*Nutrient content.*—The patterns of diet and the modifications outlined in Tables 13, 13A, 13B, and 13C for a calorie-restricted diet for an adult, an adolescent, or for use during pregnancy and lactation are all based upon amounts of the essential food groups which approximate levels of protein, minerals, and vitamins indicated in the Recommended Dietary Allowances, 6th Revised Edition, 1964 (Table 3). These plans have the advantage of being the most likely to provide for the maintenance of good nutritional health, and as such, they provide the basis for a long-term dietary program of weight control.

If, in each instance, foods for the dietary program are derived from well-liked, familiar foods which suit various ethnic and cultural habits, the likelihood of the patient's maintaining a permanent program of weight control and a feeling of well being is greatly increased. This individualization should be possible in large degree with the wide variety of alternates suggested within each essential food group; if, however, any changes are made in the amounts of the essential food groups, the nutrient content of the total diet should be reassessed by reference to Tables 2, 7, 8, or 9.

The dietitian's efforts in assisting patients call for a well-coordinated program that begins with insight gained from an adequate dietary history, and provides the modification needed for weight control and the long-term guidance which will lead to new food preferences, new methods of food preparation, and a new way of life which includes satisfying and enjoyable meals. The widening areas of responsibility of the dietitian are described by Kaufman and Mead (see Chaps. 12 and 13).

*Preparation.*—It will be necessary to take advantage of ways of cooking and flavoring foods that do not depend on the use of fats and sweets, unless these have been planned as part of the regimen. The suggestions (p. 55) are only a few of many possibilities for obtaining flavorful food.

TABLE 13

DESCRIPTION OF FOOD PLAN FOR CALORIE-RESTRICTED DIETS FOR AN ADULT
(70 Gm. Protein; 1,415 Calories; Derived from Normal Diet, Table 2)

| Daily Food Plan | Description |
|---|---|
| MILK GROUP<br>1 pt. milk | *One pint milk* contains 340 calories. One pint skim milk contains 180 calories, 18 gm. protein, and important amounts of calcium, phosphorus, and the B complex. One pint of buttermilk made from skim milk or $\frac{1}{2}$–$\frac{2}{3}$ cup non-fat dry milk (depending on brand) may be substituted for this. |
| MEAT GROUP<br>5 meat equivalents | *One meat equivalent* is approximately equal to 1 oz. (edible portion, weighed after cooking) beef, veal, lamb, pork, poultry, fish, cheese, or 1 egg. The five equivalents may be distributed throughout the day as desired. Liver and other variety meats are exceptional sources of vitamin A, iron, and the B complex. One ounce of cooked meat or 1 egg may contain approximately 7 gm. protein and 75 calories. |
| VEGETABLE AND<br>FRUIT GROUP<br>5 servings | *A dark-green or deep-yellow vegetable* is important each day for its vitamin A value. Asparagus, green beans, broccoli, carrots, green peppers, winter squash, pumpkin, and other greens make up this group. Carrots, winter squash, and pumpkin contain about 35 calories per $\frac{1}{2}$ cup serving. The others will be negligible.<br>*Other vegetables,* such as beets, cabbage, cauliflower, celery, cucumber, eggplant, lettuce, tomatoes, mushrooms, onions, peas, or turnips, contribute varied amounts of all nutrients. Beets, onions, peas, or turnips may contribute about 35 calories per $\frac{1}{2}$ cup serving. Others will be negligible.<br>*Citrus fruit or other fruit* rich in vitamin C is important each day. One orange or $\frac{1}{2}$ cup juice or $\frac{1}{2}$ grapefruit or $\frac{1}{2}$ cup juice or 1 cup tomato juice or 1 cup strawberries or 1 cup red raspberries or $\frac{1}{4}$ cantaloupe or 1 large tangerine contains about 40 calories per serving and important amounts of vitamin C.<br>*Other fruits,* such as 1 apple or 1 peach or 1 pear or 2 prunes or 4 apricot halves or 12 grapes or $\frac{1}{2}$ banana, contribute varied amounts of nutrients and contain about 40 calories per serving. For equivalent amounts of other fruits see Table 26. If sugar or syrup is included, additional calories must be calculated. |

TABLE 13—*Continued*

Daily Food Plan                                       Description
BREAD-CEREAL-POTATO-
  LEGUME GROUP
8 servings                          *One serving provides approximately 70 calories,* important
                                    amounts of the B complex, and iron. One serving is
                                    equal to 1 slice enriched or whole-grain bread, ½ cup
                                    white potato, ¼ cup sweet potato, ⅓ cup corn, ½ cup
                                    cooked macaroni, noodles, spaghetti, rice, cornmeal,
                                    ½ cup cooked dried beans or peas, ½ cup cooked cereal,
                                    ¾ cup flake-type cereal, 2 Graham crackers, or
                                    5, 2-inch-square soda crackers. For other equiva-
                                    lents see Table 27.

FATS AND SWEETS

                                    *Without this group* the calories for the day approximate
                                    1,415. If 1 level teaspoon fat or oil is used on bread,
                                    in vegetables, or in cooking, about 45 calories will be
                                    added. One thin slice crisp bacon, 2 tablespoons light
                                    cream or 1 tablespoon heavy cream, 1 teaspoon
                                    mayonnaise or oil, 1 tablespoon cream cheese or
                                    French dressing, 5 small olives, or 6 small nuts con-
                                    tain about 45 calories each.
                                    *One level teaspoon sugar, jelly, or honey* in cooking, on
                                    cereal, on fruit, or in coffee adds 20 calories. One-half
                                    cup ice cream, pudding, or gelatin dessert may add be-
                                    tween 150 and 300 calories; and 1 serving cake or pie
                                    between 300 and 700 calories (see Table 36 for addi-
                                    tional caloric values).

## MODIFICATIONS OF THE CALORIE-RESTRICTED DIET

1,200-*calorie diet for an adult.*—If 3 servings of the bread-potato-cereal-
legume group are omitted from the Daily Food Plan indicated above, the diet
will become approximately 1,200 calories. Iron and the B complex will be correspondingly lowered. Reference may be made to Table 3, Recommended Dietary Allowances to determine whether this reduction is appropriate.

If 1 pint skim milk is used instead of whole milk, the diet will approximate
1,245 calories.

1,415 *calories, using additional meat.*—If more meat is desired, 1 additional
meat equivalent (1 oz. edible portion, cooked meat) may be substituted for 1
serving of the bread group without a significant change in calories. Other rearrangements or omissions should be assessed by reference to Table 2.

1,800-*calorie diet.*—In this case 350 calories may be added from any of the
food groups desired by the patient: 350 calories may be added from the use of
4 oz. meat group, or from 4 servings of the bread group, or from additional fats
and sweets. Additional caloric values may be noted from Table 36.

## TABLE 13A

### MENU PATTERN AND SAMPLE MEALS FOR A CALORIE-RESTRICTED DIET FOR AN ADULT

(70 Gm. Protein; 1,245–1,415 Calories; Derived from Table 2)

| DAILY FOOD PLAN† | SAMPLE MENU PATTERN | SAMPLE MEALS |
|---|---|---|
| | **A.M.** | |
| MILK GROUP<br><br>1 pt. whole milk*<br><br><br>MEAT GROUP<br><br>5 equivalents‡<br>(One equivalent equals 1 oz. edible portion of cooked beef, veal, lamb, pork, poultry, fish, cheese, or 1 egg) | 1 citrus fruit or ½ cup juice<br>1 egg<br>2 slices toast<br>Coffee or tea if desired | Sliced orange<br>Poached egg<br>2 slices toast<br>Milk<br>Coffee or tea if desired |
| | **Noon** | |
| VEGETABLE AND FRUIT GROUP<br><br>5 servings<br>A dark-green or deep-yellow vegetable daily for vitamin A value<br>A citrus fruit or other fruit rich in vitamin C daily | 2 oz. (2 equivalents) lean meat, poultry, or fish<br>½ cup potato or substitute<br>Dark-green or deep-yellow vegetable<br>Other vegetable<br>2 slices enriched or whole-grain bread or alternate<br>1 glass milk<br>1 fruit | Broiled ground lean meat<br>Baked potato<br>Spinach<br>Tomato and lettuce salad with special dressing§<br>2 hot rolls<br>1 glass milk<br>¼ cantaloupe |
| | **P.M.** | |
| BREAD-CEREAL-POTATO-LEGUME GROUP<br><br>8 servings<br><br><br>FATS AND SWEETS<br><br>(Without this group the diet contains 1,415 calories)‖ | 2 oz. (2 equivalents) lean meat, poultry, fish, cheese or 2 eggs<br>Vegetable<br>1 glass milk<br>3 slices enriched or whole-grain bread or alternate | Sandwich:<br>  1 slice cheese<br>  1 slice meat<br>  2 slices bread<br>Tossed salad with special dressing§<br>1 glass milk<br>2 Graham crackers |

* If skim milk is used, 160 calories may be deducted.

† See Tables 21–29 for alternates or equivalents within each food group.

‡ If additional meat is desired, 1 meat equivalent (1 oz. lean meat) may be added, and 1 serving from bread group omitted. Other rearrangements or omissions should be reassessed by reference to Tables 2 and 3.

§ See text, p. 55, for discussion of food preparation.

‖ If 1 level teaspoon sugar, jelly, or honey is used, approximately 20 calories will be added. If 1 level teaspoon fat or oil is included, approximately 45 calories will be added. A dessert, such as ice cream, pudding, or gelatin dessert, may add 150–300 calories; pie or cake may add 300–700 calories (see Table 36 for additional caloric values).

MENU PATTERN AND SAMPLE MEALS FOR A CALORIE-RESTRICTED
DIET DURING ADOLESCENCE
(80 Gm. Protein; 1,650 Calories; Derived from Table 9)

| DAILY FOOD PLAN* | SAMPLE MENU PATTERN | SAMPLE MEALS |
|---|---|---|
| | A.M. | |
| MILK GROUP | 1 citrus fruit or ½ cup juice | ½ grapefruit |
| | 1 egg | Poached egg on toast |
| 1 qt. whole milk‖ | ½ cup cooked, enriched, or whole-grain cereal or ¾ cup flake-type cereal or alternate | ¾ cup flake-type cereal |
| | | 1 glass milk |
| MEAT GROUP | | |
| 5 equivalents† | One slice enriched or whole-grain toast | |
| (One equivalent equals 1 oz. edible portion cooked beef, veal, lamb, pork, poultry, fish, cheese, or 1 egg) | 1 glass milk | |
| | Noon | |
| VEGETABLE AND FRUIT GROUP | 2 oz. (2 equivalents) lean meat, poultry, fish, cheese or 2 eggs | Sandwich: 2 slices lean meat 2 slices bread |
| 5 servings A dark-green or deep-yellow vegetable daily for vitamin A value A citrus fruit or other fruit rich in vitamin C daily | Vegetable 1 fruit 2 slices enriched or whole-grain bread or alternate 1 glass milk | Heart of lettuce with special dressing‡ Fresh pear 1 glass milk |
| | P.M. | |
| BREAD-CEREAL-POTATO-LEGUME GROUP | 2 oz. (2 equivalents) lean meat, poultry, fish, or cheese | Lean roast beef Potato |
| 7 servings | ½ cup potato or substitute Dark-green or deep-yellow vegetable | Frozen green beans with sweet-sour sauce‡ 1 small hot roll |
| FATS AND SWEETS§ | 1 slice bread or substitute 1 fruit | Baked apple 1 glass milk |
| (Without this group the diet contains 1,650 calories) | 1 glass milk | |
| | Between | |
| | 1 glass milk with 2 Graham crackers | 1 glass milk with 2 Graham crackers |

* See Table 13 for variety in selection within each food group.

† If additional meat is desired, 1 oz. lean meat may be added and 1 serving of the bread group omitted without alteration in calories. Other rearrangements or omissions should be reassessed by reference to Tables 2, 3, and 36.

‡ See text, p. 55, for discussion of food preparation.

§ If 1 level teaspoon sugar, jelly, or honey is used, 20 calories will be added. If 1 level teaspoon fat or oil is used, 45 calories will be added (see Table 36 for additional caloric values).

‖ If skim milk is used, calories in diet may be reduced to approximately 1,300.

## TABLE 13C

### Menu Pattern and Sample Meals for a Calorie-restricted
### Diet During Pregnancy and Lactation
(80 Gm. Protein; 1,300–1,650 Calories; Derived from Table 7)

| Daily Food Plan* | Sample Menu Pattern | Sample Meals |
|---|---|---|
| | A.M. | |
| Milk Group<br><br>1 qt. whole milk‖<br><br><br>Meat Group<br><br>5 equivalents†<br>(One equivalent equals 1 oz. edible portion cooked beef, veal, lamb, pork, poultry, fish, cheese, or 1 egg) | 1 citrus fruit or ½ cup juice<br>1 egg<br>½ cup cooked, enriched, or whole-grain cereal or ¾ cup flake-type cereal or alternate<br>One slice enriched or whole-grain toast<br>1 glass milk<br>Coffee or tea if desired | ½ grapefruit<br>Poached egg on toast<br>¾ cup flake-type cereal<br>1 glass milk<br>Coffee or tea if desired |
| | Noon | |
| Vegetable and Fruit Group<br><br>5 servings<br>A dark-green or deep-yellow vegetable daily for vitamin A value<br>A citrus fruit or other fruit rich in vitamin C daily | 2 oz. (2 equivalents) lean meat, poultry, fish, cheese or 2 eggs<br>Vegetable<br>2 slices enriched or whole-grain bread or alternate<br>1 glass milk | Sandwich:<br>  2 slices lean meat<br>  2 slices bread<br>Heart of lettuce with special dressing‡<br>1 glass milk |
| | P.M. | |
| Bread-Cereal-Potato-Legume Group<br><br>7 servings<br><br><br>Fats and Sweets<br><br>(Without this group the diet contains approximately 1,650 calories)§ | 2 oz. (2 equivalents) lean meat, poultry, fish, or cheese<br>½ cup potato or substitute<br>Dark-green or deep-yellow vegetable<br>Other vegetable<br>1 slice bread or substitute<br>1 fruit<br>1 glass milk | Lean roast beef<br>Potato<br>Frozen green beans with sweet-sour sauce‡<br>Raw carrot sticks<br>A small hot roll<br>Baked apple<br>1 glass milk |
| | Between | |
| | 1 glass milk with 2 Graham crackers | 1 glass milk with 2 Graham crackers |

\* See Table 13 for variety in selection within each food group.

† If additional meat is desired, 1 oz. lean meat may be added and 1 serving of the bread group omitted without alteration in calories. Other rearrangements or omission should be reassessed by reference to Tables 2, 3, and 36.

‡ See text, p. 55, for discussion of food preparation.

§ If 1 level teaspoon sugar, jelly, or honey is used, 20 calories will be added. If 1 level teaspoon fat or oil is used, 45 calories will be added (see Table 36 for additional caloric values).

‖ If skim milk is used, calories in diet may be reduced to approximately 1,300.

Aluminum foil serves to protect meat, poultry, or fish from fat and oil during baking or roasting or in frying in the same pan used for the family. Salt, pepper, spices, and herbs, onion, garlic, or green pepper may be used as desired. Meat or fish simmered or baked in a tomato sauce (canned tomatoes, green pepper, mushrooms, onions, garlic, salt, spices, or herbs) also is a convenient method of cooking without added fat or oil.

Vegetables may be cooked together for flavor or boiled in bouillon. Mint, spices, or herbs provide variety in flavor; or small amounts of dried cheese, such as Parmesan, Romano, or American, may be added to the vegetable at the table. A hot, French-type dressing may also be used to add interest to cooked vegetables. This may be made from tomato juice or tomato puree flavored with lemon or vinegar, grated onion, celery, garlic, salt, horse-radish, spices, and herbs to suit the taste. Artificial sweetener may be added if desired. This dressing serves as a good French-type dressing on salads also. The calories are negligible. Mineral oil is not a satisfactory product for use in salad dressing. Curtis (1) has calculated that each ounce of mineral oil will dissolve 140,000 I.U. of carotene at body temperature and 120,000 I.U. at room temperature. Since it has been shown also that the ingestion of liquid petrolatum or mineral oil is capable of interfering with absorption of vitamin D, calcium, phosphorus, and vitamin K, it has been concluded by the Council on Foods and Nutrition of the American Medical Association (2) that there can be no justification for the incorporation of mineral oil in foods.

Desserts may be prepared by combining the milk and eggs from the food allowance into eggnog, flavoring with extract, and sweetening with an artificial sweetener. This may be baked as custard or frozen as eggnog ice cream. The addition of the fruit allowance to this dessert will add further variety. Rennet tablets added to flavored milk will also provide attractive milk desserts. Fruit whips may be made from the fruit allowance, unsweetened gelatin, or egg white.

If a patient must eat in a restaurant or cafeteria, it is generally more satisfactory to select plain foods such as roasted or broiled meat rather than stews or fricassees, to select salads without dressing and plain fresh fruits rather than other desserts.

*Maintenance diet.*—After reaching the desirable weight, it will become necessary to establish a level of calories on which weight is maintained. Obviously, it will not be possible to go back to the old habits of eating and inactivity without regaining weight. A gross guide to the level of calories needed may be deduced from the rate of weight loss and the caloric intake during the final period of reducing. For example, if the patient has been losing at the rate of $\frac{1}{2}$ pound per week in the final weeks of reducing, it is probable that an additional 200–300 calories per day will be sufficient to maintain his weight.

The following sources of supplementary material for popular use are available from The American Dietetic Association, 620 North Michigan Avenue, Chicago, Illinois 60611.

*The Best of Health to You* contains meal patterns for adults with suggestions for modifications which will reduce calories. Fifty copies cost $1.25.

*Step Lively and Control Weight* includes foods for an adult for one day and sample meals illustrating 1,800 calories, 1,500 calories, and 1,200 calories. Fifty copies cost $1.25.

*Give Yourself a Break*, provides questions and answers on food for the teen-ager. Hints on weight control are outlined. Fifty copies cost $1.25.

Available from the U.S. Department of Agriculture, Superintendent of Documents, Government Printing Office, Washington, D.C. 20402, is *Food and Your Weight*, Home and Garden Bulletin No. 74, revised, 1964. This pamphlet contains suggestions for reducers as well as for those who want to gain weight. Caloric needs, meals and menus, and calories are included.

### HIGH-CALORIE DIET

The high-calorie diet is a prescribed food allowance which has a caloric value above the total energy requirement per day, thus providing for storage of fat. Proteins, minerals, and vitamins are at or above the levels in the normal diet.

*Appraisal of the home dietary intake.*—A deficit in the caloric content of the patient's customary food intake is frequently accompanied by a deficiency in proteins, minerals, or vitamins. This means that the dietitian is faced with the problem of obtaining reliable information regarding the over-all nutritive content of the usual food intake.

*Caloric allowance.*—The levels of caloric intake to be recommended may vary, depending upon the individual's energy requirement for maintenance and the rate of weight gain desired. A guide to caloric allowances for the normal individual at moderate activity has been recommended by the Food and Nutrition Board of the National Research Council (Table 3). More specific estimates under various conditions of work, recreation, and exercise have been compiled by Passmore and Durnin (3). (See Table 44.)

A gross guide to the number of calories that must be added above the level of calories required for maintenance of body weight is the allowance of 500 additional calories per day. This increase may permit a gain of approximately 1 pound of body tissue per week. However, the exact gain may vary, depending upon the degree of activity and upon factors affecting metabolism, heat loss, the water balance, and the presence of disease.

*Dietary recommendations.*—Since food habits are most easily and permanently changed when consideration is given to the ethnic and cultural pattern of eating, the simplest place to start is with a food diary in which the patient has recorded his self-chosen food intake. The sufficiency of this diet for various nutrients may be assessed by reference to the outlines of normal diet in Tables 2, 7, 8, and 9.

The next step that will be of the greatest nutritional advantage to the patient will involve the addition of any foods from the essential four groups which may be in deficit and which are sufficiently acceptable to the patient to permit the use of additional amounts. Several practical suggestions for supplementing the diet by 500 calories are listed here.

MILK GROUP
500 calories

> *A milk beverage* containing about 500 calories may be prepared by adding ½–¾ cup (depending on the brand) non-fat dry milk solids (180 calories) to 1 pint of whole milk (340 calories). The addition of flavoring, such as 1 tablespoon sugar (60 calories) and 2 teaspoons cocoa (35 calories), will add another 100 calories.
>
> If the milk is preferred plain, the non-fat dry milk solids may be incorporated into such foods as cottage cheese, mashed potato, macaroni, and cereals.

*Or*

MEAT-EGG-BREAD
GROUP
500 calories
     *A sandwich* containing approximately 500 calories may be prepared by using two slices of meat or cheese (150 calories); 1 tablespoon mayonnaise or fat spread for bread (135 calories); and 2 slices bread (140 calories). One egg in beverage, dessert, or plain will add about 75 calories.

*Or*

CEREAL-AND-MILK
GROUP
500 calories
     *Cereal and milk* with a banana or other fruit may provide about 500 calories if used as follows:

*One cup cooked cereal* or 1½ cups flake-type cereal (140 calories) may be served with 1 cup whole milk (170 calories) to which ¼–⅓ cup (depending on the brand) non-fat dry milk solids (90 calories) has been added. One tablespoon sugar (60 calories) and a sliced banana (80 calories) will bring the total to approximately 500 calories. For some individuals this serves as an enjoyable bedtime snack.

*Or*

FATS AND SWEETS
     *For calories obtained* from additional desserts and sweets or from fat and oils see Table 36.

*Distribution of meals throughout the day.*—In some instances, an increase in the number of feedings may be indicated. In others, a decrease in the number of feedings per day will result in a better appetite and an increase in total food consumption. Lundgren and Hammarsten (4) report that the amount of edible tray waste decreased significantly when the quantity of between-meal nourishment was reduced. Keeton (5) has also reported highly significant increases in caloric intake when the number of meals was reduced to one or two per day.

*Plan of diet.*—For a sample menu and plan of meals see the appropriate plan of normal diet. Supplements as suggested above may then be added; or other possibilities may be developed by reference to Table 36.

If a high-caloric modification of a therapeutic or a liquid or soft diet is desired, the respective evaluations, menu patterns, and meal plans should be noted, and adaptations made to suit individual needs.

## REFERENCES

1. CURTIS, A. C. The mineral oil vitamin A problem, Virginia M. Monthly, **69**:235–36, 1942.
2. COUNCIL ON FOODS AND NUTRITION, AMERICAN MEDICAL ASSOCIATION. Mineral oil (liquid petrolatum) in foods, J.A.M.A., **123**:967–69, 1943.
3. PASSMORE, R., and DURNIN, J. V. G. A. Human energy expenditure, Physiol. Rev., **35**:801–40, 1955.
4. LUNDGREN, E. M., and HAMMARSTEN, J. F. Effect of between-meal nourishments on tray food waste, J. Am. Dietet. A., **25**:873–74, 1949.
5. KEETON, R. W. Influence of distribution of meals on appetite in the sick, J. Am. Dietet. A., **26**:336–44, 1950.

*Chapter 6* | *Modifications*

*in Fat Intake*

A food allowance may be modified in terms of a prescribed level of fat, in terms of the percentage of fat calories, or in terms of the amount of, or ratio between, fatty acids. Other nutrients should remain at a level suitable for nutritive sufficiency.

"AVERAGE" FAT CONSUMPTION IN THE UNITED STATES

The kind and extent of the changes that would be necessary in making modifications in the level of fat, the proportion of calories from fat, or the amounts of and ratio between fatty acids may be judged in some degree from the contribution of various food groups in the average diet in the United States (Table 14).

An average of 155 gm. fat per person per day was available for consumption in the United States, according to data collected in the 1955 food consumption survey (1), thus accounting for approximately 44 per cent of the total calories. It should be noted, however, that no deductions were made in the survey for food discarded.

Stiebeling (2) has estimated the nutritive content of the average diet to be as follows: calories, 3,200; fat, 155 gm.; protein, 103 gm.; calcium, 1.2 gm.; iron, 18 mg.; vitamin A value, 8,540 I.U.; thiamine, 1.6 mg.; riboflavin, 2.3 mg.; niacin, 10 mg.; ascorbic acid, 106 mg. This "average," however, should be regarded only as a statistical average. Obviously, wide differences will occur in individual food habits.

BASIC DIET: 20–35 GM. FAT

The reduction of fat to approximately 20 gm. may be accomplished by omission of separated fats and oils; by the use of lean meat; by substitution of poultry and fish low in fat for part of the customary meat and cheese; by use of skim milk; and by reduction of nuts and baked goods.

The basic plan in Table 15 indicates the kinds and amounts of the food groups that will provide approximately 20 gm. fat, 80 gm. protein, and 1,200 calories. By following values indicated in Table

TABLE 14*

TOTAL FAT AND SELECTED FATTY ACIDS IN DIETS, BY FOOD
GROUP, HOUSEHOLDS IN THE UNITED STATES
(Average per Person per Day from Food Used at Home in Week,
April–June, 1955)

| Food Group† | Total Fat (Gm.) | Saturated Fatty Acids (Gm.) | Oleic Acid (Gm.) | Linoleic Acid (Gm.) |
|---|---|---|---|---|
| Beef, veal, lamb..................... | 22.1 | 11.0 | 8.8 | 0.4 |
| Pork (excluding bacon, salt pork).... | 15.1 | 6.0 | 7.6 | 1.5 |
| Poultry, fish...................... | 4.4 | 1.2 | 1.6 | 0.8 |
| Bacon, salt pork................... | 13.4 | 5.4 | 6.7 | 1.3 |
| Lard.............................. | 9.2 | 3.7 | 4.6 | 0.9 |
| Other shortening.................. | 9.0 | 2.2 | 5.8 | 0.7 |
| Oils, salad dressing............... | 9.3 | 1.9 | 2.8 | 4.6 |
| Margarine........................ | 10.4 | 2.6 | 6.4 | 0.8 |
| Butter............................ | 10.6 | 7.0 | 2.9 | 0.4 |
| Milk, cream, ice cream, cheese...... | 28.0 | 18.5 | 7.6 | 1.0 |
| Eggs............................. | 5.6 | 2.0 | 2.5 | 0.4 |
| Other foods (purchased baked goods, nuts, fruits, vegetables, etc.)...... | 18.0 | 3.6 | 9.0 | 3.6 |
| Total...................... | 155.1 | 65.1 | 66.3 | 16.4 |

* From *Food Consumption and Dietary Levels of Households in the United States: Some Highlights from the Household Food Consumption Survey, Spring, 1955* (U.S. Department of Agriculture, Agricultural Research Service, ARS 62-6 [Washington: Government Printing Office, 1957], 0-433306).
† Estimates of quantities of foods "brought into the kitchen" appear on p. 5 in text.

15, the total fat may be reduced from 155 gm. in the average diet to 20 gm.; the saturated fatty acids from 65 to 5 gm.; and the polyunsaturated acids (chiefly linoleic acid) from 16.4 to 2.0. To increase the calories without significant alterations in the fat or fatty acid levels, further additions would have to be made in sugar and sweets, fruits, vegetables, and grains.

Totals or ratios of saturated, oleic, and polyunsaturated fatty acids may be varied by using different kinds and amounts of fats and oils. Modifications may be made by reference to typical fatty acid analyses of some fats and oils of animal and plant origin in Table 16.

## TABLE 15

### Fat, Fatty Acids, and Cholesterol in a Basic Diet Containing 1,215–1,350 Calories and 20–35 Gm. Fat

| Daily Food Intake‖‖ | Quantity — Wt. (Gm.) | Quantity — Approximate Measure | Calories | Protein (Gm.) | Fat (Gm.) | Fatty Acids — Saturated (Gm.) | Fatty Acids — Unsaturated Oleic (Gm.) | Fatty Acids — Unsaturated Linoleic (Gm.) | Carbohydrate (Gm.) | Ca (Mg.) | Fe (Mg.) | A I.U. | Ascorbic Acid (Mg.) | Thiamine (Mg.) | Riboflavin (Mg.) | Niacin (Mg.) | Cholesterol (Mg.) |
|---|---|---|---|---|---|---|---|---|---|---|---|---|---|---|---|---|---|
| Skim milk.......... | 492 | 1 pint | 180 | 18 | Tr. | .... | .... | Tr. | 26 | 596 | 0.2 | 20 | 4 | 0.20 | 0.88 | 0.4 | 15 |
| Egg*.............. | 25 | ½ egg | 40 | 3 | 3 | 1.0 | 1.5 | Tr. | Tr. | 14 | 0.6 | 295 | .... | 0.03 | 0.08 | Tr. | 140 |
| Cooked lean meat, poultry, fish or cottage cheese†.. | 180 | 6 oz. E. P. | 295 | 42 | 9 | 3.2 | 3.1 | 1.2 | .... | 88 | 3.4 | 140 | .... | 0.21 | 0.34 | 11.3 | 105 |
| Bread, white enriched or cereal#‡.. | 180 | 6 or 7 slices | 490 | 16 | 6 | 1.2 | 3.2 | 0.8 | 90 | 125 | 4.4 | Tr. | 16 | 0.45 | 0.31 | 4.2 | .... |
| Potato, white.... | 100 | 1 small | 70 | 2 | .... | .... | .... | .... | 15 | 5 | 0.5 | Tr. | 32 | 0.09 | 0.03 | 1.1 | .... |
| Vegetable (A)‡.. | 150 | 2 servings | 20 | 1 | .... | .... | .... | .... | 4 | 43 | 1.2 | 2,180 | 5 | 0.10 | 0.10 | 0.9 | .... |
| Vegetable (B)§.. Including deep-green and yellow | 50 | | | | .... | .... | .... | .... | | 12 | 0.5 | 1,660 | | 0.03 | 0.03 | 0.4 | .... |
| Fruit, citrus‖.... | 100 | 1 serving | 40 | .... | .... | .... | .... | .... | 10 | 18 | 0.1 | 140 | 40 | 0.05 | 0.01 | 0.1 | .... |
| Other fruit#.... | | 2 servings | 80 | .... | .... | .... | .... | .... | 20 | 14 | 0.8 | 945 | 9 | 0.04 | 0.06 | 0.8 | .... |
| Subtotal.......... | | | 1,215 | 82 | 18 | 5.4 | 7.8 | 2.0 | 165 | 915 | 11.7 | 5,380 | 106 | 1.20 | 1.84 | 19.2 | 260 |
| Fat or oil** | | | | | | | | | | | | | | | | | |
| "Special" margarine‡‡... | 5 | 1 teaspoon | 45 | .... | 4 | .7–1 | 1–2 | 1–1.7 | .... | | | | | | | | |
| Corn oil.......... | 10 | 2 teaspoons | 90 | .... | 10 | .7 | 2.6 | 5 | .... | | | | | | | | |
| Total††.......... | | | 1,350 | 82 | 32 | 6.8–7.1 | 11.4–12.4 | 8–8.7§§ | 165 | 915 | 11.7 | 5,380 | 106 | 1.20 | 1.84 | 19.2 | 260 |

* Egg 4 times weekly.

† The average figure was derived from an assumed intake of 175 gm. beef, 70 gm. lamb, 105 gm. pork or ham, 175 gm. fish, 525 gm. poultry, 210 gm. cottage cheese per week.

‡ Commonly used vegetables selected from the vegetable A group of the exchange lists were: tomatoes, snap beans, spinach, asparagus, broccoli, cabbage, lettuce, and cucumber. It was estimated that these vegetables might be used 10 times weekly, averaging 150 gm. daily. Weighting was adapted from Agriculture Handbook No. 215, *Consumption, Trends and Patterns for Vegetables* (U.S. Department of Agriculture, Economic and Statistical Analysis Division, Economic Research Service [July, 1961]).

§ It was assumed that the most commonly used vegetables from the vegetable B group of the exchange lists were peas, carrots, beets, and squash. It was estimated that these vegetables might be used 4 times weekly averaging 50 gm. daily. Weighting was adapted from Agriculture Handbook No. 215, *Consumption Trends and Patterns for Vegetables* (U.S. Department of Agriculture, Economic and Statistical Analysis Division, Economic Research Service [July, 1961]).

‖ Fresh orange, fresh grapefruit, canned orange juice, blended grapefruit and orange, and frozen citrus juice were considered to be commonly used citrus fruits or juice. Weighting was adapted from *Consumption of Food in the United States*, Supplement for 1962 to Agriculture Handbook No. 62 (U.S. Department of Agriculture, Agricultural Marketing Service (October, 1963)).

# Apples, bananas, canned peaches, pineapples, pears, apricots, and plums were considered commonly used. Weighting was adapted from *Consumption of Food in the United States*, Supplement for 1962 to Agriculture Handbook No. 62 (U.S. Department of Agriculture, Agricultural Marketing Service (October, 1963)).

** For additional values on saturated fatty acids, oleic, and linoleic acids, see Tables 16, 36.

†† Meets Recommended Dietary Allowances (Table 3) for adult in good health except for iron level for women.

‡‡ "Special" margarine differs from regular in having a higher polyunsaturated fatty acid content (3).

§§ Polyunsaturated: saturated fatty acids = 8/6.8 and 8.7/7.1 = 1.2, approximately.

‖‖ Values from Table 36, page 154, in text for skim milk, egg, meat, and bread.

## Values from Agriculture Handbook No. 8, *Composition of Foods, Raw, Processed, Prepared* (U.S. Department of Agriculture, [revised 1963]). Weight of one slice bread may vary from 23 to 30 gm.

DESCRIPTION OF DAILY FOOD PLAN: BASIC DIET—*20–35* GM. FAT
(80 Gm. Protein; 1,215–1,350 Calories; Derived from Table 15)

| Daily Food Plan* | Description |
|---|---|
| **MILK**<br>1 pt. skim | *One pint skim milk* contains 180 calories, 18 gm. protein, and important amounts of calcium, phosphorus, and the B complex vitamins. One pint buttermilk, made from completely skim milk, or $\frac{1}{2}$–$\frac{2}{3}$ cup (depending on brand) of non-fat milk solids is equivalent. |
| **EGG**<br>4 per week | *One egg* contributes approximately 7 gm. protein and 75 calories. |
| **MEAT GROUP** | *The fat and fatty acid levels* indicated in Table 15 may be attained by the weekly use of approximately 12 oz. of *lean* beef, pork, or lamb; 18 oz. poultry; 6 oz. low-fat fish and 7 oz. cottage cheese. For methods of preparation, see p. 64. |
| **VEGETABLE AND FRUIT GROUP**<br>5 servings | *A dark-green or deep-yellow vegetable* is important each day for its vitamin A value. Asparagus, green beans, broccoli, carrots, green pepper, winter squash, pumpkin, and other greens make up this group. Carrots, winter squash, and pumpkin may contain about 35 calories per serving. The others will be negligible.<br>*Other vegetables,* such as beets, cabbage, cauliflower, celery, cucumber, eggplant, lettuce, mushrooms, onions, peas, tomatoes, or turnips, contribute various amounts of all nutrients. Beets, onions, peas, or turnips may contribute about 35 calories per $\frac{1}{2}$-cup serving. Others will be negligible.<br>*Citrus fruit* or other fruit rich in vitamin C is important each day. One orange or $\frac{1}{2}$ cup juice or $\frac{1}{2}$ grapefruit or 1 cup tomato juice or 1 cup strawberries or 1 cup red raspberries or $\frac{1}{4}$ cantaloupe or 1 large tangerine contains about 40 calories per serving and important amounts of vitamin C.<br>*Other fruits,* such as 1 apple or 1 peach or 1 pear or 4 halves of apricots or 12 grapes or $\frac{1}{2}$ banana, contribute various amounts of all nutrients and contain about 40 calories per serving. For other fruits see Table 26 in text. If sugar or syrup is included, add between 25 and 50 calories per serving. |

* See p. 64 in text for food preparation.

TABLE 15A—*Continued*

| Daily Food Plan* | Description |
|---|---|
| BREAD OR CEREAL | |
| 6 or 7 servings | *One serving provides approximately 70 calories,* important amounts of the vitamin B complex, and iron: One |
| POTATO OR | slice enriched or whole-grain bread, ½ cup white |
| SUBSTITUTES | potato, ¼ cup sweet potato, ½ cup cooked macaroni, |
| 1 serving | spaghetti, or noodles, rice, cornmeal, cooked dried peas or beans, ¾ cup flake-type cereal, 2 Graham crackers, or 4 arrowroot cookies. |
| FAT OR OIL | |
| | *One teaspoon "special" margarine and 2 teaspoons oil* will add approximately 135 calories bringing the total diet to 1,350 calories. |
| SWEETS | |
| | *If sugar, jelly, or honey* are included approximately 20 calories must be added for each teaspoon. |

For additional values on fatty acid composition see Table 36 in the Appendix. These values have been selected from a more complete listing which appears in *Composition of Foods—Raw, Processed, Prepared* (U.S. Department of Agriculture, Agriculture Handbook No. 8 [December, 1963]).

#### FOOD PREPARATION

*Diet containing 20 gm. fat.*—Separated fats and oils must be eliminated entirely; and meat should be well trimmed to eliminate fat. Cooking must be limited to boiling or simmering with bouillon or tomato juice and broiling or roasting without added fat. Seasoning may be done with lemon, vinegar, wines, onion, garlic, salts, spices, and herbs instead of fats and oils. Meat tenderizers may be useful. Wrapping fat-trimmed meat, skinned poultry, or fish in aluminum foil also serves as a convenient method for cooking individual servings which must remain fat-free. In this way meat remains moist and well flavored in addition to being protected from fat, even if placed in the same frying pan with meat for the family.

Salad dressing may be prepared without added oil. Tomato juice or tomato puree may be used as a base, with lemon or vinegar, grated onion, grated celery, garlic, horse-radish, sugar, salt, and pepper added to suit the taste. Other seasoning may be used as desired, but oil must be avoided completely. This dressing may be used to marinate meat or may be served hot as a flavoring for cooked vegetables.

# TABLE 15B

## Menu Pattern and Sample Meals: Basic Diet—20–35 Gm. Fat
### (80 Gm. Protein; 1,215–1,350 Calories;* Derived from Tables 15 and 15A)

| Daily Food Plan† | Sample Menu Pattern‡ | Sample Meals§ |
|---|---|---|
| | **A.M.** | |
| **Milk** | | |
| 1 pt. skim | ½ cup citrus fruit juice or substitute | ½ cup orange juice |
| **Egg** | 1 egg | Poached egg |
| | ½ cup cooked enriched or | Toast—2 slices |
| One, 4 times weekly | whole-grain cereal or ¾ | Coffee or tea |
| | cup flake-type cereal, | Skim milk |
| **Meat Group** | and 1 slice enriched or | "Special margarine"# |
| | whole-grain toast | |
| 12 oz. (cooked weight of edi- | Coffee or tea if desired | |
| ble portion) *lean* beef, pork, | Skim milk | |
| or lamb; 18 oz. poultry; 6 | 1 teaspoon "special" | |
| oz. low-fat fish; 7 oz. cot- | margarine | |
| tage cheese per week‖ | | |
| | **Noon** | |
| **Vegetable and Fruit Group** | | |
| | 3 oz. lean meat, poultry, or | Baked chicken |
| 5 servings | fish | Potato |
| Dark-green or deep-yellow | ½ cup potato, rice, | Frozen greens |
| vegetable is important for | spaghetti, or noodles | Honeydew melon |
| vitamin A value | Green or yellow vegetable | Skim milk |
| Citrus fruit or other fruit rich | Fruit | Bread |
| in vitamin C is important | Skim milk | "Special margarine"# |
| daily | 1 slice enriched or whole- | |
| | grain bread | |
| **Bread or Cereal** | | |
| 6 or 7 servings | **P.M.** | |
| **Potato or Substitute** | | |
| | 3 oz. lean meat, poultry, or | Salmon, baked in tomato |
| 1 serving | fish | sauce§ |
| | ½ cup potato, rice, | Rice with chives |
| **Fat or Oil#** | spaghetti, or noodles | Tossed salad with special |
| | Vegetable | dressing§ |
| (Without fat or oil, the diet | Fruit | Baked apple |
| will approximate 1,215 cal- | Skim milk | Skim milk |
| ories. With 3 teaspoons | 1 slice enriched or whole- | Bread |
| fat or oil the diet becomes | grain bread | "Special margarine"# |
| 1,350 calories) | | |
| **Sugar*** | | |

\* If more calories are needed, the following may be included without significant alteration of fatty acids. 1 teaspoon sugar, jelly, or honey, 20 calories; ½ cup plain gelatin dessert or 1 serving sweetened fruit, 100 calories. 3 teaspoons special margarine will add 135 calories and increased amounts of linoleic acid.

† For variety within each food group see Table 15A for alternates.

‡ For foods to avoid, see p. 66 in text.

§ See p. 64 in text for discussion of food preparation.

‖ The average figure was derived from an assumed intake of 175 gm. beef, 70 gm. lamb, 105 gm. pork or ham, 175 gm. fish, 525 gm. poultry, 210 gm. cottage cheese per week.

# See "special margarine," Table 15.

Baked goods must be limited to those prepared without added fat, such as angel-food cake, arrowroot cookies, and Graham crackers. Desserts may include gelatin, fruit, fruit whips made from egg white or gelatin, ices, and puddings or frozen desserts prepared from skim milk. Bread may be spread with jam, jelly, or honey.

Olives, potato chips, popcorn, cheese, gravy, or soups containing fat, avocado, nuts, cream, chocolate, and coconut must be restricted. Labels on canned or processed foods must be examined carefully to note any fat content.

TABLE 16

SELECTED FATTY ACIDS IN COMMON FATS AND OILS
(Per 100 Grams, Edible Portion)*

| Food | Total Fat (Gm.) | Total Saturated Fatty Acids (Gm.) | Unsaturated Fatty Acids | |
|---|---|---|---|---|
| | | | Oleic (Gm.) | Linoleic (Gm.) |
| Animal fats: | | | | |
| Lard............. | 100.0 | 38 | 46 | 10 |
| Butter.......... | 81.0 | 46 | 27 | 2 |
| Vegetable oils: | | | | |
| Corn oil......... | 100.0 | 10 | 28 | 53 |
| Cottonseed oil.... | 100.0 | 25 | 21 | 50 |
| Olive oil......... | 100.0 | 11 | 76 | 7 |
| Peanut oil....... | 100.0 | 18 | 47 | 29 |
| Safflower oil..... | 100.0 | 8 | 15 | 72 |
| Sesame oil....... | 100.0 | 14 | 38 | 42 |
| Soybean oil...... | 100.0 | 15 | 20 | 52 |
| Chocolate, bitter or baking...... | 53.0 | 30 | 21 | 1 |

* Selected from *Composition of Foods—Raw, Processed, Prepared* (U.S. Department of Agriculture, Agriculture Handbook No. 8 [December, 1963]).

*Fatty acid modifications.*—If the prescribed levels of saturated or unsaturated fatty acids permit adding fats and oils in the diet, these may be incorporated in cooking, in the salad dressing, as a spread for bread and potatoes, or in a beverage made from the egg and skim milk allotted in the basic diet. Two plans for the use of fat-controlled meals have been prepared by the American Heart Association in cooperation with The American Dietetic Association and the Heart Disease Control Program, U.S. Public Health Service: "Planning Fat-Controlled Meals" for 1,200 and 1,800 calories; and "Planning

Fat-Controlled Meals" for unrestricted calories. These booklets may be obtained through a physician or nutritionist from the American Heart Association, 44 East 23d Street, New York, New York.

Numerous special-purpose cookbooks have also been published. However, the suitability of a recipe depends on the particular level of fat, the percentage of fat calories, or the proportion of saturated and unsaturated fatty acids prescribed in the individual diet. For this reason, the physician, dietitian, or nutritionist should aid in selecting appropriate recipes.

For a description of a daily food plan, a sample menu pattern, and sample meals containing 20–35 gm. fat, see Tables 15, 15A, 15B. Modifications from this basic diet may be made to suit individual needs.

Those who wish to read further may refer to "The Regulation of Dietary Fat," a report of the Council on Foods and Nutrition of the American Medical Association published in J.A.M.A. (August 4, 1962), **181**:411–29.

## REFERENCES

1. Household food consumption survey, 1955. (U.S. Department of Agriculture, Agricultural Research Service Reports, Nos. 1–10.) 1957.
2. STIEBELING, HAZEL K. (Director, Institute of Home Economics, U.S. Department of Agriculture, Agricultural Research Service). Food and nutrient consumption trends and consumer problems. Talk at the American Institute of Nutrition, Chicago, Illinois, April 17, 1957. (Mimeo.)
3. Composition of certain margarines. A council statement. J.A.M.A. (March 3, 1962) **179**:719.

The normal food allowance may be modified in terms of a prescribed level of protein, the kind and amount of amino acids, or the character of the protein fraction. Other nutrients should remain at a level suitable for nutrient sufficiency.

### 125-GM. PROTEIN DIET

A level of protein above the normal allowance may be indicated most clearly if it is prescribed in terms of grams of protein per kilogram of desirable weight. For the normal, healthy adult, 1 gm. protein per kilogram of desirable weight has been recommended (Table 3). For children, the level will be correspondingly higher per unit of weight (Table 3). For therapeutic purposes, appropriate increases should be specified.

In evaluating proteins, one considers two general aspects: (*a*) digestibility and (*b*) biologic value. By digestibility is meant the percentage of the consumed protein, measured in terms of nitrogen, that is absorbed. Biologic value means the percentage of absorbed nitrogen that is retained by the body and not excreted in the urine. The body requires a definite combination or pattern of amino acids, each in proper amount, for the formation of tissue proteins. If any essential amino acid is supplied in insufficient amounts, then this amino acid will limit the amount of tissue protein made; other amino acids, regardless of the amount present, can be used only to the extent that is required for this tissue protein, and the remainder will be metabolized and the nitrogen excreted in the urine; therefore, the proteins deficient in essential amino acids will have low biologic values. Although there are exceptions, most vegetable proteins have lower digestibilities and biologic values than do animal proteins. For this reason, most nutritionists and dietitians recommend some source of animal protein in each meal. The dietetic practice of providing half or more of the protein from animal sources permits a wide margin of safety in the normal diet for an adult. In diets for children and in most convalescent diets it is a common practice to provide two-thirds of the protein from animal sources.

As an example of a protein allowance for an adult which has been increased above normal, a diet containing 125 gm. protein and 2,000 calories has been evaluated in Table 17. This daily food plan has been derived from the Normal Diet for an Adult (Tables 2, 2A, and 2B), with the addition of 1–1$\frac{1}{3}$ cups (depending on the brand) of non-fat milk solids to 1 quart of fluid skim milk. The total protein for the day then becomes 125 gm. In this illustration, the increase may be obtained by a high-protein drink. Sugar and flavoring could be added as appropriate. If the non-fat milk solids are more acceptable in other forms than a drink, they may be added as a dry ingredient to cottage cheese, mashed potatoes, cereal, milk soups, macaroni or spaghetti, puddings, cake, or cookies.

The possibilities of using other of the essential food groups to increase the protein content may be noted by reference to the protein values indicated in Table 17. If a therapeutic modification of a high-protein diet is desired, such as a liquid or soft diet, see the respective tables.

### AMINO ACIDS

A renewed interest in requirements has come about in part from the recognition of amino acid deficiencies in various parts of the world, particularly as *kwashiorkor* in infants and young children (1). Holt (2) and Albanese (3) have made observations on amino acid requirements of infants; Reynolds (4) of young women; and Rose and his associates (5, 6) have indicated tentative minimum quantities necessary for maintenance of nitrogen equilibrium in young adult males. Tentative minimum requirements for amino acids by young adults appear in Table 45. In addition, a committee of the Food and Agriculture Organization of the United Nations (7) has recently appraised protein requirements.

## TABLE 17

### NUTRIENT EVALUATION OF 125-GM. PROTEIN DIET
#### (1,990 Calories)

| Daily Food Intake | Weight (Gm.) | Approximate Measure | Calories* | Protein* (Gm.) | Fat* (Gm.) | Carbohydrate* (Gm.) | Ca (Mg.) | Fe (Mg.) | A (I.U.) | Ascorbic Acid (Mg.) | Thiamine (Mg.) | Riboflavin (Mg.) | Niacin (Mg.) |
|---|---|---|---|---|---|---|---|---|---|---|---|---|---|
| Milk, skim, fluid§§ | 970 | 1 quart | 360 | 36 | Tr. | 52 | 1,102 | 0.4 | 40 | 8 | 0.40 | 1.76 | 0.8 |
| Milk, dry, non-fat instant§§ | 100 | 1¼ cups | 360 | 36 | 1 | 52 | 1,293 | 0.6 | 30 | 7 | 0.35 | 1.78 | 0.9 |
| Egg | 50 | 1 medium | 75 | 7 | 5 | | 27 | 1.1 | 590 | | 0.05 | 0.15 | Tr. |
| Meat, poultry, fish, cooked† | 120 | 4 oz. E.P.§ | 300 | 28 | 20 | | 16 | 3.4 | 35 | | 0.40 | 0.25 | 5.9 |
| Bread, whole-grain or enriched white‡ | 180 | 6 slices | 420 | 12 | | 90 | 123 | 4.6 | Tr. | | 0.46 | 0.31 | 4.0 |
| Cereal, whole-grain or enriched | 20 | ½ cup | 70 | 2 | | 15 | 21 | 0.7 | Tr. | | 0.07 | 0.05 | 0.7 |
| Potato, cooked | 100 | 1 small | 70 | 2 | | 15 | 5 | 0.5 | Tr. | 16 | 0.09 | 0.03 | 1.1 |
| Vegetable (A)‖ | 150 | 2 servings | | 1 | | | 43 | 1.2 | 2,180 | 32 | 0.10 | 0.10 | 0.9 |
| Vegetable (B)# | 50 | | | | | 4 | 12 | 0.5 | 1,660 | 5 | 0.03 | 0.03 | 0.4 |
| Including deep-green and yellow | | | | | | | | | | | | | |
| Citrus fruit** | 100 | 1 serving | 40 | | | 10 | 18 | 0.1 | 140 | 40 | 0.05 | 0.01 | 0.1 |
| Other fruit† | | 2 servings | 80 | | | 20 | 14 | 0.8 | 945 | 9 | 0.04 | 0.06 | 0.8 |
| Subtotal | | | 1,795 | 124 | 26 | 258 | 2,764 | 13.9 | 5,620 | 117 | 2.04 | 4.53 | 15.6 |
| Sugar | 15 | 3 level teaspoons | 60 | | | 15 | | | | | | | |
| Fats or oils | 15 | 3 level teaspoons | 135 | | 15 | | | | 165 | | | | |
| Total‡‡ | | | 1,990 | 124 | 41 | 273 | 2,764 | 13.9 | 5,785 | 117 | 2.04 | 4.53 | 15.6 |

* Values for calories, carbohydrate, protein, and fat from the Food Exchange Lists, Table 20, have been used to evaluate foods and food groups.

† Weighting was adapted from *Meat Consumption Trends and Patterns* (U.S. Department of Agriculture, Agriculture Handbook No. 187, Agricultural Marketing Service, Agricultural Economics Division [Washington, D.C., July, 1960]). Weekly consumption estimated as 350 gm. beef, 280 gm. pork, 140 gm. poultry, and 70 gm. fish.

‡ 30 gm. (1 oz.) has been the weight assigned to one slice of bread in the exchange lists. It is recognized that variation is common. Adjustments should be made where usage varies.

§ Edible portion.

‖ Commonly used vegetables selected from the vegetable A group of the exchange lists were: tomatoes, snap beans, spinach, asparagus, broccoli, cabbage, lettuce, and cucumber. It was estimated that these vegetables might be used 10 times weekly averaging 150 gm. daily. Weighting was adapted from Agriculture Handbook No. 215, *Consumption Trends and Patterns for Vegetables* (U.S. Department of Agriculture, Economic and Statistical Analysis Division, Agricultural Marketing Service, Economic Research Service [July, 1961]).

# It was assumed that the most commonly used vegetables from the vegetable B group of the exchange lists were peas, carrots, beets, and squash. It was estimated that these vegetables might be used 4 times weekly averaging 50 gm. daily. Weighting was adapted from Agriculture Handbook No. 215, *Consumption Trends and Patterns for Vegetables* (U.S. Department of Agriculture, Economic and Statistical Analysis Division, Economic Research Service [July, 1961]).

** Fresh orange, fresh grapefruit, canned orange juice, blended grapefruit and orange and frozen citrus juice were considered to be commonly used citrus fruits or juice. Weighting was adapted from *Consumption of Food in the United States,* Supplement for 1962 to Agriculture Handbook No. 62 (U.S. Department of Agriculture, Agricultural Marketing Service [October, 1963]).

†† Apples, bananas, canned peaches, pineapples, pears, apricots, and plums were considered commonly used. Weighting was adapted from *Consumption of Food in the United States,* Supplement for 1962 to Agriculture Handbook No. 62 (U.S. Department of Agriculture, Agricultural Marketing Service [October, 1963]).

‡‡ Meets Recommended Dietary Allowances (Table 3) for adult in normal good health except for iron level for women.

§§ Values from Table 36 in text for skim milk and dry milk.

‖‖ Caloric needs should be adjusted to individual requirements. For variations in need, see Tables 3 and 5.

Tryptophan has become the first amino acid for which an allowance has been indicated by the Food and Nutrition Board in *Recommended Dietary Allowances*, Revised, 1964 (Table 3). Its sparing action on the need for niacin has been quantitated in terms of tryptophan where 60 mg. tryptophan represents 1 mg. niacin. Horwitt (8) has discussed the basis for this assumption and its application to the evaluation of dietaries. This may be of particular importance in situations where food patterns have become skewed either for therapeutic reasons or from unusual food habits on the part of the patient.

The term "niacin equivalent" is used to apply to the potential niacin value—that is, to the sum of the preformed niacin and the amount of niacin that could be derived from tryptophan (25). There is a need for tryptophan over and above its use as a precursor of niacin, however, and this need has not been established. The average diet in the United States, provides enough tryptophan to increase the niacin value by approximately a third.

### PHENYLALANINE-RESTRICTED DIET

A small but significant number of infants are born without the ability to metabolize phenylalanine properly, as a result of a deficiency of the enzyme phenylalanine hydroxylase. This enzyme normally converts phenylalanine to tyrosine. In its absence the accumulation of phenylalanine and abnormal metabolites interferes with normal brain development. Improvement has been brought about in many instances by reducing the phenylalanine in the diet to the minimal levels necessary to permit normal growth and development. Koch (10) has reviewed this topic briefly. More comprehensive reviews have been made by Centerwall (9), Lyman (13), and the Conference on Phenylketonuria called by the British Medical Research Council (14). Also a recent Statement on Treatment of Phenylketonuria by the Committee of the Handicapped Child of the American Academy of Pediatrics has been published (24). An up-to-date, selected, and annotated bibliography on phenylketonuria is available from the U.S. Department of Health, Education, and Welfare, Children's Bureau (12).

Management of the diet requires a reduction of phenylalanine, which is an essential amino acid, to the point where it is low enough to avoid excessive blood levels but high enough to provide for good growth and development. At the same time other nutrients must remain at a level for nutritive sufficiency. Experience seems to indicate wide variations in nutritional requirements both from one individual to another and from time to time in the same infant or child. For this reason constant surveillance of clinical responses, dietary intake, and the blood levels of phenylalanine and other nutrients are necessary to avoid too rigorous or prolonged restrictions. Present experience (24) seems to indicate that phenylalanine requirements for children with phenylketonuria lie somewhere between 20 and 40 mg. per pound of body weight per day, infants needing the upper values, small children the medium values, and children over 5 the lower values. The initial phenylalanine prescription serves only to assess phenylalanine tolerance. From this point, management must be carefully individualized, frequently monitored, and appropriately readjusted as required.

In planning a phenylalanine-restricted diet particular attention must be given to the protein portion of the diet since natural protein has been assumed to contain between 4 and 6 per cent phenylalanine. The basis for the diet must therefore be a specially prepared food from which most of the phenylalanine has been removed. Such a product is Lofenalac, developed by the Mead Johnson Laboratories (16). Phenylalanine has been removed by the passage of an enzymic hydrolysate of casein through a column of activated charcoal. In this way, the phenylalanine is removed, as well as other aromatic acids. The hydrolysate is then supplemented with DL-methionine, L-tryptophan, L-tyrosine, and minerals and vitamins. The powder contains 0.06 to 0.1 per cent phenylalanine in contrast to approximately 5 per cent in natural food proteins. The amount of this powder commonly prescribed for young infants may roughly approximate one measuring cup (150 gm.) per day depending upon the infant's age and condition. Between one and two years of age approximately one-and-one-half to two cups powder may be used daily. Fluid intake should be equivalent to that of healthy normal infants. The composition of 100 gm. Lofenalac powder is indicated in Table 18.

The physician will establish the amounts of phenylalanine, pro-

## TABLE 18

### Composition per 100 Grams of Lofenalac Powder*

Approximate Analysis

| | |
|---|---|
| Calories | 460 |
| Total nitrogen (equivalent to approximately 15 gm. protein) | 2.4 |
| Fat, gm. | 18 |
| Carbohydrate, gm. | 57 |

Minerals

| | |
|---|---|
| Calcium, gm. | 0.65 |
| Phosphorus, gm. | 0.5 |
| Iron, gm. | 0.01 |
| Sodium, gm. | 0.4 |
| Potassium, gm. | 1 |
| Chlorine, gm. | 0.65 |
| Magnesium, gm. | 0.087 |
| Copper, mg. | 0.1 |
| Zinc, gm. | 0.0005 |

| | |
|---|---|
| Phenylalanine content of powder, mg.† | 80 |

Vitamin Content

| | |
|---|---|
| A, U.S.P. units | 1,080 |
| D, U.S.P. units | 286 |
| Ascorbic acid, mg. | 22 |
| Thiamine hydrochloride, mg. | 0.33 |
| Riboflavin, mg. | 1.32 |
| Niacin amide, mg. | 2.86 |
| Pyridoxine hydrochloride, mg. | 0.35 |
| Calcium D-panthothenate, mg. | 2.31 |
| Folic acid, mg. | 0.033 |
| Biotin, mg. | 0.02 |
| Vitamin E, mg. | 3.53 |
| Inositol, mg. | |
| Choline chloride, mg. | 108 |
| Vitamin $B_{12}$, mcg. | 3.3 |
| Vitamin K | |

Amino Acids

| | |
|---|---|
| L-tyrosine, gm. | 0.8 |
| L-tryptophan, gm. | 0.2 |
| DL-methionine, gm. | 0.2 |
| L-methionine, gm. | 0.25 |
| L-arginine, gm. | 0.3 |
| L-histidine, gm. | 0.25 |
| L-lysine, gm. | 1.6 |
| L-leucine, gm. | 1.4 |
| L-isoleucine, gm. | 0.75 |
| L-threonine, gm. | 0.81 |
| L-valine, gm. | 1.1 |

* Dilutions: "Normal dilution" for infant formula (20 calories per fl. oz.) is 1 packed "measure" (9.5 gm.) to each 2 fluid oz. water or 1 level measuring cup (150 gm.) to a quart of water. This dilution supplies about 3.5 mg. phenylalanine per fl. oz. and 0.6 gm. protein. A more concentrated preparation (for children) of 1 cup Lofenalac powder to 2½ cups water supplies about 30 calories, 5 mg. phenylalanine per fl. oz., and 1 gm. protein.

† Range 60–100 mg.

tein, and calories to be used by the patient. Since Lofenalac may constitute 85–100 per cent of the total diet depending upon the age and condition of the child, it is important to recommend additional foods carefully to supplement the diet properly. To facilitate selection, foods have been grouped into equivalents representing 15 mg. phenylalanine (see Table 19). Additional considerations concerning the phenylalanine assay of foods have been reported by Miller (15), however, indicating a need for more precise information on phenylalanine content of foods.

Parents, of course, have many questions and problems relating to the diet. To aid professional persons in counseling patients, a publication entitled *The Low Phenylalanine Diet* has been prepared by the State of California, Department of Public Health, Bureau of Public Health Nutrition, Berkeley 4, California. Suggestions for recipes, meal planning, and recording of the daily food intake are included.

MAPLE-SYRUP URINE DISEASE

Another hereditary metabolic aberration in amino metabolism for which dietary alteration has been attempted has been named "maple syrup urine disease," owing to the maple syrup urine odor that appears within two months after birth. The biochemical manifestations of this disease are attributed to a deficiency in the oxidative decarboxylation of the branched chain amino acids—leucine, iso-leucine, and valine—that results in an accumulation of alpha keto-acids in the urine. Westall (17) and Snyderman (26) have reported on dietary treatment of children with this disease.

Recently, new and less costly methods of assay of the amino acid content of foods have resulted in a substantial accumulation of data. These have been compiled by Orr and Watt (18) for eighteen amino acids in 202 food items in terms of amino acids per gram of total nitrogen and in terms of amino acids in 100 gm. food. A portion of the original table on the average amount of amino acids per 100 gm. food appears in Table 40 (p. 191), including the eight "essential amino acids" that are necessary for maintenance of body tissue plus arginine and histidine, which have been found to be important for growth.

An excellent guide for public health nurses entitled *Feeding Mentally Retarded Children* (U.S. Department of Health, Education,

## TABLE 19

FOOD EQUIVALENTS FOR LOW-PHENYLALANINE DIET (11)

| FOOD | AMOUNT |
|---|---|
| **List I—Lofenalac: 30 Mg. Phenylalanine—2 Equivalents*** | |
| Lofenalac† (dry) | 4 Tbsp. |
| Lofenalac (reconstituted) | 1 c. |
| **List II—Vegetables: 15 Mg. Phenylalanine—1 Equivalent** | |
| Beans, green | |
|     Strained and junior | 1½ Tbsp. |
|     Regular | 3 Tbsp. |
| Beets | |
|     Strained | 2 Tbsp. |
|     Regular | 3 Tbsp. |
| Cabbage, raw, shredded | 4 Tbsp. |
| Carrots | |
|     Strained and junior | 3 Tbsp. |
|     Raw | ¼ large |
|     Canned | 4 Tbsp. |
| Celery, raw | 1½ small stalks |
| Cucumber, raw | ⅓ medium |
| Lettuce, head | 2 leaves |
| Spinach, creamed—strained and junior | 1½ Tbsp. |
| Squash | |
|     Winter | |
|         Strained | 3 Tbsp. |
|         Junior | 6 Tbsp. |
|         Cooked | 4 Tbsp. |
|     Summer, cooked | 4 Tbsp. |
| Tomato | |
|     Raw | ¼ small |
|     Canned | 2 Tbsp. |
|     Juice | 2½ Tbsp. |
| **List III—Fruits; 15 Mg. Phenylalanine—1 Equivalent‡** | |
| Banana | 4 Tbsp. |
| Dates, dried | 2 |
| Fruit cocktail, canned | 2½ Tbsp. |
| Grapefruit | |
|     Sections | ⅓ c. |
|     Juice | ⅓ c. |
| Orange | |
|     Sections | 3 Tbsp. |
|     Juice | 3 Tbsp. |
| Grape juice | ⅓ c. |
| Lemon juice | 3 Tbsp. |

\* One equivalent may be defined as providing 15 mg. phenylalanine.

† Mead Johnson Laboratories, Evansville, Indiana.

‡ Newer assays for phenylalanine content of fruits indicate a lower value than the ones used in this report (15).

TABLE 19—*Continued*

Peaches
  Raw................................⅔ medium
  Canned in syrup......................1½ halves
  Strained...........................5 Tbsp.
  Junior............................7 Tbsp.
Pears
  Raw...............................⅓ medium
  Canned in syrup.....................3 halves
  Strained and junior..................10 Tbsp.
Pears and pineapple, strained and junior...7 Tbsp.
Pineapple
  Raw...............................⅓ c.
  Canned in syrup....................1½ small slices
  Juice..............................½ c.
Plums, canned in syrup................1½ medium
Plums with tapioca
  Strained............................5 Tbsp.
  Junior............................7 Tbsp.
Prunes
  Cooked............................2 medium
  Juice..............................⅓ c.
  Strained............................3 Tbsp.
Raisins..............................1½ Tbsp.
Strawberries...........................3 large
Tangerine............................⅔ small
Watermelon...........................⅔ c.

### List IV—Breads: 30 Mg. Phenylalanine—2 Equivalents

Barley cereal, Gerber's, dry...............2⅓ Tbsp.
Biscuits§...............................1 small
Cereal food, Gerber's, dry...............2 Tbsp.
Cookies, arrowroot.....................1½
Corn.................................2 Tbsp.
Cornflakes............................⅓ c.
Crackers
  Barnum animal.......................6
  Saltines............................3
Cream of Wheat, cooked................2 Tbsp.
Farina, cooked.........................2½ Tbsp.
Ice cream§‖
  Chocolate...........................⅓ c.
  Pineapple...........................⅓ c.
  Strawberry..........................⅓ c.
  Vanilla.............................⅓ c.
Mixed cereal, Pablum, dry...............1⅔ Tbsp.
Oatmeal
  Gerber's strained.....................1⅔ Tbsp.
  Pablum, dry.........................1⅔ Tbsp.

§ Special recipe must be used.
‖ Milk is very high in phenylalanine (1 oz. contains 55 mg.), but it may on occasion be ordered to bring phenylalanine blood levels up to normal.

TABLE 19—*Continued*

LIST IV—*Continued*

| | |
|---|---|
| Potatoes, Irish | 2½ Tbsp. |
| Rice Flakes, Quaker | ⅓ c. |
| Rice Krispies, Kellogg's | ⅓ c. |
| Rice, Puffed, Quaker | ½ c. |
| Sugar Crisps | ¼ c. |
| Sweet potatoes or yams | |
|     Cooked | 3 Tbsp. |
|     Strained | 4 Tbsp. |
| Wafers, sugar, Nabisco | 6 |
| Wheat, Puffed, Quaker | ⅓ c. |

List V—Fats: 5 Mg. Phenylalanine—⅓ Equivalent

| | |
|---|---|
| Butter | 1 tsp. |
| Cream, heavy | 1 tsp. |
| Margarine | 1 Tbsp. |
| Mayonnaise | 1½ Tbsp. |
| Olives, ripe | 1 large |

List VI—Desserts: 15 Mg. Phenylalanine—1 Equivalent

| | |
|---|---|
| Cookies | |
|     Rice-flour (19) | 1 |
|     Corn starch (19) | 1 |
| Ice creams—see List IV, Breads | |
| Puddings‡ | ½ c. |
| Sauce, Hershey syrup | 1 Tbsp. |

List VII—Free Foods: Little or No Phenylalanine; May Be Used as Desired

| | |
|---|---|
| Candy | |
|     Butterscotch | — |
|     Cream mints | — |
|     Fondant | — |
|     Gum drops | — |
|     Hard | — |
| Jelly beans | — |
| Lollipops | — |
| Cornstarch | — |
| Guava butter | — |
| Honey | — |
| Jams, jellies, and marmalades | — |
| Molasses | — |
| Oil | — |
| Sauces | — |
|     Lemon‡ | — |
|     White‡ | — |
| Syrups | |
|     Corn | — |
|     Maple | — |
| Sugar | |
|     Brown | — |
|     White | — |
| Tapioca | — |

TABLE 19—*Continued*

List VIII—Foods to Avoid: High Phenylalanine Content; May Be Used
Only Occasionally in Very Small Portions

Breads, most.......................... —
Cheeses of all kinds.................... —
Eggs................................. —
Legumes, dried....................... —
Meat, poultry, fish................... —
Nuts................................. —
Nut butters.......................... —

and Welfare, Children's Bureau, 1964) is available from the Government Printing Office, Washington, D.C., 20402, at a price of 15 cents per copy. This booklet includes guidance in taking a dietary history, assessment of feeding methods, and techniques and teaching for development of skills by the family and child.

### PROTEIN FRACTIONS: GLIADIN RESTRICTION

Various fractions of protein have long been of interest in connection with allergic manifestations. As a result, certain foods have been eliminated, the most common being eggs, milk, and various grain products. This has posed a problem in constructing acceptable recipes for breads, desserts, sauces, and so forth, in which the offending products are avoided. Recipes have been collected and tested for this purpose by committees of the Diet Therapy Section of The American Dietetic Association and are now compiled and available in the booklet entitled *Allergy Recipes* (1957).

More recently the gliadin, or glutamine-bound fraction of protein in wheat, rye, oats, and barley has become of particular interest in the treatment of certain malabsorption syndromes (19–22). In this instance, in which wheat, rye, oats, and barley are omitted, other grains and cereal products must be substituted, leaving corn flour, cornmeal, potato flour, rice flour, soybean flour, wheat-starch flour ("gliadin-free") as the alternates.

The wheat-rye-oat-free diet has been described by Sleisenger, Rynbergen, Pert, and Almy (23). Several recipes are included for corn muffins, corn pone, rice-flour bread, rice-flour muffins, rice-flour sponge cake, and rice-flour brownies. Additional recipes may be found in a new booklet by Margaret Abowd, *Low Gluten Diet with*

*Recipes* (Ann Arbor: University of Michigan, University Hospital, 1958).

*Luncheon with Laurie* by Carolyn Busbee Carpenter is also an excellent collection of recipes. It is available from the State Printing Company, Columbia, South Carolina at $1.75 per copy postpaid from 237 Pinewood Lane, Rock Hill, South Carolina.

For additional information on the protein fractions in some of the principal proteins of common foodstuffs, reference may be made to W. H. Peterson and F. M. Strong, *General Biochemistry* (Englewood Cliffs, N.J.: Prentice-Hall, Inc., 1953).

## REFERENCES

1. BROCK, J. F. Survey of world situation on kwashiorkor, Ann. New York Acad. Sci., **57**:696–713, 1954.
2. HOLT, L. E., JR. "Nutrition in infancy and adolescence," in Modern nutrition in health and disease, eds. M. G. WOHL and R. S. GOODHART. Philadelphia: Lea & Febiger, 1955, chap. 34.
3. ALBANESE, A. A. Protein and amino acid requirements of infants, Pediatrics, **8**:455–62, 1951.
4. REYNOLDS, M. S. Amino acid requirements of adults, J. Am. Dietet. A., **33**:1015–18, 1957.
5. ROSE W. C. The amino acid requirements of adult man, Nutrition Abstr. & Rev., **27**:631–47, 1957.
6. ROSE, W. C., WIXOM, R. L., LOCKHART, H. B., and LAMBERT, G. F. The amino acid requirements of man, J. Biol. Chem., **217**:987–95, 1955.
7. FOOD AND AGRICULTURE ORGANIZATION OF THE UNITED NATIONS. Report of the FAO Committee on Protein Requirements. Rome, 1957.
8. HORWITT, M. K. Niacin-tryptophan requirements of man, J. Am. Dietet. A., **34**:914–19, 1958.
9. CENTERWALL, WILLARD R. Phenylketonuria–A general review, J. Am. Dietet. A., **36**:201–5, 1960.
10. KOCH, R., ACOSTA, P., RAGSDALE, N., and DONNELL, G. Nutrition in the treatment of phenylketonuria, J. Am. Dietet. A., **43**:212–5, 1963.
11. ACOSTA, P. B., and CENTERWALL, W. R., Phenylketeonuria; Dietary Management Special Low Phenylalanine Recipes, J. Am. Dietet. A., **36**:206–11, 1960.
12. Phenylketonuria—A selected Bibliography. U.S. Department of Health, Education, and Welfare, Children's Bureau, 1963.
13. LYMAN, FRANK (ed.). Phenylketonuria. Springfield, Ill.: Charles C Thomas, 1963, 318 pp.
14. REPORT TO THE MEDICAL RESEARCH COUNCIL OF THE CONFERENCE ON PHENYLKETONURIA. Treatment of Phenylketonuria, Brit. Med. J. (June 29, 1963), 1691–97.
15. MILLER, G. T., WILLIAMS, V. R., and MOSCHETTE, D. S. Phenylalanine content of fruit, J. Am. Dietet. A., **46**:43–45, 1965.

16. MEAD JOHNSON LABORATORIES. Phenylketonuria—Low Phenylalanine Dietary Management with Lofenalac-low Phenylalanine, Food (March, 1965), Evansville, Indiana.

17. WESTALL, R. G. Dietary treatment of a child with maple sugar urine disease (branched-chain-keto-aciduria), Arch. diseases childhood **38**:485–91, 1963.

18. ORR, M. L., and WATT, B. K. Amino acid content of foods, (U.S. Department of Agriculture, "Home Economic Research Reports," No. 4.) 1957.

19. ADLERSBERG, D. Problems of management of idiopathic sprue, New York State J. Med., **55**:3575–82, 1955.

20. DICKE, W. K., WEIJERS, H. A., and VAN DE KAMER, J. H. Coeliac disease. 2. The presence in wheat of a factor having a deleterious effect in cases of coeliac disease, Acta paediat., **42**:34–42, 1953.

21. VAN DE KAMER, J. H., WEIJERS, H. A., and DICKE, W. K. Coeliac disease. 4. An investigation into the injurious constituents of wheat in connection with their action on patients with coeliac disease, Acta paediat., **42**:223–31, 1953.

22. VAN DE KAMER, J. H., and WEIJERS, H. A. Coeliac disease. 5. Some experiments on the cause of the harmful effect of wheat gliadin, Acta paediat., **44**:465–69, 1955.

23. SLEISENGER, M. H., RYNBERGEN, H. J., PERT, J. H., and ALMY, T. P. A. Wheat-rye-and-oat-free diet, J. Am. Dietet. A., **33**:1137–40, 1957.

24. COMMITTEE ON THE HANDICAPPED CHILD, AMERICAN ACADEMY OF PEDIATRICS. Statement on treatment of phenylketonuria, Pediatrics, **35**:501–3, 1965.

25. Composition of Foods—Raw, Processed, Prepared, U.S. Department of Agriculture, Agriculture Handbook No. 8 (December, 1963).

26. SNYDERMAN, S. E., NORTON, P. M., ROITMAN, E., HOLT, L. E., JR. Maple syrup urine disease, with particular reference to diet therapy. Pediatrics, **34**:454–72, 1964.

# Chapter 8 | Modifications in Protein-Fat-Carbohydrate[1]

Modifications in protein-fat-carbohydrate have been simplified in three ways: first, by combining foods into six groups comparable in protein-fat-carbohydrate content as well as approximate mineral and vitamin worth; secondly, by describing these groups in commonly measured or purchased units of food; and third, by limiting foods in each group to those in common usage. These food groups were originally developed by the Committee on Diabetic Diet Calculations, The American Dietetic Association working co-operatively with the Committee on Education, American Diabetes Association, and the Diabetes Section, U.S. Public Health Service, and were named "Food Exchange Lists."

Since 1950, when the first report was published, there has been a wide acceptance of the Food Exchange Lists that have brought simplification, flexibility, and standardization into the selection of values and foods used in quantitative diets. The diet for patients with diabetes is a prime example.

Inevitably new data on food composition have accumulated, new food products have appeared on the market, and special considerations relating to ethnic groups and educational programs have arisen. In order that appropriate guidelines for adaptations of the exchange lists can be brought into perspective, the original report, which appeared in 1950, is reproduced below.

1. Report of the Committee on Diabetic Diet Calculations, The American Dietetic Association. Prepared co-operatively with the Committee on Education, American Diabetes Association, and the Diabetes Section, U.S. Public Health Service. Compiled by Elizabeth K. Caso.

For the purpose of working toward the standardization of values on food composition in the dietary management of diabetes, the American Diabetes Association in 1947 invited The American Dietetic Association to select a committee to work jointly with its Committee on Education. Since the work of the Diabetes Section of the U.S. Public Health Service is so intimately concerned with these matters, it joined in this project to become the third co-operating organization. The objectives of this joint committee were to prepare a set of representative values suitable for use in dietary calculation and to develop a simplified method for planning the diet, including several "exchange lists" of foods of similar food value.

The joint committee was faced with many difficulties due in part to a lack of uniformity in the composition of food occurring as a result of varietal differences, variations in conditions of growth, degree of maturity, and methods of harvesting, storage, or preparation. For example, two different types of peaches may vary as much as 125 per cent in carbohydrate content. The composition of a piece of well-done meat will be roughly 25 per cent higher in protein than a piece which is rare, owing to a difference in water content. The carbohydrate content of bread will fluctuate, depending upon its age and the way it has been stored (1). McCance and Widdowson (2) have pointed out that an appreciable amount of carbohydrate may be lost in the cooking of vegetables. American food tables (3, 4) report "total carbohydrate" values which are considered to contain a varying percentage of unavailable carbohydrate (5). All these factors had to be considered carefully and weighted in preparing figures for calculating diabetic diets.

On the other hand, there is a great variation from day to day in bodily requirements and utilization of food which is dependent on such factors as activity, emotional status, and insulin dosage. In fact, differences in bodily needs far exceed differences in food composition and therefore minimize the problem of the inevitable variation in food content. Thus nothing more than reasonable detail is justifiable in calculating diabetic diets. As a result, foods have been grouped in terms of similarity in composition.

FOOD EXCHANGE LISTS

Recognizing these facts, the joint committee has submitted the food values given in Table 20. As mentioned above, the list is greatly abbreviated by combining foods of similar composition into food exchange lists.

TABLE 20

FOOD VALUES FOR CALCULATING DIABETIC DIETS

| Group | Amount | Weight (Gm.) | Carbo-hydrate (Gm.) | Protein (Gm.) | Fat (Gm.) | Energy (Calories) |
|---|---|---|---|---|---|---|
| Milk, whole.......... | ½ pt. | 240 | 12 | 8 | 10 | 170 |
| Vegetable, group A... | As desired | ........ | ........ | ........ | ........ | ........ |
| Vegetable, group B... | ½ cup | 100 | 7 | 2 | ........ | 36 |
| Fruit................ | Varies | ........ | 10 | ........ | ........ | 40 |
| Bread exchanges...... | Varies | ........ | 15 | 2 | ........ | 68 |
| Meat exchanges...... | 1 oz. | 30 | ........ | 7 | 5 | 73 |
| Fat exchanges........ | 1 teaspoon | 5 | ........ | ........ | 5 | 45 |

*Milk.*—In rounded figures, the composition of 1 cup (8 oz.) of whole fresh milk averages 12 gm. carbohydrate, 8 gm. protein, and 10 gm. fat (4). One cup or ½ pt. is purposely used as the unit of measurement, since milk in most sections of this country is purchased by the quart. Thus ½ pt. is relatively easy for the patient to measure, and any multiple of ½ pt. can be figured into the meal plan for the day. This is much simpler than prescribing odd amounts, such as 7 or 14 oz. per day.

Several forms of cow's milk are available, such as evaporated, dried, or skim milk. These types of milk have been combined into one table called "List 1—Milk Exchanges" (Table 21). In the amounts listed, one may be substituted for another, since they are all approximately equal in composition.

*Problems of measuring carbohydrate.*—Innumerable lists have been prepared which classify vegetables according to the amount of carbohydrate they contain. In some instances, vegetables have been divided into lists containing approximately 3, 6, 9, and 12 per cent

cent vegetables. One author might place a vegetable in the 6 per cent group while another might include it in the 3 per cent list. There has been little uniformity in this matter. In addition, the percentage classification has been difficult for the patient to comprehend and to put into practical use.

TABLE 21

LIST 1—MILK EXCHANGES
(Per Serving: Carbohydrate, 12 Gm.; Protein, 8 Gm.; Fat, 10 Gm.)

| Type of Milk | Approximate Measure | Weight (Gm.) |
|---|---|---|
| Whole milk (plain or homogenized)... | 1 cup (8 oz.) | 240 |
| Skim milk*...................... | 1 cup | 240 |
| Evaporated milk................. | ½ cup | 120 |
| Powdered whole milk............. | ¼ cup | 35 |
| Powdered skim milk (nonfat dried milk)*........................ | ¼ cup | 35 |
| Buttermilk (from whole milk)........ | 1 cup | 240 |
| Buttermilk (from skim milk)*........ | 1 cup | 240 |

* Since these forms of milk contain no fat, two fat exchanges may be added to the diet when they are used.

In seeking some simpler manner of grouping the vegetables, the committee took into account the controversy regarding "total" and "available" carbohydrate. According to the Department of Agriculture (3), " 'total' carbohydrate in the majority of cases is reckoned as carbohydrate by difference, that is, as the difference between 100 per cent and the sum of the percentages of water, protein, fat, and ash. This measure includes starch, dextrin, and sugars, and is to this extent an approximate measure of the total carbohydrate that can be utilized by the body. However, it tends to over-estimate the available carbohydrate since it also includes crude fiber and organic acids, when present, and any undetermined solids." The American Diabetes Association, upon the recommendation of W. H. Olmsted, has defined available carbohydrate as follows (5): "This term includes starch, dextrin, glycogen, glucose, fructose, galactose, sucrose, lactose, and maltose. It represents the portion of the carbohydrate of foods available to the human body for glycogen formation." That organization feels that available carbohydrate is the preferred value for computing diabetic diets. carbohydrate. In others, they have been grouped as 5, 10, or 15 per

There is evidence to show that cellulose, hemicellulose, and gums are broken down by bacterial action in the human intestinal tract to form volatile fatty acids (5, 6) which do enter into glycogen formation. However, isotopic studies of the intermediary metabolism of volatile fatty acids (7–10) seem to indicate that they do not cause a *net* increase in the body's supply of glycogen.

The organic acids, chiefly malic and citric, are converted to glucose. In each case, two molecules of citrate or malate form one of glucose. Altogether, the total amount of glucose formed from organic acids is variable. Some workers believe that it is negligible. More studies in this field are needed (5).

These studies of the availability of fractions making up "total-carbohydrate-by-difference" are very complex. Bernice K. Watt, of the Bureau of Human Nutrition and Home Economics, Department of Agriculture, feels that it may be a long time before the ideal in food analysis is reached, with not only quantitative data but data on human utilization available for the separate components of the so-called "carbohydrate-by-difference."

The question then arises as to the advisability of using values for starch and sugar alone as the measure of the carbohydrate content of vegetables and fruits. Dr. Watt has stated, after reviewing data in the bureau files, that, for a fair number of fruits, the analyses for sugar and starch appear to be as representative of the product as were estimates of total carbohydrate. For some fruits and many vegetables this is not the case, since products selected for study of sugar or starch content were not always ordinary products but were often selected for study because of some particular characteristic or condition of growth. The Department of Agriculture is currently accumulating considerable data on the carbohydrate fractions of foods.

Furthermore, McCance and Widdowson (2) report a loss of carbohydrate in the cooking process. Although the analyses were done on English foods and have not been, to any extent, carried out on American foods, at least the findings are significant and would tend to justify the use of lower values for carbohydrate content.

This whole problem resolves itself into the need for some practical basis to use for the calculation of carbohydrate in diabetic diets. After some consideration, the joint committee finally recommended the figures for starch and sugar as representative of available carbohydrate, even though they may be short of the ideal.

*Classification of vegetables.*—In Table 22 are summarized the data used to arrive at a simplified grouping of the more commonly used vegetables.

The first group of vegetables (group A) contains 3 gm. or less of carbohydrate per 100-gm. serving. Therefore, the committee recommends that these vegetables be grouped in one list (Table 23), and that the negligible amount of carbohydrate which they contain need not be figured in the diet unless more than 200 gm. is used at a meal.

The second group of vegetables in Table 22 contains more carbohydrate. Some of them are more popular than others. Therefore, a weighted average was taken (Table 24), and, based on these data, the committee decided to figure the composition of these vegetables as 7 gm. carbohydrate and 2 gm. protein per 100-gm. serving.

Although the list of group B vegetables is short, it contains some of the more popular vegetables. However, it is not likely that more than one of these vegetables would be eaten in one day. The dietitian who has previously figured three or more vegetables in the diet may now find that she needs to calculate only one group B vegetable and allow the patient other vegetables from group A as desired.

The remainder of the vegetables in Table 22 contains appreciably more carbohydrate. For simplicity they are included in the list of bread exchanges and will be considered later. None of the other lists represents as major a change as this new classification of vegetables (Table 23).

*Fruit.*—The carbohydrate content of fruit differs with the variety as in vegetables, and fruits have been classified into groups according to their carbohydrate content. To avoid the confusion of having several groups and to simplify dietary instruction for the patient, the practice in the past few years (13, 14) has been to list all fruits together in *amounts* that would supply either 10 or 15 gm. carbohydrate. The committee working on the material was in favor of the list (Table 25) which contained 10 gm. carbohydrate, since it presented the majority of the more common fruits in serving sizes that are easy to purchase, economical to serve, and relatively satisfying in amount. The carbohydrate values of the fruits are based on the starch and sugar analyses of the Department of Agriculture (3). For practicality the figures were rounded.

TABLE 22

CARBOHYDRATE CONTENT OF VEGETABLES PER 100-GM. SERVING

| FOOD | SOURCE OF REFERENCE | | |
|---|---|---|---|
| | U.S. Dept. of Agriculture (3) (Sugar and Starch) (Gm/100 Gm) | McCance and Widdowson (2) (Gm/100 Gm) | Williams et al. (11) (Gm/100 Gm) |
| List 2, Group A—Vegetable Exchanges | | | |
| Asparagus............ | 1.7 | 1.1 | .......... |
| Beans, string, young... | 2.6 | 2.9 | 5.8 |
| Beet greens.......... | 0.5 | .......... | .......... |
| Broccoli............. | 1.9 | 0.4 (tops) | 1.1 |
| Brussels sprouts....... | .............. | 1.7 | 2.6 |
| Cabbage............. | 3.5 | 3.0 | 2.5 |
| Cauliflower.......... | 2.6 | 1.2 | 1.0 |
| Celery.............. | 1.2 | 1.3 | .......... |
| Chard............... | 0.8 | .......... | .......... |
| Chicory............. | 0.2 | .......... | .......... |
| Cucumber........... | 2.6 | 1.8 | .......... |
| Dandelion greens...... | 0.9 | .......... | .......... |
| Eggplant............. | .............. | 3.1 | .......... |
| Kale................ | 1.4 | .......... | .......... |
| Lettuce.............. | 1.6 | 1.8 | 1.4 |
| Mushrooms.......... | 0 | 0 | .......... |
| Mustard greens....... | 0.4 | 0.9 | .......... |
| Radishes............ | 3.4 | 2.8 | .......... |
| Spinach............. | 0.3 | 1.4 | 0.7 |
| Squash, summer....... | 1.2 | .......... | .......... |
| Tomatoes........... | 3.4 | 2.8 | 1.6 |
| List 2, Group B—Vegetable Exchanges | | | |
| Beets............... | 9.6 (total CHO) | 9.9 | 7.3 |
| Carrots............. | 7.5 | 5.4 | 6.0 |
| Onions.............. | 7.2 | 5.2 | .......... |
| Peas, greens......... | 9.0 | 10.6 | 8.3 |
| Pumpkin............ | 5.1 | 3.4 | .......... |
| Rutabaga........... | 6.7 | .......... | .......... |
| Squash, winter....... | 4.9 | .......... | .......... |
| Turnip.............. | 4.6 | 3.8 | 3.5 |
| List 4—Bread Exchanges | | | |
| Beans, baked........ | 18.8 | 17.3 | .......... |
| Beans, dried......... | 62.1 (total CHO) | .......... | .......... |
| Beans, Lima......... | 23.5 | .......... | .......... |
| Corn............... | 18.9 | .......... | 14.8 |
| Parsnips............ | 11.9 | 11.3 | .......... |
| Peas, dried......... | 45.1 | 50.0 (raw) 19.1 (cooked) | .......... |
| Potato, white........ | 15.6 | 18.3 | 16.4 |
| Potato, sweet........ | 25.6 | 20.1 | 23.7 |

## TABLE 23

### LIST 2—VEGETABLE EXCHANGES
### Group A

Negligible Carbohydrate, Protein, and Calories if 1 Cup
(200 Gm.) or Less Is Used

| | | |
|---|---|---|
| Asparagus | Eggplant | Lettuce |
| Beans, string, young | Greens* | Mushrooms |
| Broccoli* | Beet | Okra |
| Brussels sprouts | Chard, Swiss* | Pepper* |
| Cabbage | Collard | Radish |
| Cauliflower | Dandelion | Sauerkraut |
| Celery | Kale | Squash, summer |
| Chicory* | Mustard | Tomatoes* |
| Cucumbers | Spinach | Watercress* |
| Escarole* | Turnip | |

### Group B

Per Serving: Carbohydrate, 7 Gm.; Protein, 2 Gm.
(1 Serving = ½ Cup = 100 Gm.)

| | | |
|---|---|---|
| Beets | Peas, green | Squash, winter* |
| Carrots* | Pumpkin* | Turnip |
| Onions | Rutabaga | |

* These vegetables have high vitamin A value. At least one serving should be included in the diet each day.

## TABLE 24

### DATA USED TO CALCULATE THE COMPOSITION OF VEGETABLES, GROUP B

| Food | Carbohydrate Content (Starch and Sugar)* (Gm/100 Gm) | Weighting (Based on Usual Rate of Consumption)† |
|---|---|---|
| Beets................. | 8.0 | 3 |
| Carrots............... | 7.5 | 4 |
| Onions... /............ | 7.2 | 1 |
| Peas, green (medium).... | 9.0 | 4 |
| Pumpkin.............. | 5.1 | .......... |
| Rutabaga............. | 6.7 | ½ |
| Squash, winter......... | 4.9 | 2 |
| Turnip............... | 4.6 | 1 |

* U.S. Department of Agriculture figures (3).

† From *Family Food Consumption in the United States, Spring, 1942* (18) and *Consumption of Food in the United States, 1909–48* (12).

In Table 26 the fruits have been listed in household measurements. Since each fruit in the amount listed contains approximately 10 gm. carbohydrate, one may be exchanged for the other. There is some variation between measured and weighed portions of fruit. Every so-called "small" apple will not weigh exactly 80 gm. Here again, however, the variation seems reasonable on the basis of the difference in actual carbohydrate content of each food.

*Bread, cereals, and vegetables of high carbohydrate content.*—Again, it was obvious that if many foods of high carbohydrate content could be included in the one list of bread exchanges, it would be much easier for all those concerned with the planning of diabetic diets. Many lists of this sort have been prepared by other groups. The joint committee agreed upon the list given in Table 27, which includes several types of breadstuffs, a number of cereals, different varieties of crackers, and the vegetables with the highest carbohydrate content, as shown in Table 22.

Although the average slice of bread may weigh 25 gm. and contain approximately 13 gm. carbohydrate, it was decided that it would be preferable to list all the foods in this group in amounts that contain approximately 15 gm. carbohydrate. A ½-cup serving of many of these foods, which is an easy quantity to measure, yields this amount of carbohydrate. During the course of a day, an individual who is allowed six bread exchanges, for example, is likely to select several different foods from List 4, such as potato, cereal, or crackers. The average typical day's consumption of bread exchanges is therefore approximately 15 gm. carbohydrate per serving.

*Meat, fish, poultry, eggs, and cheese.*—The foods which are high in protein have been listed in amounts that are equal in protein and fat content to approximately 1 oz. meat. It was noted that the method or preparation or the cut of the meat (rib or rump) will influence the protein and fat content. Also, some forms of cheese are higher in fat than others as a result of the type of milk (whole or skim) used in their preparation. Some varieties of fish (cod versus mackerel) contain more fat than others. In a mixed diet, these differences become minimized. After reviewing the dietary analyses of these foods, the committee recommended the list of meat exchanges given in Table 28 and the figures of 7 gm. protein and 5 gm. fat per unit of exchange.

# TABLE 25

## AMOUNT OF FRUIT SUPPLYING
### 10 GM. CARBOHYDRATE

| FOOD | SOURCE OF REFERENCE | |
| --- | --- | --- |
| | U.S. Dept. of Agriculture (3) (Gm.) | Joint Committee's Recommendations (Gm.) |
| Apple.................. | 97 | 80 |
| Applesauce............. | 126 | 100 |
| Apricots, fresh........... | 96 | 100 |
| Apricots, dried.......... | 22 | 20 |
| Banana................. | 52 | 50 |
| Blackberries............. | 164 | 150 |
| Blueberries ............. | 103 | 100 |
| Canteloupe............. | 238 | 200 |
| Cherries................ | 75 | 75 |
| Dates.................. | 16 | 15 |
| Figs, fresh.............. | 62 | 50 |
| Figs, dried.............. | 18 | 15 |
| Grape juice............. | 60 | 60 |
| Grapefruit.............. | 154 | 125 |
| Grapefruit juice......... | 118 | 100 |
| Grapes................. | 67–87 | 75 |
| Honeydew melon........ | 143 | 150 |
| Mango................. | 73 | 70 |
| Orange................. | 113 | 100 |
| Orange juice............ | 111 | 100 |
| Papaya................. | 111 | 100 |
| Peach.................. | 114 | 100 |
| Pear................... | 112 | 100 |
| Pineapple.............. | 84 | 80 |
| Pineapple juice.......... | 83 | 80 |
| Plums.................. | 120 | 100 |
| Prunes, dried........... | 24 | 25 |
| Raisins................. | 16 | 15 |
| Raspberries............. | 139 | 150 |
| Strawberries............ | 189 | 150 |
| Tangerines.............. | 115 | 100 |
| Watermelon............. | 167 | 175 |

## TABLE 26

### LIST 3—FRUIT EXCHANGES*
(Carbohydrate—10 Gm. per Serving)

| Food | Approximate Measure |
|---|---|
| Apple (2-in. diameter) | 1 |
| Applesauce | $\frac{1}{2}$ cup |
| Apricots | |
|     Fresh | 2 medium |
|     Dried | 4 halves |
| Banana | $\frac{1}{2}$ small |
| Blackberries | 1 cup |
| Blueberries | $\frac{2}{3}$ cup |
| Cantaloupe (6-in. diameter)† | $\frac{1}{4}$ |
| Cherries | 10 large |
| Dates | 2 |
| Figs, fresh | 2 large |
| Figs, dried | 2 |
| Grape juice | $\frac{1}{4}$ cup |
| Grapefruit† | $\frac{1}{2}$ small |
| Grapefruit juice† | $\frac{1}{2}$ cup |
| Grapes | 12 |
| Honeydew melon (7-in. diameter) | $\frac{1}{8}$ |
| Mango | $\frac{1}{2}$ small |
| Orange† | 1 small |
| Orange juice† | $\frac{1}{2}$ cup |
| Papaya | $\frac{1}{3}$ medium |
| Peach | 1 medium |
| Pear | 1 small |
| Pineapple | $\frac{1}{2}$ cup |
| Pineapple juice | $\frac{1}{3}$ cup |
| Plums | 2 medium |
| Prunes, dried | 2 medium |
| Raisins | 2 tablespoons |
| Raspberries | 1 cup |
| Strawberries† | 1 cup |
| Tangerine | 1 large |
| Watermelon | 1 cup |

* Unsweetened canned fruits may be used in the same amount as listed for the fresh fruit.

† These fruits are rich sources of ascorbic acid. At least one serving should be included in the diet each day.

## TABLE 27

### LIST 4—BREAD EXCHANGES
(Per Serving: Carbohydrate, 15 Gm.; Protein, 2 Gm.)

| Food | Approximate Measure | Weight (Gm.) |
|---|---|---|
| *Bread:* | 1 slice | 25 |
| biscuit, roll (2-in. diameter).......... | 1 | 35 |
| muffin (2-in. diameter).............. | 1 | 35 |
| cornbread (1½-in. cube).............. | 1 | 35 |
| Flour............................. | 2½ tablespoons | 30 |
| *Cereal:* | | |
| cooked......................... | ½ cup | 100 |
| dry (flake and puffed).............. | ¾ cup | 20 |
| rice and grits, cooked.............. | ½ cup | 100 |
| Spaghetti and noodles, cooked......... | ½ cup | 100 |
| *Crackers:* | | |
| graham (2½-in. square).............. | 2 | 20 |
| oysterettes....................... | 20 (½ cup) | 20 |
| saltines (2-in. square).............. | 5 | 20 |
| soda (2½-in. square)............... | 3 | 20 |
| round, thin (1½-in. diameter)........ | 6–8 | 20 |
| *Vegetables:* | | |
| beans and peas, dried, cooked....... | ½ cup | 100 |
| (Lima, navy, split pea, cowpeas) | | |
| beans, Lima, fresh................. | ½ cup | 100 |
| beans, baked, no pork.............. | ¼ cup | 50 |
| corn, sweet....................... | ⅓ cup | 80 |
| corn, popped..................... | 1 cup | 20 |
| parsnips......................... | ⅔ cup | 125 |
| potatoes, white—baked or boiled (2-in. diameter)....................... | 1 | 100 |
| potatoes, white—mashed........... | ½ cup | 100 |
| potatoes, sweet or yams............ | ¼ cup | 60 |
| Sponge cake, plain (1½-in. cube)........ | 1 | 25 |
| Ice cream (omit 2 fat exchanges)........ | ½ cup | 70 |

Diets which include odd amounts of meat, such as 75 or 105 gm., are difficult to measure. Servings of 1, 2, or 3 oz., for example, are more practical for the patient, since the food is usually purchased in these amounts. This factor was taken into consideration in preparing this list.

*Fats.*—The problem of arriving at a figure for the composition of

TABLE 28

LIST 5—MEAT EXCHANGES
(Per Serving: Protein, 7 Gm.; Fat, 5 Gm.)

| Food | Approximate Measure | Weight (Gm.) |
|---|---|---|
| Meat and poultry, medium fat (beef, lamb, pork, liver, chicken).......... | 1 oz. | 30 |
| Cold cuts (4½ in. square, ⅛ in. thick)... | 1 slice | 45 |
| Frankfurter (8 or 9 per lb.)........... | 1 | 50 |
| *Fish:* | | |
| cod, mackerel..................... | 1 oz. | 30 |
| salmon, tuna, crab................ | ¼ cup | 30 |
| oysters, shrimp, clams............. | 5 small | 45 |
| sardines......................... | 3 medium | 30 |
| *Cheese:* | | |
| Cheddar or American............. | 1 oz. | 30 |
| cottage......................... | ¼ cup | 45 |
| Eggs.............................. | 1 | 50 |
| Peanut butter*..................... | 2 tablespoons | 30 |

* Limit use or adjust carbohydrate (deduct 5 gm. carbohydrate per serving when used in excess of one exchange).

fats was relatively simple, since there are fewer variable factors involved. The joint committee accepted the value of 5 gm. fat per fat exchange. The list (Table 29) contains foods that are approximately equal in fat content.

These six exchange lists (Tables 21, 23, 26, 27, 28, and 29) will allow the patient great variety in his diet and permit him to select foods from the different groups that may suit his income and food habits. The lists should also help to establish some uniformity in dietary instruction and counteract a practice that has no scientific basis, that of excluding various foods, such as potato, certain fruits, and some other foods, from the diet.

TABLE 29

LIST 6—FAT EXCHANGES
(Fat—5 Gm. per Serving)

| Food | Approximate Measure | Weight (Gm.) |
|---|---|---|
| Butter or margarine......... | 1 teaspoon | 5 |
| Bacon, crisp.............. | 1 slice | 10 |
| *Cream:* | | |
| light, 20%............. | 2 tablespoons | 30 |
| heavy, 40%............ | 1 tablespoon | 15 |
| Cream cheese............ | 1 tablespoon | 15 |
| French dressing........... | 1 tablespoon | 15 |
| Mayonnaise............... | 1 teaspoon | 5 |
| Oil or cooking fat.......... | 1 teaspoon | 5 |
| Nuts.................... | 6 small | 10 |
| Olives................... | 5 small | 50 |
| Avocado (4-in. diameter)..... | ⅛ | 25 |

*Special considerations.*—The following foods contain negligible amounts of carbohydrate, protein, and fat and may therefore be used as desired in the diet:

Coffee
Tea
Clear broth
Bouillon
Gelatin, unsweetened
Rennet tablets
Cranberries
Lemon

Rhubarb
Mustard
Pickles, sour
Pickles, dill—unsweetened
Saccharin
Pepper
Spices
Vinegar

"Specialty" foods for diabetic patients are not recommended. They are expensive, the information on the package is often misleading, and the patient can usually eat all the natural foods (breads, cereals, unsweetened fruits, vegetables) in the amount specified in his diet outline.

### CALCULATION OF THE DIABETIC DIET

By using the short list of food values given in Table 20, it will be possible to calculate diet prescriptions with considerable ease and simplicity, taking into account the amount of each of these food groups which the patient should eat. This simplicity in calculating a diet will result in the saving of time for both the physician and the dietitian. The patient will also benefit immeasurably by a diet that is made to suit his food habits. Variety in the diet will be achieved by using the food exchange lists (Tables 21, 23, 26, 27, 28, and 29).

The nutritive adequacy of the diet will be assured by including the same *basic foods* that are recommended for the normal individual. These include the following:

Milk..............................1 pt. for adults; 1 qt. for children
Meat, fish, poultry, eggs, and cheese... 4–5 oz.
Whole-grain or enriched cereal or bread. To meet caloric needs
Fruit—one a citrus fruit or tomato.... 2 servings
Vegetables—one green or yellow...... 2 servings
Fat or oil......................... To meet caloric needs

The actual calculation of the diet can be reduced to a simple formula, as shown in the tabulation on p. 84. To determine the number of servings of bread, meat, and fat exchanges required to complete the diet prescription, it is necessary only to:

*a)* Subtract the number of grams of carbohydrate (61 in the example in the table) furnished by the other sources of carbohydrate from the amount prescribed (180) and divide the result by 15, the number of grams of carbohydrate in one serving of bread exchange, as noted in List 4.

*b)* Adjust the amount of protein in the diet to the prescription by subtracting the number of grams of protein (34 in the example) supplied by milk, vegetables, and bread exchanges from the amount prescribed (80) and dividing the remainder by 7, the amount of protein in each meat exchange.

*c)* Follow the same procedure with regard to fat, except to divide the result by 5, the number of grams of fat in one serving, as noted in List 6.

The diet is figured to coincide as closely as possible with the prescription. However, it is not practical to split bread or meat exchanges into halves or to add extra fruits and vegetables if the patient does not care for larger amounts. Therefore, the carbohydrate may vary as much as 7 gm. from the amount ordered, and the protein may differ by 3 gm. The fat will agree closely with the prescription, since the figures for fat are all in multiples of 5.

## DIVISION OF FOOD INTO MEALS

Division of the total amount of food prescribed into meals should be worked out with the patient. In doing this, several factors must be considered:

*a*) Present meal patterns, which are usually related to such factors as occupation, working hours, and place of eating.

## PROCEDURE FOR CALCULATING A DIABETIC DIET (15)

Sample Prescription

| | |
|---|---|
| Carbohydrate.................. | 180 gm. |
| Protein...................... | 80 gm. |
| Fat.......................... | 70 gm. |
| Calories..................... | 1,700 |

| | Amount | Carbohydrate (Gm.) | Protein (Gm.) | Fat (Gm.) |
|---|---|---|---|---|
| Milk, whole (List 1)........................... | 1 pt. | 24 | 16 | 20 |
| Vegetables (List 2, Group A).................... | As desired | ... | .. | .. |
| Vegetables (List 2, Group B)................... | 1 serving | 7 | 2 | .. |
| Fruit (List 3)............................... | 3 servings | 30 | .. | .. |
| Total carbohydrate from sources other than bread exchanges........................ | ......... | 61 | | |

180 gm. carbohydrate in prescription
— 61 gm. from sources other than bread exchanges
___
119 ÷ 15 = 8 bread exchanges

| | Amount | Carbohydrate (Gm.) | Protein (Gm.) | Fat (Gm.) |
|---|---|---|---|---|
| Bread exchanges (List 4)...................... | 8 servings | 120 | 16 | |
| Total protein from sources other than meat exchanges.................................. | ......... | ... | 34 | |

80 gm. protein in prescription
− 34 gm. from sources other than meat exchanges
___
46 gm. ÷ 7 = 7 meat exchanges

| | Amount | Carbohydrate (Gm.) | Protein (Gm.) | Fat (Gm.) |
|---|---|---|---|---|
| Meat exchanges (List 5)...................... | 7 servings | | 49 | 35 |
| Total fat from sources other than fat exchanges | ......... | ... | .. | 55 |

70 gm. fat in prescription
−55 gm. from sources other than fat exchanges
___
15 gm. ÷ 5 = 3 fat exchanges

| | Amount | Carbohydrate (Gm.) | Protein (Gm.) | Fat (Gm.) |
|---|---|---|---|---|
| Fat exchanges (List 6)........................ | 3 servings | | | 15 |
| | | 181 | 83 | 70 |

*b)* Diabetic condition, i.e., tendency to excrete more or less sugar at varying times during the day.

*c)* Type of insulin—regular, protamine zinc, globin, or Lente.

The carbohydrate content of the diet should be divided between the meals, avoiding too large a proportion of the total at any one meal. When protamine insulin is used, nourishment at bedtime (perhaps one-seventh of the day's allowance of carbohydrate) should be recommended. When globin insulin is used, also give an afternoon lunch (approximately one-seventh) and reduce the carbohydrate of the breakfast to about the same amount.

A good source of protein should be included at each meal (milk, eggs, meat, fish, or cheese). The fat is apt to divide itself naturally with fairly even distribution throughout the meals.

### SAMPLE MEAL PLANS

The simplified method of calculating a diabetic diet just described is recommended, since it is the procedure most likely to make certain that the diet is adjusted to the food preferences of the individual. "Diet lists" prepared in advance can be used for convenience, provided that they are modified to suit the special needs of the individual. For this reason nine sample meal plans (Tables 30 and 31) were prepared by the committee to fit various needs.

Each of these nine diets has been outlined and illustrated with sample menus in small leaflets which may be distributed to patients. It is expected that these will be used in conjunction with the booklet *Meal Planning with Exchange Lists* which has also been prepared for the use of patients. In addition, two other leaflets for patients have been prepared in one of which appropriate changes in the exchange lists have been made to fit the need for modifications in sodium content. The other leaflet indicates adaptations of the exchange lists to fit those who may need to use bland-flavored foods.

For the physician, a special leaflet has been prepared, containing the carbohydrate, protein, fat, and caloric content of each food exchange, tables of prescriptions for various levels of dietary intake, desirable weights for men and women, and notes regarding the selection of diet prescriptions for adults and children.

The twelve leaflets and the *Meal Planning with Exchange Lists* are available from The American Dietetic Association, 620 North Michigan Avenue, Chicago 11, Illinois.

CONSIDERATIONS IN ADAPTING THE FOOD EXCHANGE LISTS

*New data on food composition.*—Since 1950 new values for some food items now included in the exchange lists have been reported in *Composition of Foods—Raw, Processed, Prepared* (U.S. Department of Agriculture, Agriculture Handbook No. 8 [December, 1963]). In

TABLE 30

CALORIC LEVELS OF SAMPLE MEALS FOR DIABETICS

| Meal Plan | Carbo-hydrate (Gm.) | Protein (Gm.) | Fat (Gm.) | Energy (Calories) |
|---|---|---|---|---|
| 1 | 125 | 60 | 50 | 1,200 |
| 2 | 150 | 70 | 70 | 1,500 |
| 3 | 180 | 80 | 80 | 1,800 |
| 4 | 220 | 90 | 100 | 2,200 |
| 5* | 180 | 80 | 80 | 1,800 |
| 6* | 250 | 100 | 130 | 2,600 |
| 7* | 370 | 140 | 165 | 3,500 |
| 8 | 250 | 115 | 130 | 2,600 |
| 9 | 300 | 120 | 145 | 3,000 |

* Planned particularly for children.

TABLE 31

SAMPLE MEAL PLANS FOR DIABETICS

| Diet | Milk | Veg. A | Veg. B | Fruits | Bread Exchange | Meat Exchange | Fat Exchange |
|---|---|---|---|---|---|---|---|
| 1 | 1 pt. | As desired | 1 | 3 | 4 | 5 | 1 |
| 2 | 1 pt. | As desired | 1 | 3 | 6 | 6 | 4 |
| 3 | 1 pt. | As desired | 1 | 3 | 8 | 7 | 5 |
| 4 | 1 pt. | As desired | 1 | 4 | 10 | 8 | 8 |
| 5* | 1 qt. | As desired | 1 | 3 | 6 | 5 | 3 |
| 6* | 1 qt. | As desired | 1 | 4 | 10 | 7 | 11 |
| 7* | 1 qt. | As desired | 1 | 6 | 17 | 10 | 15 |
| 8 | 1 pt. | As desired | 1 | 4 | 12 | 10 | 12 |
| 9 | 1 pt. | As desired | 1 | 4 | 15 | 10 | 15 |

* These diets contain more milk and are especially suitable for children.

most instances, however, the change has been small and when related to the usual frequency of consumption of the varied items in an exchange list, no real impact is made on the representative value for carbohydrate, protein, and fat now assigned.

An exception may occur, however, if the frequency of use of certain items is altered. For example, in certain areas of the country, more lean cuts of meat are available on the market, reflecting in part a demand for lower calories and less saturated fat. If this increased consumption of lean meat were coupled with increased use of fish and poultry and a concomitant reduction in the use of items higher in fat such as bologna, frankfurters, peanut butter, and most cheeses, the present value of the meat exchange might be closer to 8 gm. protein and 2 gm. fat than the present value of 7 gm. protein and 5 gm. fat. These considerations have been pointed up by Parente *et al.* (19) in "Adaptation of Exchange Lists—Use in Planning Metabolic Ward Diets."

Various ratios of polyunsaturated to saturated fats, percentages of fats, and reduced levels of cholesterol may easily be incorporated for therapeutic purposes. For an assessment of a basic diet that may be used for this purpose, see Table 15.

Some variations are also known to occur from state to state in the fat content of milk. In addition, convenience foods and numerous special purpose foods vary from market to market and from time to time in the same market, necessitating continuous alertness on the part of the dietitian and special compilations of data on food composition representing foods available in the local market.

*Total nutrient worth.*—Since the integrity of the total diet depends upon the nutrient merit of the component food groups, a critical appraisal by the dietitian not only of carbohydrate, protein, and fat, but also of minerals and vitamins is in order. With these criteria alone, the frequent substitution, for example, of a candy bar for a glass of milk, or of a soft drink for orange juice would be unjustified —in spite of any "equivalence" in carbohydrate, protein, or fat. For a gross comparison of the nutrient worth of a food item not on the exchange list, reference may be made to Tables 2 and 36.

*Frequency of use.*—If a wide variety of the food items enumerated in any one food group is consumed, and if this food intake represents some proximity to the proportions indicated in the per capita consumption of foods reported by the U.S. Department of Agriculture (20), the present values for carbohydrate, protein, and fat in the exchange lists will be approximated. If the patient narrows his food intake to one or two items, however, or if intentional changes are recommended, a reassessment of the selection should be made to determine the effect of the bias introduced on the nutrient quality of the diet as a whole.

*Ethnic food habits.*—Some adaptations of the exchange list may be advisable in those situations where nationality, religious, or regional food preferences represent foods not now included in the exchange lists. Many of these items may be of equal or superior nutrient merit. Information on nutrient content, methods of food preparation, and appropriateness for therapeutic use should be determined in conference with the physician.

*Sweets and alcohol.*—Concentrated sweets and alcohol will reduce the total nutrient merit of the diet and in some cases alter the utilization of medication. The inclusion of either in the diet should be determined in conference with the physician.

### EDUCATIONAL PROGRAM

Stone (21) has directed an excellent paper to the dietitian entitled "A Rational Approach to Diet and Diabetes in 1964." He defines a rational diet as one that has been made to fit the individual patient with the first step being a careful assessment of the diet history. From this point, the dietitian can plan appropriate meals from familiar foods, from foods within the income of the patient, and in line with the therapeutic goals established by the physician. In counseling the patient, factors of motivation, educational level, and appropriate materials become of major concern.

The expanding range of responsibilities of the dietitian for patient care is described by Kaufman (see chap. 13). More sophisticated means are now available to present information needed by the patient. After an appropriate diet history has been obtained and an individual meal plan has been discussed with him by the dietitian, programmed instruction in book form or teaching machines serve to amplify in effective detail the basic background information needed by every patient and his family. For individual or group instruction, film strips or slide sets in color together with sound recordings are also available and serve as another sophisticated medium for hospital and community service (22, 23). Information regarding available materials of this nature may be obtained from the U.S. Public Health Service, Diabetes and Arthritis Program, Division of Chronic Diseases, Washington, D.C. The series covers practical presentations of the Food Exchange Lists, as well as the other aspects of patient care.

For professional reference, an up-to-date volume entitled *Dia-*

*betes Mellitus Diagnosis and Treatment* has been published by the American Diabetes Association, Inc. 18 East 48th Street, New York, New York 10017.

*Nutritional evaluation.*—An appraisal of the various nutrient, mineral, and vitamin contents of the diet may be made simply by comparison with the normal dietary plans. As previously stated, an evaluation of the vitamin A and the carotene content of various diets has been made by a committee of the Diet Therapy Section (17). It was found that low-caloric and low-fat diets frequently served to diabetics contained between 91 and 2,600 I.U. of vitamin A when liver was not served once a week. These same diets were high in carotene, however, owing to the large amount of fruits and vegetables present. These facts become of importance where there is a dysfunction in the assimilation and metabolism of carotene, as frequently occurs in diabetes and liver damage. In these cases it will be desirable to use liver one or more times per week or to add vitamin A supplements.

### THE GALACTOSE-FREE DIET

A review of the current concepts of the basic defects in galactosemia has been presented by Koch *et al.*, and a method of monitoring dietary control is suggested (25). The chief dietary modification involves the elimination of milk, of galactose-storing organ meats such as liver, pancreas, and brain, and possibly of the oligosaccharides, raffinose, and stachyose that occur in legumes and beets. A list of foods to include, those to exclude, and galactose-free recipes are reported.

The Children's Bureau, U.S. Department of Health, Education, and Welfare has prepared a selected and annotated bibliography entitled *Galactosemia, A Selected Bibliography*, 1963. This may be obtained from the Government Printing Office for 30 cents a copy.

Also, an excellent guide to the feeding of mentally retarded children has been prepared by the Children's Bureau, U.S. Department of Health, Education, and Welfare, Washington, D.C. This booklet includes guidance in taking a dietary history, assessment of feeding methods, and techniques and teaching for development of skills by the family and child. The booklet entitled, *Feeding Mentally Retarded Children*, 1964, may be obtained from the Government Printing Office, Washington, D.C. for 15 cents.

## REFERENCES

1. Calculation of diabetic diets, J. Am. Dietet. A., **24**:218–19, 1948.
2. McCANCE, R. A., and WIDDOWSON, E. M. Chemical composition of foods. 2d ed. Brooklyn, N.Y.: Chemical Publishing Co., 1947.
3. CHATFIELD, C., and ADAMS, G. Proximate composition of American food materials. (U.S. Department of Agriculture Circular No. 549.) 1940.
4. BUREAU OF HUMAN NUTRITION AND HOME ECONOMICS in co-operation with the NATIONAL RESEARCH COUNCIL. Tables of food composition in terms of eleven nutrients. ("U.S. Department of Agriculture Miscellaneous Publications," No. 572.) 1945.
5. OLMSTED, W. H. The available carbohydrate of fruits and vegetables, Proc. Am. Diabetes A., **9**:385–406, 1950.
6. HUMMEL, F. C., SHEPHERD, M. L., and MACY, I. G. Disappearance of cellulose and hemicellulose from the digestive tracts of children, J. Nutrition, **25**:59–70, 1943.
7. BUCHANAN, J. M., and HASTINGS, A. B. The use of isotopically marked carbon in the study of intermediary metabolism, Physiol. Rev., **26**:120–55, 1946.
8. BLOCH, K. The metabolism of acetic acid in animal tissues, Physiol. Rev., **27**:574–620, 1947.
9. WOOD, H. G. The fixation of carbon dioxide and the inter-relationships of the tricarboxylic acid cycle, Physiol. Rev., **26**:198–246, 1946.
10. STADIE, W. C. The intermediary metabolism of fatty acids, Physiol. Rev., **25**:395–441, 1945.
11. WILLIAMS, R. D., WICKS, L., BIERMAN, H. R., and OLMSTED, W. H. Carbohydrate values of fruits and vegetables, J. Nutrition, **19**:593–604, 1940.
12. BUREAU OF HUMAN NUTRITION AND HOME ECONOMICS. Consumption of food in the United States, 1909–48. ("U.S. Department of Agriculture Miscellaneous Publications," No. 691.) 1949.
13. STERN, F. Applied dietetics. 3d ed. Baltimore: Williams & Wilkins Co., 1949.
14. TURNER, D. Handbook of diet therapy. 1st ed. Chicago: University of Chicago Press, 1946.
15. CASO, E. K., and STARE, F. J. Simplified method for calculating diabetic diets, J.A.M.A., **133**:169–71, 1947.
16. Revised tables of food values, Proc. Am. Diabetes A., **9**: 403–6, 1950.
17. JOHNSON, D. Vitamin A versus carotene content of low-fat diets in obesity, cholecystitis, and liver disease, J. Am. Dietet. A., **25**:873–74, 1942.
18. BUREAU OF HUMAN NUTRITION AND HOME ECONOMICS. Family food consumption in the United States, spring, 1942. ("U.S. Department of Agriculture Miscellaneous Publications," No. 550.) 1944.
19. PARENTE, B. P., GAFFIELD, B. E., HILL, R. B., and OHLSON, M. A. Adaptation of Exchange Lists—Use in Planning Ward Diets, J. Am. Dietet. A., **46**:267–75, 1965.
20. ECONOMIC RESEARCH SERVICE. Consumption of Food in the United States, Supplement for 1961. (U.S. Department of Agriculture, Agriculture Handbook No. 62.) 1962.

21. STONE, DANIEL B. A. rational approach to diet and diabetes in 1964, J. Am. Dietet. A., **46**:30–35, 1965.
22. KAUFMAN, M. Programmed instruction materials on diabetes J. Am. Dietet. A., **46**:36–38, 1965.
23. DOWNING, C. B. What is programmed instruction? J. Am. Dietet. A., **46**:39–42, 1965.
24. Composition of Foods—Raw, Processed, Prepared. (U.S. Department of Agriculture, Agriculture Handbook No. 8 [December, 1963].)
25. KOCH, R., ACOSTA, P., RAGSDALE, N., and DONNELL, G. N. Nutrition in the treatment of galactosemia. J. Am. Dietet. A., **43**:216–22, 1963.

The sodium-restricted diet is an allowance of food and drink in which the sodium content is restricted to a prescribed level. Other nutrients remain as nearly as possible on a level satisfactory for nutritive sufficiency.

Sodium restriction is most often prescribed in the control of edema accompanying congestive heart failure, and has been shown also to be of benefit in the treatment of some cases of hypertension, cirrhosis of the liver, toxemias of pregnancy, and certain kidney diseases.

Physicians vary in their use of sodium-restricted diets and the levels prescribed. Some prescribe them in conjunction with drug therapy, such as diuretics, thereby making it possible to use a less restricted level of sodium. Certain patients experience toxic reactions or other complications with drug therapy; and for these, dietary restriction of sodium remains the safest treatment.

Since it is the sodium ion that is significant in sodium-restricted therapy such terms as "low salt," "salt poor," and "salt free" are inadequate. A prescribed level of dietary sodium should be indicated and with due consideration for the sodium content of drinking water and medications.

The person on an unrestricted diet may consume ordinarily between 5 and 10 gm. sodium daily. Water varies in sodium content from source to source and from time to time depending in part upon the water softeners added at the treatment plant or at home. Foods in their natural state contain widely differing amounts of sodium; and the amount of sodium added in food preparation and in commercial processing is significant. Bills *et al.* (2) have pointed out:

Many manufactured food products which are not intentionally salted contain somewhat more sodium than the natural foods from which they are prepared. The source of this sodium is found in the numerous special uses of sodium compounds in the food industry. Sodium chloride is employed for many purposes besides seasoning, preserving, pickling, and koshering. As brine it is used (*a*) in the flotation process of sorting green peas from hardened peas and heavy extraneous matter, (*b*) for preventing enzymic discoloring of freshly sliced apples and pears which are to be canned, (*c*) as a heat transfer and blanching agent in freezing foods, and (*d*) for regenerating base-exchange water softeners (the sodium appears in the softened water as bicarbonate, and water thus treated is used in canning to prevent toughening of vegetables).

Sodium alginate is employed as a stabilizer for ice cream and chocolate milk drinks. Sodium aluminum sulphate is the alum of baking powders. Sodium benzoate is used as a preservative in fruit juice concentrates, confectionery, margarine, and so on. Sodium bicarbonate is the gas source in baking powders and self-rising flours. It is also used with cocoa in the "Dutching" process, for tenderizing vegetables, and for neutralizing. Sodium carbonate is used for Dutching, neutralizing, and water softening. It has a special use in removing hop resins from brewers' yeast in the debittering process. Sodium citrate is used as a stabilizing agent in evaporated milk and jellies. Sodium glutamate is an important flavoring adjunct. Sodium hydroxide is used for Dutching cocoa, neutralizing corn syrup, debittering ripe olives, and hulling corn in the old lye process of hominy manufacture. It is also widely used in peeling apricots, peaches, grapefruit segments, carrots, and sweet potatoes, for canning, and for dipping fruits prior to drying. Sodium acid phosphate is used as an acidulating agent. The secondary phosphate is used for emulsifying process cheese, for stabilizing evaporated milk, and as the quickening agent in quick-cooking farina. Sodium acid sulphite is employed for sulphuring fruits prior to drying. These few examples may serve to explain the almost ubiquitous occurrence in processed foods of sodium in amounts greater than are present in the corresponding natural products.

In planning a regimen, reference should be made to sodium since equal weights of different sodium compounds do not contain equal weights of sodium. With respect to sodium chloride, 58.5 gm. or one gram-molecule is composed of 23 gm. sodium (one gram-atom) and 35.5 gm. chlorine (one gram-atom). To convert a specified weight of sodium chloride to sodium, multiply by 0.393; thus 10 gm. of sodium chloride contains 3.93 gm. of sodium.

The millimolecular weight (mmole) and milliequivalent weight (mEq.) are one thousandth of the gram molecular weight and the equivalent gram-atomic weight, respectively.

$$\text{1 mEq. of sodium} = 23 \text{ mg.}$$

To derive the sodium content in mEq. divide the weight of sodium in mg. by 23. For example, if the sodium content of milk is 50 mg. per

100 gm. or approximately 500 mg. per liter, the mEq. weight is $\frac{500}{23}$ or about 22 mEq. per liter. The following conversions may be useful (6):

1,000 mg. (1 gm.) of sodium = 43.5 mEq.

100 mg. of sodium = 4.35 mEq.

10 mg. of sodium = 0.44 mEq.

1 mg. of sodium = 0.04 mEq.

100 mEq. of sodium = 2,300 mg. (2.3 gm.)

10 mEq. of sodium = 230 mg.

1 mEq. of sodium = 23 mg.

10 gm. of sodium chloride $= \dfrac{10,000}{58.5} =$ 171 mEq. of sodium chloride, sodium, or chloride.

1 gm. of sodium chloride = 17.1 mEq. of sodium chloride, sodium, or chloride.

Selected values for sodium and potassium content of foods appear in Table 41, pages 209–20. A more extensive list of values may be found in *Composition of Foods* (U.S. Department of Agriculture, Agricultural Research Service, Agriculture Handbook No. 8), 1963.

### NUTRIENT CONTENT

Since the level of sodium prescribed for therapy may vary from 200 mg. daily to 2,000 mg. or more, depending upon the needs of the individual patient, it becomes desirable to have a basic plan in which protein, mineral, and vitamin needs may be at a level for nutritive sufficiency but from which modifications may be made to suit the level of sodium prescribed. For this reason, adaptations of the plans of normal diet described, are recommended as the basic pattern of diet. For example, if the patient is an adult, the appropriate basic pattern (Table 2) may be used for making modifications. If the patient is a pregnant woman, the respective plan of diet (Table 7) should be used. In the case of an adolescent or a child, normal patterns of diet (Tables 8 and 9) should be used as a basis for the sodium modifications. In planning a 500-mg. sodium diet for an adult, an illustration of the kind and amount of the food groups which might be used are described in Table 32A. The meal pattern and sample menus appear in Table 32B.

TABLE 32

500-MG. SODIUM DIET FOR AN ADULT

(70 Gm. Protein; 1,500 Calories; Adapted from Normal Diet, Table 2)

| Daily Food Plan | Sodium† (Mg.) | Protein (Gm.) | Calories |
|---|---|---|---|
| MILK GROUP* | | | |
| 1 pt. whole.............................. | 244 | 16 | 340 |
| MEAT AND EGG GROUP | | | |
| 1 egg................................. | 60 | 7 | 75 |
| 4 oz. cooked meat, poultry or fish (edible portion), *no sodium added*.................. | 70 | 28 | 300 |
| VEGETABLE AND FRUIT GROUP | | | |
| 5 servings (*no sodium added*) | | | |
| Dark-green or yellow (1 serving)............ | 9 | ............ | ............ |
| Other vegetable (1 serving)................. | 4 | ............ | 35 |
| Citrus fruit or other fruit rich in vitamin C (1 serving)............................ | 1 | ............ | 40 |
| Other fruit (2 servings).................... | 5 | ............ | 80 |
| BREAD-CEREAL-POTATO-LEGUME GROUP | | | |
| 8 servings (*no sodium added*) | | | |
| Bread, 6 slices (*no sodium added*)........... | 54 | 12 | 420 |
| Potato, ½ cup, or ½ cup cooked rice, white or red beans, cornmeal, noodles, spaghetti, ⅓ cup corn or ¼ cup sweet potato (*no sodium added*) | 5 | 2 | 70 |
| Cereals, cooked, ½ cup, such as farina, rolled oats, rolled wheat cereal (*no sodium added*). | 5 | 2 | 70 |
| FATS AND SWEETS‡ | | | |
| 1 teaspoon butter or margarine (*no sodium added*)................................ | 1 | ............ | 45 |
| 1 teaspoon sugar, jelly, or jam.............. | 1 | ............ | 20 |
| WATER† | | | |
| Total............................ | 459 ᵗ | 67 | 1,495‡ |

* During pregnancy, adolescence, and childhood, 1 quart of milk may be used, thus increasing calories to 1,800, protein to 83 gm., and sodium to 700 mg. If less sodium is desired, low-sodium milk may be used.

† For additional values on sodium (and potassium) content of foods, see Table 41. Sodium content of water should be added to the total. Local health department should be contacted for information on current sodium content of municipal water supplies.

‡ For substitutions or additions to suit caloric needs see Table 36. For a sample menu pattern and sample meals see Table 32B.

*Modification for 250-mg. sodium diet.*—The use of low-sodium milk may reduce the sodium content by about 90 per cent. This change alone will reduce the diet to about 250 mg. sodium.

*Modification for 1,000-mg. sodium diet.*—Numerous choices are possible in making substitutions where an additional amount of sodium is permitted on the 500-mg. sodium diet. One slice of ordinary salted bread may contain approximately 180 mg. sodium; and 1 teaspoon of ordinary salted butter or margarine may provide approximately 50 mg. sodium; thus totaling 230 mg. sodium per one slice of ordinary bread and butter or margarine. If ordinary canned vegetables are an item of choice, approximately 250 mg. sodium per one-half cup serving may be expected if no salt is added at the table. These and other items may be substituted for items in the 500-mg. sodium diet by reference to the values for sodium content of foods in Table 41.

*Modification for 2,000-2,500-mg. sodium diet.*—If the eight servings of the bread group were from ordinary salted bread, approximately 1,500 mg. sodium would be added, making the diet 2,000 mg. sodium. If 8 teaspoons ordinary salted butter or margarine were used with the bread, 400 more mg. sodium would be added, making the total sodium approximately 2,400 mg. Alternates, sample menu patterns, and sample meals appear in Tables 32, 32A, and 32B.

DAILY FOOD PLAN OF DIET CONTAINING 500 MG. SODIUM
(70 Gm. Protein; 1,500 Calories; Derived from Table 32)

| Daily Food Plan | Description |
|---|---|
| **MILK GROUP** | |
| 1 pt. | *One pint of whole milk* contains approximately 16 gm. protein, 340 calories, and 244 mg. sodium. It is also an important source of minerals and vitamins of the B complex. One pint skim milk may contain approximately 180 calories and similar protein and sodium to whole milk. |
| | *Palatable milks* prepared by an ion-exchange process are available in some areas. Sodium is reduced by 90 per cent; thiamine, niacin, and vitamin $B_{12}$ by about 50 per cent; and calcium and vitamin $B_6$ by about 75 per cent. Potassium may be increased to about twice ordinary milk. |
| **MEAT AND EGG GROUP** | |
| 1 egg | *One egg* will contain approximately 60 mg. sodium, 7 gm. protein, and 75 calories. |
| 4 oz. cooked meat, poultry, or fish | *One ounce (edible portion) of cooked beef, veal, lamb, pork, poultry or fish (no sodium added)* contains about 18 mg. sodium, 7 gm. protein, and 75 calories. Meat, poultry, or fish salted at any stage of processing will not be suitable for use; therefore, ordinary canned or smoked and seasoned meat and cheese should be omitted. All products must be specially canned or prepared without added sodium, to be suitable for this diet. Four ounces meat contain approximately 70 mg. sodium. |
| **VEGETABLE AND FRUIT GROUP** | |
| 5 servings | |
| A dark-green or yellow vegetable is important daily for vitamin A value | *A dark-green or yellow vegetable* is important each day for vitamin A value. This group includes asparagus, green beans, peppers, yellow squash, pumpkin. Each serving may be estimated at 9 mg. sodium. Carrots, kale, beet greens, chard, and spinach have been excluded. One-half cup squash and pumpkin may contain 35 calories. Others are negligible. |
| | *Other vegetables* to which no sodium has been added may be used, such as cauliflower, cucumber, eggplant, onion, radishes, summer squash, and tomatoes. Each serving will contain about 4 mg. sodium. Calories are negligible. Beets, celery, and white turnips have been excluded. |
| A citrus fruit or other fruit rich in vitamin C daily | *One orange or $\frac{1}{2}$ grapefruit or 1 large tangerine or $\frac{1}{2}$ cup citrus juice* is considered one serving of citrus fruit. One cup strawberries, or 1 cup red raspberries, or $\frac{1}{4}$ cantaloupe is a satisfactory substitute. Sodium content of fruit is approximately 1 mg. per serving and 40 calories per serving. |
| Other fruit, 2 servings | *Will contribute 5 mg. sodium and 80 calories for 2 servings.* |

Daily Food Plan                    Description

BREAD-CEREAL-POTATO-
   LEGUME GROUP
(no sodium added)
8 servings            *One slice of bread* or substitute (*no sodium added*) con-
                      tains about 70 calories and 9 mg. sodium or less; i.e.,
                      ½ cup cooked potato, rice, dried beans, cornmeal,
                      noodles, spaghetti, ⅓ cup corn, or ¼ cup sweet potato
                      will contain less than 5 mg. sodium. Certain cooked
                      cereals, such as farina, rolled oats, rolled wheat
                      cereal, and wheat meals are low in sodium (avoid
                      "quick-cooking" cereals to which a sodium salt has
                      been added). Certain prepared cereals which have no
                      sodium added are Puffed Rice, Puffed Wheat, and
                      Shredded Wheat. Avoid any prepared cereals with
                      sodium added.

FATS AND SWEETS

                      *If 1 teaspoon sugar, jelly, or honey* is included, approxi-
                      mately 20 calories are added. No sodium need be
                      estimated for this.
                      *If 1 teaspoon fat or oil* is included, approximately 45
                      calories are added. Oils are not ordinarily salted.
                      Bacon, ham fat, salt pork, sausage fat, margarine,
                      and butter will have considerable amounts of sodium.
                      Two teaspoons ordinary, salted butter or margarine
                      contain about 100 mg. sodium. Unsalted butter and
                      margarine to which no sodium has been added will be
                      a negligible source of sodium.

SALT SUBSTITUTES

                      *Salt substitutes* should be used only upon recommenda-
                      tion of a physician.

ARTIFICIAL SWEETENERS

                      *Sodium cyclamate or saccharin* may be significant sources
                      of sodium.

IODINE                *A source of iodine* may become necessary, since iodized
                      sodium chloride cannot be used.

WATER                 *Drinking water* may be an important source of sodium.
                      Check with local health department regarding sodium
                      content of municipal water supplies.

500-MG. SODIUM DIET—MENU PATTERN AND SAMPLE MEALS FOR AN ADULT
(70 Gm. Protein; 1,500 Calories; Derived from Table 32A)

| DAILY FOOD PLAN* | SAMPLE MENU PATTERN‡ | SAMPLE MEALS‡ |
|---|---|---|
| | A.M. | |
| MILK GROUP<br><br>1 pt.<br><br><br>MEAT AND EGG GROUP<br><br><br>1 egg and 4 oz. (edible portion) meat, poultry, or fish<br>*No sodium added* | 1 citrus fruit or ½ cup juice<br>1 egg<br>½ cup low-sodium cooked cereal or ¾ cup flake-type with milk*<br>1 slice low-sodium, enriched, or whole-grain bread or toast<br>Spread†<br>Coffee or tea if desired<br>Sugar | Sliced tangerine<br>1 egg<br>Oatmeal with milk and sugar†<br>Toast with spread†<br>Coffee<br>Sugar |
| | Noon | |
| VEGETABLE AND FRUIT GROUP<br><br>5 servings<br>A dark-green or deep-yellow vegetable daily<br>Citrus fruit or other fruit rich in vitamin C daily<br>*No sodium added* | 2 oz. (edible portion) meat, poultry, or fish<br>3 servings of the bread-potato-cereal group*<br>Fresh or cooked vegetable<br>Fruit<br>Milk<br><br>Tea or coffee if desired | Club sandwich:<br>Sliced chicken<br>Sliced tomato<br>Lettuce<br>Spread†<br>Fresh mixed fruits<br>Milk |
| BREAD-CEREAL-POTATO-GROUP<br><br>8 servings<br>*No sodium added* | P.M. | |
| FATS AND SWEETS†<br><br>*No sodium added*<br>(Without this group the diet contains 1,500 calories) | 2 oz. (edible portion) meat, poultry, or fish<br>3 servings from potato-bread-cereal group*<br>Dark-green or deep-yellow vegetable<br>Other vegetable<br>Fruit<br>Milk | Roast pork<br>Sweet potato<br>Frozen green beans<br>Baked apple<br>Hot roll (*no sodium added*)<br>Spread†<br>Milk |

\* See Table 32A for alternates or substitutes in each food group.

† If 1 teaspoon fat or oil is included in addition to the basic diet of 1,500 calories, 45 calories per teaspoon should be added. This may be used on bread or in cooking.
If 1 teaspoon sugar, jelly, or honey is included in addition to the basic diet, approximately 20 calories should be added. These may be added in amounts suitable to meet caloric needs of individual patients.

‡ For discussion of food preparation see pp. 111–12.

### FOOD PREPARATION

Meat, poultry, and fish may be enhanced in flavor by using fruit combinations. Cranberry sauce with poultry, applesauce with pork, mint jelly with lamb, and lemon with fish are standbys. For those who like meat or fish cooked in tomato sauce, unsalted canned tomatoes, juice, or puree may be combined with garlic, onion, green pepper, and mushrooms and flavored with such herbs as oregano if desired. Meat and fish may be simmered or baked in this sauce. Low-sodium wines, French-type dressings, lemon, and vinegar provide excellent marination for meat.

Some additional flavor combinations are as follows:

Beef—dry mustard, marjoram, nutmeg, onion, sage, thyme, pepper, bay leaf, grape jelly

Lamb—mint, garlic, rosemary, curry, broiled pineapple rings, lemon juice, and oregano

Veal—bay leaf, ginger, marjoram, curry, currant jelly, spiced apricots

Chicken—paprika, mushroom, thyme, sage, parsley, cranberry sauce

Fish—dry mustard, paprika, curry, bay leaf, lemon juice, mushrooms, and sherry

Eggs—pepper, green pepper, mushrooms, dry mustard, paprika, curry, jelly, or pineapple omelet

Vegetables may be flavored with a sweet-sour sauce (diluted vinegar and sugar, seasoned with grated onion, spices, and herbs as desired) or with hot low-sodium salad dressing made as follows: canned tomatoes, tomato juice, or puree (no sodium added) may be flavored with lemon or vinegar, sugar, grated horse-radish root, onion, garlic, spices, and herbs as desired. Calories will be negligible. Other possible flavor combinations are as follows:

Asparagus—lemon juice

Beans, green—marjoram, lemon juice, nutmeg, dill seed

Broccoli—lemon juice

Cabbage—mustard dressing, dill seed, unsalted butter with lemon and sugar

Cauliflower—nutmeg

Corn—green pepper, tomatoes

Peas—mint, mushroom, parsley, onion

Potatoes—parsley, unsalted butter, mace, chopped green pepper, chives, onion

Squash—ginger, mace

Sweet potatoes—candied, or glazed with cinnamon or nutmeg, or escalloped with apples

Tomatoes—basil, oregano

Vegetable aspics may be concocted with plain gelatin, tomato juice (no sodium added), and lemon, grated cabbage, cucumber, and green pepper. Low-sodium dressing or mayonnaise with no added sodium may be used. Vegetables canned without added sodium are available. Frozen Lima beans or peas may have sodium added. Labels should be carefully read, and information sought from commercial firms.

*Baked goods* pose a special problem because usual products may contain added salt, salted shortening, baking powder, or soda. Such products might exceed 300 mg. sodium per 100 gram. This can be reduced greatly by preparation with unsalted shortening and with a low-sodium baking powder, possibly as low as 20 to 40 mg. sodium per 100 gm. On the other hand, the potassium content of products made with the low-sodium baking powder may increase by one-and-a-half to three-and-a-half times more than if sodium aluminum sulfate baking powder were used.

Low-sodium products may be prepared from combinations of foods permitted on the diet. Unsalted fats and oils are available. Leavening may be obtained from yeasts or sodium-free baking powder. The following formula for sodium-free baking powder may be obtained from a pharmacist:

Potassium bicarbonate........ 39.8 gm.
Cornstarch................. 28.0 gm.
Tartaric acid............... 7.5 gm.
Potassium bitartrate......... 56.1 gm.

Bread and rolls also pose special problems. Ordinary bread might contain approximately 600 mg. per 100 gm. In low-sodium bread, the sodium content might be reduced to approximately 60 mg. per 100 gm. of product. Ranges are wide, however, and it is important to read the labels of commercial products purported to be low in sodium to assess the mg. of sodium per 100 gm. of product. The same admonition applies to cereal products, since such items as puffed wheat, and shredded wheat, for example, appear in both the salted and unsalted form.

Low-sodium milk is available. In many parts of the country a palatable product has been obtained by passing fluid milk through an ion-exchange resin at 35°–40° F. The result is the replacement of sodium with an equivalent amount of potassium. The taste and flavor of the milk are only slightly affected. However, this product contains only about 50 per cent of the thiamine, niacin, and vitamin $B_{12}$ of the original milk and about 75 per cent of the calcium and vitamin $B_6$. The potassium is doubled but is still within the normal physiologic intake of 3–5 gm. for adults. The Council on Foods and Nutrition of the American Medical Association (3) recommends the following levels per quart:

| | | |
|---|---|---|
| Sodium, less than | 50 | mg. |
| Potassium, less than | 2.5 | gm. |
| Thiamine, at least | 0.15 | mg. |
| Riboflavin, at least | 1.0 | mg. |
| Niacin, at least | 0.4 | mg. |
| Vitamin $B_6$, at least | 300 | μg. |
| Vitamin $B_{12}$, at least | 3 | μg. |

Dried, low-sodium milk products are also available.

*Other low-sodium dietetic foods* are available. Such foods as vegetables canned without added salt, specially processed cheeses and meat add variety, save time, and increase the acceptance of the diet by the patient. Two federal regulations relating to labeling provide protection and information to persons on sodium-restricted therapy. One regulation requires that all labels on low-sodium, dietetic foods must indicate the sodium content in milligrams of sodium per 100 grams of food as well as in an average serving of food. The other regulation relates to frozen vegetables. If salt has been used either directly or indirectly during processing, the label must state that salt has been added or is present.

### SUPPLEMENTARY MATERIALS

Numerous special cookbooks have been prepared for patients on low-sodium diets. However, the value of any recipe depends upon an accurate estimate of the sodium content per serving and the proper substitution within each individual diet. This usually requires guidance from a dietitian, nutritionist, or physician. A critical review of low-sodium cookbooks, booklets, and materials on meal planning has been prepared at the request of the Nutrition Committee, American Heart Association, and published in the *Journal of the American Dietetic Association* (5).

Three booklets (4) for patients have been prepared by a Subcommittee on Sodium Restricted Diets, American Heart Association. Whys and wherefores of a sodium-restricted diet are discussed; diet plans limited in sodium and calories are described; and questions regarding food preparation are answered. The plans are limited to 500 mg., 1,000 mg., and 2,400–4,500 mg. sodium diets, since it was felt that prescriptions between these levels are usually unnecessary for therapeutic purposes. These booklets are available from the American Heart Association, 44 East Twenty-third Street, New York, New York, to physicians, dietitians, nutritionists, and nurses without charge. Simplified leaflets have been derived from the booklets as well as a recipe booklet for the patient.

*The Food You Eat and Heart Disease* (Public Health Service Publication No. 537), revised 1963, is a 12-page pamphlet for the layman on the importance of diet as specific therapy in some forms of heart disease. It counteracts the popular misconception of diet as a cure-all or preventive of cardiac diseases. Single copies are available without charge from the U.S. Department of Health, Education, and Welfare, Washington, D.C., 20402. Up to 50 copies may be obtained free by professional persons.

For professional persons, the publication entitled *Sodium Restricted Diets: The Rationale, Complications, and Practical Aspects of Their Use* ("Food and Nutrition Board–National Research Council Publications," No. 325 [1954]) continues to provide an excellent reference on the normal physiology of sodium metabolism, the use of sodium-restricted diets in congestive cardiac failure, hypertension, renal disease, cirrhosis of the liver, toxemias of pregnancy, Ménière's disease, and hormone therapy, as well as contra-indications for the use of low-sodium diets and salt substitutes.

Since sodium is closely related to other extra- and intra-cellular ions, particularly potassium, a limited number of values for both potassium and sodium have been included in Table 41, page 209. A more complete listing of sodium and potassium values appears in *Composition of Food—Raw, Processed, Prepared* (U.S. Department of Agriculture, Agricultural Research Service, Agriculture Handbook No. 8), 1963. Additional mineral elements (1) appear in Table 42.

## REFERENCES

1. PETERSON, W. H., SKINNER, J. T., and STRONG, F. M. Elements of food biochemistry. New York: Prentice-Hall, Inc., 1953, pp. 262–65.
2. BILLS, C. E., McDONALD, F. G., NIEDERMEIER, W., and SCHWARTZ, M. C. Sodium and potassium in foods and water, J. Am. Dietet. A., 25:304–14, 1949.
3. COUNCIL ON FOODS AND NUTRITION. Low sodium milk, J.A.M.A., 163:739, 1957.
4. HEAP, B., and ROBINSON, C. New diet booklets for cardiac patients and sodium restriction, J. Am. Dietet. A., 34:277–79, 1958.
5. REIMER, A., JOHNSON, D., and ROBINSON, C. Sodium restricted diets, J. Am. Dietet. A., 33:104–7, 1957.
6. Sodium Restricted Diets: The Rationale, Complications, and Practical Aspects of Their Use. (Food and Nutrition Board–National Research Council Publications, No. 325.) 1954.

The low-purine diet is a food allowance in which sources of purines, such as glandular organs, dried legumes and lentils, and meat extractives are eliminated, and other meat and fish are restricted to 4 oz. weekly, thus reducing the daily intake of uric acid equivalent to approximately 35 mg. If a high-carbohydrate, low-fat regimen is imposed in addition, as has been suggested by Bartels (1), further modifications may be made as outlined in the discussion of the low-fat diet (p. 60).

The following discussion of the purine content of foods and the outline for the low-purine diet is taken from a report of a committee of the Diet Therapy Section of The American Dietetic Association (2):

A review of the available literature regarding the purine content . . . of foods revealed a distressing paucity of usable figures and consistent values. The committee felt itself incompetent to evaluate the data inasmuch as the sources used and methods of analyses could not be satisfactorily compared.

In an attempt to obtain the most recent figures available, aid was solicited from outstanding authorities throughout the United States. It was found that none were using purine calculations or could add to the common list of references, or would attempt to evaluate comparatively the tables given in current texts.

An outline has been prepared by this committee as a guide for practical use in planning a low-purine diet. When protein-rich foods have been omitted because of their relatively high purine content, increases have been made in milk, eggs, and cheese to maintain normal protein levels.

## BREAKFAST

Fruit—citrus fruit or tomato juice
Cereal (except oatmeal), with cream or milk and sugar
Eggs—2
Toast (whole-grain or enriched white), with butter or enriched margarine. Jelly, jam, honey, or marmalade if desired
Beverages—decaffeinated coffee or cereal coffee with cream and sugar

## LUNCH AND DINNER

Soup—milk soups made with any vegetables except those forbidden (see special instructions below)
Meat, fish, or fowl—only 2-oz. portion twice weekly, omitting glandular meats entirely; 2-oz. portion of cheese daily on days meat is not served
Vegetables—potato daily if desired; 2–4 additional vegetables (any except those on forbidden list)
Bread—whole-grain or enriched, with butter or enriched margarine
Dessert—fruit, puddings, cake, ice cream, gelatin desserts, or pie
Beverage—milk or buttermilk and decaffeinated coffee or cereal coffee

## SPECIAL INSTRUCTIONS

1. Avoid liver, sweetbreads, brains, and kidney. A 2-oz. portion of any other meat, fish, or fowl may be served twice weekly.
2. Serve cheese and eggs as meat substitutes. Fish roe and caviar may be used as desired.
3. Use 1–2 pt. of milk daily to meet the protein need.
4. Omit all meat extracts, broth soups, and gravies.
5. Eliminate the following vegetables entirely from the diet: dried beans, lentils, dried peas, spinach.
6. Avoid coffee, tea, chocolate, and cocoa. Use decaffeinated coffee or a cereal coffee if desired. (There is some question as to whether or not caffeine can be converted into uric acid in the body.)
7. Omit alcoholic beverages of all kinds.
8. Allow fruits of all kinds—fresh, canned, and dried.
9. Allow cereals of all kinds except oatmeal.
10. Serve sugar as desired with amounts adjusted to caloric needs. Cream and butter may be restricted when a low-caloric allowance is needed or when a low-fat regimen is desired.

### TABLE 33

PURINE CONTENT OF FOODS PER 100 GM.

| Group I (0–15 Mg.) | Group II (50–150 Mg.) | Group III (150–800 Mg.) |
|---|---|---|
| Vegetables | Meats | Sweetbreads |
| Fruits | Fish | Anchovies |
| Milk | Sea food | Sardines |
| Cheese | Beans, dry | Liver |
| Eggs | Peas, dry | Kidney |
| Cereals | Lentils | Meat extracts |
| | Spinach | |

## TABLE 34

### EVALUATION OF A BASIC PLAN FOR A LOW-PURINE DIET
#### (1,885 Calories; 70 Gm. Protein)

| DAILY FOOD INTAKE | QUANTITY | | FOODSTUFFS | | | | MINERALS | | VITAMINS | | | | |
|---|---|---|---|---|---|---|---|---|---|---|---|---|---|
| | Weight (Gm.) | Approximate Measure | CALORIES* | Protein* (Gm.) | Fat* (Gm.) | Carbohydrate* (Gm.) | Ca (Mg.) | Fe (Mg.) | A (I.U.) | Ascorbic Acid (Mg.) | Thiamine (Mg.) | Riboflavin (Mg.) | Niacin (Mg.) |
| Milk, whole | 976 | 1 quart | 680 | 32 | 40 | 48 | 1,152 | 0.4 | 1,400 | 8 | 0.32 | 1.68 | 0.4 |
| Egg | 50 | 1 medium | 75 | 7 | 5 | ..... | 27 | 1.1 | 590 | ..... | 0.05 | 0.15 | Tr. |
| Cheese, cheddar | 60 | 2 oz. | 240 | 15 | 20 | 2 | 450 | 0.6 | 785 | ..... | 0.02 | 0.28 | 0.1 |
| Bread, whole-grain or enriched white† | 150 | 5 slices | 350 | 10 | ..... | 75 | 102 | 3.9 | Tr. | ..... | 0.38 | 0.26 | 3.3 |
| Cereal, whole-grain or enriched | 20 | ½ cup, cooked | 70 | 2 | ..... | 15 | 21 | 0.7 | Tr. | ..... | 0.07 | 0.05 | 0.7 |
| Potato, cooked | 100 | 1 small | 70 | 2 | ..... | 15 | 5 | 0.5 | Tr. | 16 | 0.09 | 0.03 | 1.1 |
| Vegetable (A)‡ | 150} | 2 servings | 20 | 1 | ..... | 4 | 43 | 1.2 | 2,180 | 32 | 0.10 | 0.10 | 0.9 |
| Vegetable (B)§ | 50} | | | | | | 12 | 0.5 | 1,660 | 5 | 0.03 | 0.03 | 0.4 |
| Including deep green or yellow | | | | | | | | | | | | | |
| Fruit, citrus|| | 100 | 1 serving | 40 | ..... | ..... | 10 | 18 | 0.1 | 140 | 40 | 0.05 | 0.01 | 0.1 |
| Other fruit# | | 2 servings | 80 | ..... | ..... | 20 | 14 | 0.8 | 945 | 9 | 0.04 | 0.06 | 0.8 |
| Subtotal | ..... | ..... | 1,625 | 69 | 65 | 189 | 1,844 | 9.8 | 7,700 | 110 | 1.15 | 2.65 | 7.8 |
| Sugar | 20 | 4 teaspoons | 80 | ..... | ..... | 20 | ..... | ..... | ..... | ..... | ..... | ..... | ..... |
| Butter, fortified margarine or oil | 20 | 4 teaspoons | 180 | ..... | 20 | ..... | ..... | ..... | 660 | ..... | ..... | ..... | ..... |
| Total** | ..... | ..... | 1,885†† | 69 | 85 | 209 | 1,844 | 9.8 | 8,360 | 110 | 1.15 | 2.65 | 7.8 |

* Values for calories, carbohydrate, protein, and fat from the Food Exchange Lists, Table 20, have been used to evaluate foods and food groups.

† 30 gm. (1 oz.) has been the weight assigned to one slice of bread in the exchange lists. It is recognized that variation is common. Adjustments should be made where usage varies.

‡ Commonly used vegetables selected from the vegetable A group of the exchange lists were tomatoes, snap beans, asparagus, broccoli, cabbage, lettuce, and cucumber. It was estimated that these vegetables might be used 10 times weekly averaging 150 gm. daily. Weighting was adapted from Agriculture Handbook No. 215, *Consumption Trends and Patterns for Vegetables* ((U.S. Department of Agriculture, Economic and Statistical Analysis Division, Economic Research Service [July, 1961]).

§ It was assumed that the most commonly used vegetables from the vegetable B group of the exchange lists were peas, carrots, beets, and squash. It was estimated that these vegetables might be used 4 times weekly averaging 50 gm. daily. Weighting was adapted from Agriculture Handbook No. 215, *Consumption Trends and Patterns for Vegetables.*

|| Fresh orange, fresh grapefruit, canned orange juice, blended grapefruit and orange and frozen citrus juice were considered to be commonly used citrus fruits or juice. Weighting was adapted from *Consumption of Food in the United States*, Supplement for 1962 to Agriculture Handbook No. 62 (U.S. Department of Agriculture, Agricultural Marketing Service [October, 1963]).

# Apples, bananas, canned peaches, pineapples, pears, apricots, and plums were considered commonly used. Weighting was adapted from *Consumption of Food in the United States*, Supplement for 1962 to Agriculture Handbook No. 62.

** Meets Recommended Dietary Allowance (Table 3) for adult in good health except for iron.

†† Caloric needs should be adjusted to individual requirements. For variations in need, see Tables 3 and 5.

The approximate content of the above diet is 11 mg. of purine nitrogen or 34 mg. of uric acid. The normal diet plan as outlined in Table 2 contains approximately 132 mg. of purine nitrogen or 265 mg. of uric acid.

Table 33, adapted from Stare and Thorn (3), gives a rough approximation of the purine content of foods. Table 34 contains an enumeration and evaluation of the mineral, vitamin, carbohydrate, protein, and fat content of a low-purine diet. Modifications may be made to meet the needs of individual patients by making adjustments in any of the components of the diet.

## REFERENCES

1. BARTELS, E. C. Successful treatment of gout, Ann. Int. Med., 18:21–28, 1943.
2. DUCKLES, D. Purine and cholesterol content of foods, J. Am. Dietet. A., 15:772–74, 1939.
3. STARE, F. J., and THORN, G. W. Protein nutrition in problems of medical interest, J.A.M.A., 127:1120–27, 1945.

KETOGENIC DIETS

A ketogenic diet is one in which the proportion of carbohydrate, protein, and fat is regulated so that the ratio of the ketogenic to the antiketogenic values equals 2 or more or until it is sufficiently high to produce a ketosis (see Glossary).

*Ketogenesis.*—The production of the ketone bodies, that is, acetone, aceto-acetic acid, and beta-oxybutyric acid, is known as ketogenesis. The precursors of the ketone bodies are the fatty acids and certain of the amino acids such as phenylalanine, tyrosine, leucine, and histidine; these are known as "ketogenic substances." For clinical purposes the ketogenic portion of the diet may be estimated as 90 per cent of the weight of the fat and 50 per cent of the protein.

*Antiketogenesis.*—Carbohydrate and the amino acids, such as alanine and glycine which are convertible to glucose in the body, tend to prevent the accumulation of ketone bodies and are said to be "antiketogenic." Approximately 10 per cent of the weight of the fat in the diet, 50 per cent of the protein, and 100 per cent of the carbohydrate may be estimated as the antiketogenic portion. When the supply of carbohydrate is inadequate, ketogenesis becomes predominant.

*Plan of daily food intake.*—If the basic plan of normal diet contains carbohydrate, 150 gm.; protein, 70 gm.; and fat, 70 gm., the ketogenic to antiketogenic ratio is 1 : 2. To reverse this ratio and produce a ketosis, it is necessary to reduce the carbohydrate and change the proportions approximately to carbohydrate, 20 gm.; protein, 70 gm.;

and fat, 125 gm. When a higher caloric intake is desired, the carbohydrate may be slightly increased. Thus, for a 1,860-calorie diet (Table 35), the distribution could be carbohydrate, 35 gm.; protein, 70 gm.; and fat, 160 gm.

*Preparation.*—This diet is likely to be unpalatable, expensive, and difficult to follow. Some degree of acceptability may be obtained, however, by the following measures:

Cream of high fat content may be used in ice cream, custards, and other desserts, as well as in salad dressings and soups. Saccharin may be used for sweetening.

The fruits and vegetables used should be those of minimum carbohydrate content and may be served in salads with oil dressings or hot in cream soups. Gelatin sweetened with saccharin may be used for desserts.

Washed-bran wafers may be offered as a bread substitute. Soybean muffins offer a low-carbohydrate bread substitute.

### ACIDIC AND BASIC ELEMENTS IN THE DIET

The major mineral elements which are evaluated when an estimate is made of the acid ash residue or the alkaline ash residue of the diet are sodium, potassium, calcium, magnesium, phosphorus, sulfur, and chlorine.

In evaluating the acid ash residue, the inorganic constituents— chlorine, sulfur, and phosphorus, which form acid ions (anions) in the body, namely, chloride, sulfate, and phosphate—are measured as the amount of tenth-normal alkali required for neutralization. In appraising the alkaline ash residue, the inorganic constituents— sodium, potassium, calcium, and magnesium, which form basic ions (cations) in the body—are measured as the amount of tenth-normal acid required for neutralization.

An acid-forming (acidogenic) diet is an allowance of foods having a total anion-forming ash content that is equivalent to 10–20 cc. of tenth-normal acid in excess of the total cation-forming ash, which will be equivalent to 30–35 cc. of tenth-normal alkali when milk, fruits, and vegetables are included as in the normal diet; proteins, minerals, and vitamins remain at levels necessary for nutritive sufficiency (see Glossary).

An alkali-forming (alkalinogenic) diet is an allowance of foods

## TABLE 35

### EVALUATION OF A BASIC PLAN FOR A KETOGENIC DIET

(Carbohydrate 35 Gm.; Protein 70 Gm.; Fat 160 Gm.; Calories 1,860)

| DAILY FOOD INTAKE | QUANTITY Weight (Gm.) | QUANTITY Approximate Measure | CALORIES | FOODSTUFFS Protein (Gm.) | FOODSTUFFS Fat (Gm.) | FOODSTUFFS Carbohydrate (Gm.) | MINERALS Ca (Mg.) | MINERALS Fe (Mg.) | VITAMINS A (I.U.) | VITAMINS Ascorbic Acid (Mg.) | VITAMINS Thiamine (Mg.) | VITAMINS Riboflavin (Mg.) | VITAMINS Niacin (Mg.) |
|---|---|---|---|---|---|---|---|---|---|---|---|---|---|
| Milk, whole* | 100 | ¾ cup | 65 | 3 | 4 | 5 | 118 | Tr. | 140 | 1 | 0.03 | 0.17 | 0.1 |
| Cream, 20 per cent* | 100 | ⅜ cup | 210 | 3 | 20 | 4 | 102 | Tr. | 840 | 1 | 0.03 | 0.15 | 0.1 |
| Eggs† | 100 | 2 medium | 150 | 14 | 10 | ......... | 54 | 2.2 | 1,180 | ......... | 0.10 | 0.30 | Tr. |
| Meat, poultry, or fish* | 180 | 6 oz. E.P. | 450 | 42 | 30 | ......... | 24 | 5.1 | 50 | ......... | 0.60 | 0.38 | 8.9 |
| Bacon* | 32 | 4 strips | 210 | 8 | 20 | ......... | 4 | 1.0 | ......... | ......... | 0.15 | 0.10 | 1.6 |
| Vegetable (A)† | 150 | 2 servings | 20 | 1 | ......... | 4 | 43 | 1.2 | 2,180 | 32 | 0.10 | 0.10 | 0.9 |
| (B)† | 50 | | | | | | 12 | 0.5 | 1,660 | 5 | 0.03 | 0.03 | 0.4 |
| Including deep-green or yellow | | | | | | | | | | | | | |
| Fruit, citrus† | 100 | 1 serving | 40 | | | 10 | 18 | 0.1 | 140 | 40 | 0.05 | 0.01 | 0.1 |
| Other fruit† | ......... | 1 serving | 40 | | | 10 | 7 | 0.4 | 475 | 5 | 0.02 | 0.03 | 0.4 |
| Butter, fortified margarine or oil† | 75 | ⅓ cup | 675 | | 75 | | | | 2,100 | | | | |
| Total‡ | ......... | ......... | 1,860 | 71 | 159 | 33 | 382 | 10.5 | 8,765 | 84 | 1.11 | 1.27 | 12.5 |

* Values for nutrients from Table 36.

† Values for carbohydrate, protein, fat from Exchange Lists (Tables 21–29).

‡ Meets Recommended Dietary Allowances (Table 3) for adult in good health except for calcium, iron, thiamine, and riboflavin.

having a total cation-forming ash content that is equivalent to 20 cc. or more of tenth-normal alkali in excess of the total anion-forming ash, which will be equivalent to 25 cc. or less of tenth-normal acid; proteins, minerals, and vitamins remain at levels necessary for nutritive sufficiency.

In general, it can be said that vegetable and fruits are predominantly basic, whereas cereals, meats, poultry, and fish are predominanantly acidic in residue. Most fruits, in spite of their acidity, exert a basic effect on the body, since a number of organic acid radicals, such as citrate and malate, may be oxidized completely to carbon dioxide and water, leaving the salts to contribute to the supply of basic elements in the residue. A few organic acids such as benzoic and quinic acids, however, are not so oxidized, and hence contribute to the total acidity. Cranberries, plums, and prunes are examples of such fruits. Exceptions have been found, however, in certain varieties of prunes and plums (1). Foods which exert no acidic or basic effect are refined sugar, butter, lard, oil, cornstarch, and tapioca. Molasses is strongly basic in residue, with an excess of 59.4 cc. of tenth-normal base per 190 gm. Information relating to the excess acid and base values may be found in Table 42, taken from Bridges and Mattice (2).

## REFERENCES

1. TURNER, D., and PARSONS, H. Not all plums and prunes acid-forming when used in human diet. In: Annual report of the director, 1930–31. Madison: Agricultural Experiment Station, University of Wisconsin, 1932 (Bull. 421), p. 121.
2. MATTICE, M. R. Bridges' food and beverage analyses, 3d revised ed. Philadelphia: Lea & Febiger, 1950, pp. 201–32.

# SECTION III | INTERVIEWING THE PATIENT

Chapter 12 | *Interviewing*

*the Patient*[1]

*by Margaret Mead*

*Formerly*
*Executive Secretary, Committee on Food Habits,*
*National Research Council, Washington, D.C.*

The modern trend in therapy is to consider the patient as a whole personality in a social setting[2] and to regard as significant and important every therapeutic contact with the physician, with medical or family caseworker, and with the dietitian. It is realized that, to obtain the best results, specialists must, in addition to performing their special tasks, co-operate in a common therapeutic task—the work and skill of one complementing that of the others. The increased emphasis upon the importance of the patient's whole personality makes new demands upon the dietitian as increased knowledge shows the many ways in which specific food behavior, as well as disease pictures requiring special diets, are themselves concomitants of deep-seated personality distortions and over-emphasis.[3]

1. This discussion draws upon materials contributed by the large group of members of The American Dietetic Association who co-operated in the project of the Diet Therapy Section on Food and Emotions during 1942–44, which was undertaken in co-operation with the Committee on Food Habits, National Research Council; and the case histories were analyzed by Dr. Margaret Mead, executive secretary of that committee. Received for publication, February 5, 1945. From *Journal of The American Dietetic Association*, Vol. 21, No. 7, July–August, 1945.

2. H. B. Richardson, *Patients Have Families* (New York: Commonwealth Fund, 1944); also G. C. Robinson, *The Patient as a Person* (New York: Commonwealth Fund, 1939).

3. F. Alexander, The influence of psychologic factors upon gastro-intestinal disturbances: a symposium: a report upon research carried on at the University of Chicago Institute for Psychoanalysis. I. General principles, objectives, and preliminary results. Summarized in Psychosom. Med., 1:429, 1939. See also the following: H. Bruch, *Ad-*

Just as at an earlier period in the development of dietetic practice the dietitian learned to understand the extent to which aspects of the patient's behavior in the dietetic interview might be referred to a need for attention, to a desire to show off, or to the gratification of long-denied needs for a relationship with another human being who appeared to take an interest in one's health and fate, now there is a need to integrate into dietetic practice the new findings based upon the work of psychiatrists exploring the new field of psychosomatic medicine. If this integration is to keep pace with the growing discoveries in this field, it must take place not only in the professional schools as new students enter dietetics and in the training for internships of recent graduates but also in the established practice within the hospital and food clinic. In the professional schools young dietitians can profit by instruction from psychiatrists; in the operating clinical situation the new methods can spread best by self-aware teamwork in which the dietitian re-evaluates her current procedures in the light of increasing knowledge of the patient's whole personality and takes it upon herself to communicate to her colleagues—the physician, the psychiatrist, the medical caseworker, and the nurse—just what the possibilities of a dietetic interview are in terms of an all-round therapy designed to meet the needs of the patient as a whole personality who emerges from the hospital to live in a real social situation.

One of the ways in which this increased awareness on the part of the dietitian may be developed is by a consideration of the different roles in which the dietitian sees herself, in which the patient sees her, and in which her professional colleagues in related professions see her. The role of the dietitian is subject to great variation in scope, from that of someone who merely works out a list of foods based

*justment to Dietary Changes in Various Somatic Disorders, in the Problem of Changing Food Habits* (Committee on Food Habits, National Research Council Bull. 108 [Washington, 1943]), p. 66; H. Bruch and G. Touraine, Obesity in childhood. V. The family frame of obese children, Psychosom. Med., 2:141–206, 1940; H. Bruch, Food and emotional security, in *The Nervous Child*, 3:165. Also M. Mead, Dietary patterns and food habits, J. Am. Dietet. A., 19:1, 1943; L. Rahman, H. B. Richardson, and H. S. Ripley, Anorexia nervosa with psychiatric observations, Psychosom. Med., 1:335, 1939; J. V. Waller, R. M. Kaufman, and F. Deutsch, Anorexia nervosa, a psychosomatic entity, Psychosom. Med., Vol. 2, No. 1, 1940; B. Mittelmann, H. G. Wolff, and M. P. Scharf, Emotions and gastroduodenal function: experimental studies on patients with gastritis, duodenitis, and peptic ulcer, Psychosom. Med., 4:5–61, 1942.

upon a physician's prescription and the age and body weight and degree of activity of the patient, through to the concepts of the worker in a food clinic (*a*) as a specialist who can *translate* for the patient-client a *regime* prescribed by the physician into exact amounts and kinds of foods prepared in specific ways; (*b*) as a specialist in the relationship between food and bodily needs who can *guide* the patient-client in making a selection of foods which will produce changes or maintain a given bodily state; (*c*) as a specialist in all the *problems of adjustment* which an individual faces in one facet of his or her existence—the consumption of food, including budgetary problems, conditions of preparation, etc.; and (*d*) as a *member of a team* of therapists—including the physician, psychiatrist, caseworker, public health nurse—in which case the specific type of help and instruction which the dietitian gives must be keyed to the treatment being given by the whole team and oriented not only to the physical needs of the patient-client but to his whole personality.

Each of these roles, or any combination of them, has to be clear to the dietitian and to the patient; and, if the referral from physician or caseworker has not indicated to the patient what role the dietitian plays, it is necessary for her to indicate it herself. This can usually be done best if the dietitian takes a minute to discover what the patient has been led to expect and then elaborates upon and corrects that impression. But a clear definition of why the dietitian is there, what the referring specialist has asked her to do, and what the patient may and may not expect is very important if the dietetic interview is to have its fullest usefulness. Roles *a* and *b* are discussed in the preceding sections. This present section is concerned primarily with roles *c* and *d*.

As growing interest and research amplify the scope of the dietitian's work and bring into it an increasing knowledge of social conditions, of personality dynamics, and of the process of therapy as an interpersonal relationship, it is important that these new emphases should not obscure the dietitian's distinctive role as a specialist in the adjustment between bodily needs and eating habits. It is important that she should include in the interview as many as possible of the insights and procedures which make for a good interview, whether conducted by physician, caseworker, or any other specialist in human relations. But it is also necessary that she do definite and concrete teaching about foods, the nature of the particular diet, how it may be calculated, and how the recommended amounts and proportions may be obtained within the framework of the patient's habit patterns. While it is true that, in the past, physicians and caseworkers have underestimated the general therapeutic implications of the dietetic interview and regarded the dietitian as an automatic source of information upon which the patient would inevitably act, it would easily be possible to err in the other direction and demand so much caseworking skill from the dietitian that her necessary and distinctive teaching function would be obscured.

This distinctive character of the dietetic interview imposes definite limitations upon its form. The dietitian must teach concrete, precise material. She must, whenever possible, also convey to the patient some sense of the principles upon which her concrete teaching is based, and in practically every instance she has to persuade the patient to do something which is painful, that is, to attend, from a new point of view, to the details of diet. This is painful because in our society the conscious application of thought—especially of measuring, counting, calculating, estimating—to an aspect of life which is ordinarily associated with gratification of the senses is regarded as reducing pleasure. Reduction in pleasure is likely to be resisted, except by those patients whose peculiar character formation makes them enjoy deprivation, and such patients will present other problems equally difficult to the therapist. However, attempts to make the following of a diet meaningful can be highly successful. The dietitian may expect the patient to feel that her advice is definitely useful if she makes the diet prescription intelligible and easier to follow, makes the goal of loss or gain in weight or a very altered pattern of intake possible of attainment, and makes the diet itself reasonably related to the patient's own bodily state and not an arbitrary set of rules. But the dietitian *cannot* expect to make the following of a diet a pleasure-giving experience, and efforts to clothe the interview in such terms are likely to be disappointing. Many instances have been reported where the patient has developed a tie to the dietitian and improved in health and functioning because someone was taking an interest in him, but this usually means that the dietitian has had to overstep her role and engage in casework for which she may not have been specially trained and at the expense of giving other patients specific dietary help.

The dietetic interview remains an interview between a specialist-in-food-adjustments and a patient-who-needs-to-learn-something-about-his-diet, and all improvements in procedure must necessarily take this core into account.

### EXTENSION OF THE DIETITIAN'S SKILL IN HELPING THE PATIENT ADJUST HIS FOOD HABITS

Recognition of the importance of treating the patient as a whole personality, with a specific cultural background and real life-situation, leads to the inclusion in the dietetic interview of an attempt to get some understanding of the patient's personality, what his reaction is to the diagnosis which has brought him there, what motives may be invoked in teaching new food patterns, and what special resistances have to be overcome. This preliminary exploration of the patient's personality can take place within the framework of the dietetic interview itself and need not wander to wider topics. The more knowledge the dietitian has of the human personality, the better. She needs to be aware of such special problems of childhood as the conflict between dependence upon the mother and the need to be independent, which is likely to express itself strongly in the field of eating, or of the adolescent desire to be like other young people, as illustrated in the following:

### EXTRACT FROM AN INTERVIEW WITH A THIRTEEN-YEAR-OLD DIABETIC GIRL

Patient had come in crying, after a two-month absence, and her tests showed sugar.

DIETITIAN: Why K, what seems to be the trouble? You've always had such a nice smile.

PATIENT: Oh, I've been hungry since school started and have eaten more than I should have—even candy sometimes. I just can't help it when all the others can have everything. I *hate* school.

D: What would you like to have to eat? We should be able to get together on this and plan your meals the way you want them.

P: Oh, *could* you? I'd love to have more bread, dessert once in a while, a little gum and candy.

D: Have you ever tried D-Zerta or candy or gum sweetened with saccharin? D-Zerta is a gelatin dessert and can be used in many ways, such as with whipped cream or with fruit. [*D. conferred with doctor.*] If you like, we might increase the amount of insulin and your food allowance to include another slice of bread and a couple of pieces of candy.

P: Why, that will make my meals practically the same as all the other girls! That's swell!

The patient came in once a month from then on. She was happy, felt well, liked school, and tests were good.

The foregoing illustrates the methods of a dietitian who responded sensitively to the evidences of distress and placed them in context against the patient's previous behavior. She estimated carefully the importance—to an adolescent—of behaving like the other girls and so evaluated correctly the phrase, "I *hate* school," treated the dietary prescriptions as flexible and capable of adjustment to a genuine need on the part of the patient, and succeeded in establishing the patient in an adequate adjustment.

Each age, each sex, has its special problems. For old age it is important to realize that the patient needs to be treated with the respect due to age and experience of life, yet protected, by written advice for instance, from a growing forgetfulness. Thus increased understanding of different regularities of this sort provides a background for a better understanding of personality.

Knowledge of the patient's cultural background—whether from a rural American home; from a foreign-born family's home; from a minority group, which almost inevitably means poor housing and limited household equipment; from a home where religious usages are observed; or from a type of home where no traditional practices may be relied upon, as when mountain people of the South are transplanted to a northern or western area where all the ways of living are unfamiliar—helps the dietitian to make her teaching realistic and relevant. The more she knows of these differences in dietary practice from one socioeconomic group to another and from one nationality background to another, the surer will be her understanding of the patient's questions or probable confusions, misunderstandings, or embarrassments.

A skilled dietitian will also take into account the patient's social situation in terms of status, occupation, income, and living arrangements—making specific allowance for the difficulties of the patient who lives in a cheap club for girls, the bus driver, or the elevator operator; the domestic servant, who is likely to nibble; the underprivileged mother of young children, who is likely to skimp her own diet to feed them better; the housewife, who must shop on a hand-to-mouth basis or who works and must leave the shopping to a small child; the three-shift household with its irregular meals; and the family in an overcrowded district that has only restricted kitchen privileges. Imaginative inclusion within the dietetic interview of the reality situation of the patient goes a long way toward insuring its success and has high general therapeutic value in increasing the patients' sense that the dietitian is someone who is treating them as they really are—people with ten minutes for lunch, people who have iceboxes but cannot afford to run them, people who are too poor to shop in chain stores where cash must be paid and who depend instead on credit.[4]

A knowledge of current prices, scarcities, and abundances, of current food fads among young people, and of the trend of radio advertising—especially for children—is also important in helping the dietitian to make it seem possible for the patient to follow her instructions easily. While every physician and every nurse should understand the basic principles of nutrition, it devolves upon the dietitian to translate this knowledge into everyday practice in terms of the needs, the intelligence, the emotional attitudes, and the actual situation of each patient.

### THE DIETITIAN AS A MEMBER OF A THERAPEUTIC TEAM

The dietitian's functioning in the therapeutic team in hospital or clinic may be considered from three points of view: (1) referral to the dietitian; (2) the dietetic interview or series of interviews; (3) referral from the dietitian, or case report to some other member of the team.

*Referral to the dietitian.*—At present, referral to the dietitian comes usually from the physician if the need is a medical one and from the caseworker if it is a matter of home management. The physician tends to limit himself to such phrases as "reducing diet," "low-fat diet," "high-caloric diet," "high-vitamin diet," "bland diet," and to omit any information on the patient's personality, capacity to

---

4. Background materials for the inclusion in dietetic practice of cultural and socioeconomic factors may be found among the materials developed at the Boston Dispensary Food Clinic by Frances Stern; at the Community Service Society, New York, by Lucy Gillett; and materials currently issued by the Massachusetts Department of Health and the Committee on Food Habits, National Research Council.

follow directions, the role that the patient's illness plays in the patient's life, etc. Upon the hospital dietitian devolves the task of developing such a working relationship with the physician that, instead of saying, "Stop in and see Miss Jones, the dietitian, and she'll give you your diet," the physician will realize the importance of an interpretative referral and say: "Now Miss X, you will need some help in planning the diet which I have prescribed for you. You'll find that Miss Y, our dietitian who specializes in helping people adjust their meals to their particular health needs, will help you work out the details." With increasingly good working relationships between other therapists and the dietitian, the physician and the caseworker also come to appreciate the importance of giving the dietitian clues about the personality of the patient, namely, summaries of what otherwise would often demand many hours of contact with the patient and experience with the way he responds to different types of suggestions; warnings about ways in which the patient will try to use a relationship; and diagnosis of the role that eating plays in the patient's life—as the only available form of sense gratification, as a reaction to mood, as a method of punishing other people or the self, etc. The interested dietitian can accustom physicians to including such suggestions in their referrals. Thus the dietetic interview will get off to a quick start, the patient will be better oriented in what to expect, and the dietitian already alert to some of the patient's most conspicuous characteristics.

*The dietetic interview.*—The extent to which the dietetic interview itself becomes an integral part of the treatment of a patient who, in addition to being cured of a specific disease condition or taught to keep the disease under control, is also being adjusted as a whole to a life-situation, depends not only on the dietitian's knowledge of personality but on the knowledge of other members of the therapeutic team concerning the character of dietetic interviews in that particular dietetic department of their own hospital or clinic. Too often physicians, caseworkers, and nurses include in their planning for patients their picture of a dietetic interview, experienced or witnessed twenty years ago, in quite another setting. They may actually seek to prepare the patient for, or seek to adjust subsequent treatment to, a dietetic interview very different from that which the patient actually experiences. This ever present danger can be guarded against by the dietitian's assuming responsibility for seeing that the other members of the therapeutic team actually know what her practice and that of her staff are, what types of alternatives are recognized in adjusting different kinds of patients to the same general dietary prescription, how much detailed instruction is actually involved, and what sorts of aids, written schedules, models, scales, slides, charts, etc., she uses. Adequate exposure of physicians and caseworkers to the procedure of a dietetic department will result in their raising questions about the possibilities inherent in the situation, which in turn will assist the dietitian in orienting her practice to their premises and deepen her knowledge of the emotional factors with which she has to deal.

*Referral from the dietitian and case reports.*—As the dietitian works more in a team, the other members of which know what her special skills actually are, both she and they will recognize ways in which material gleaned in the dietetic interview may be used as an indicator of the patient's problems or progress. A series of dietetic interviews is sometimes an excellent device for maintaining contact with a patient, especially if the dietitian is alert to signs of improvement or deterioration, of indications of developing conditions—as when a problem which at first looked like simple malnutrition begins to show signs of anorexia nervosa. Attempts to fit the dietetic interview into an integrated pattern of treatment are an excellent device for focusing more attention upon the whole personality of the patient, thereby making the treatment more effective.

## REFERENCES

1. ALDRICH, C. K. Prescribing a diet is not enough, J. Am. Dietet. A., **33**: 785–87, 1957.
2. BABCOCK, CHARLOTTE G. Psychologically significant factors in the nutrition interview, J. Am. Dietet. A., **23**:8–12, 1947.
3. ———. Food and its emotional significance, *ibid.*, **24**:390–93, 1948.
4. ———. Problems in sustaining the nutritional care of the patient, *ibid.*, **28**:222–27, 1952.
5. ———. Comments on human interrelations, *ibid.*, **33**:871–79, 1957.
6. BAYLES, S., and EBAUGH, F. G. Emotional factors in eating and obesity, J. Am. Dietet. A., **26**:430–34, 1950.
7. BERGEVIN, P. Telling vs. teaching—learning by participation, J. Am. Dietet. A., **33**:781–84, 1957.
8. BRENER, R. Dietitian and patient: evaluation of an interpersonal relationship, J. Am. Dietet. A., **28**:515–19, 1952.

9. BRUCH, HILDE. The importance of overweight. New York: W. W. Norton & Co., Inc., 1957.
10. COWING, A. G. Readable writing, J. Am. Dietet. A., **23**:1036–40, 1947.
11. ———. Writing that sells good diet, *ibid.*, **24**:592–94, 1948.
12. DONAHUE, W. T. Psychologic aspects of feeding the aged, J. Am. Dietet. A., **27**:461–66, 1951.
13. ENGLISH, O. SPURGEON. Psychosomatic medicine and dietetics, J. Am. Dietet. A., **27**:721–25, 1951.
14. EPPRIGHT, E. S. Factors influencing food acceptance, J. Am. Dietet. A., **23**:579–87, 1947.
15. FLESCH, R. The art of plain talk. New York: Harper & Bros., 1946.
16. ———. The art of readable writing. New York: Harper & Bros., 1949.
17. GALDSTON, IAGO. Motivation in health education, J. Am. Dietet. A., **25**:745–51, 1949.
18. ———. Nutrition from the psychiatric viewpoint, *ibid.*, **28**:405–9, 1952.
19. GARRETT, ANNETTE. Interviewing: its principles and methods. New York: Family Service Association of America, 1950.
20. GEBHARD, B. Exhibit planning and analysis, J. Am. Dietet. A., **24**:394–98, 1948.
21. HALL, DOROTHY. The dietetic interview as a tool in changing food habits, J. Am. Dietet. A., **22**:999–1002, 1946.
22. HAMBURGER, W. W. The psychology of weight reduction: the initial nutritional interview; the nutritionist-patient relationship; and complications of weight reduction, J. Am. Dietet. A., **34**:17–22, 1958.
23. HOULE, C. O. The dietitian as a teacher of adults, J. Am. Dietet. A., **24**:837–40, 1948.
24. HYMES, J. L. Significance of feeding from the viewpoint of child development, J. Am. Dietet. A., **25**:611–12, 1949.
25. ILG, F. L. The child's idea of what and how to eat, J. Am. Dietet. A., **24**:658–60, 1948.
26. KREITLOW, B. W. Teaching adults democratically, J. Am. Dietet. A., **33**:788–92, 1957.
27. LEACH, J. M. Motivating people to use educational material, J. Am. Dietet. A., **29**:245–47, 1953.
28. MEAD, MARGARET. Cultural patterning of nutritionally relevant behavior J. Am. Dietet. A., **25**:677–80, 1949.
29. MILLER, C. D. Food and food habits in the Hawaiian Islands, J. Am. Dietet. A., **27**:461–66, 1951.
30. MITCHELL, HELEN S., and JOFFE, NATALIE F. Food patterns of some European countries: background for study programs and guidance of relief workers, J. Am. Dietet. A., **24**:676–87, 1944.
31. POSZ, A. C. Do you irritate others when you listen? J. Am. Dietet. A., **34**:730–32, 1958.
32. PRAGOFF, HALE. Areas of cooperation between medical social workers and dietitians, J. Am. Dietet. A., **24**:485–90, 1948.
33. RABINOVITCH, R. D., and FISCHHOFF, J. Feeding in childhood to meet emotional needs: a survey of the psychologic implications of eating, J. Am. Dietet. A., **28**:614–21, 1952.
34. RADKE, MARIAN, and CASO, E. K. Experiments in changing food habits, J. Am. Dietet. A., **23**:403–9, 1947.

35. ———. Lecture and discussion—decision as method of influencing food habits, *ibid.*, 24:23–31, 1948.
36. SPENCER, M. E. An educator talks about motivating people, J. Am. Dietet. A., 25:209–12, 1949.
37. TOWLE, C. Common human needs. ("Public Assistance Reports," No. 8.) Washington: Federal Security Agency, 1945.
38. TRULSON, M., WALSH, E. D., and CASO, E. K. A study of obese patients in a nutrition clinic, J. Am. Dietet. A., 23:941–46, 1947.
39. WALSH, ETHEL. Nutritionists and social workers cooperate on mutual problems, J. Am. Dietet. A., 25:681–83, 1949.
40. WHITE, G. The patient as the focus of attention, J. Am. Dietet. A., 30:25–28, 1954.
41. DEPARTMENT OF PEDIATRICS, UNIVERSITY OF CHICAGO. Liberal infant feeding, J. Am. Dietet. A., 22:622–24, 1946.
42. Motivation in health education. (The 1947 Health Education Conference of the New York Academy of Medicine.) New York: Columbia University Press, 1948.
43. MARGARET MEAD. Food Habits Research: Problems of the 1960's. NAS-NRC Publication 1225, Washington, D.C. 1964.
44. The Problem of Changing Food Habits (1943), Bull. 108.
45. Manual for the Study of Food Habits (1945), Bull. 111 from Printing and Publishing Office, NAS, Washington, D.C. 20418.

# SECTION IV | EXPANDING OPPORTUNITIES IN THE PRACTICE OF DIET THERAPY

Chapter 13 | *Expanding Opportunities in the*

*Practice of Diet Therapy*

*by Mildred Kaufman*

*Nutrition Consultant, Diabetes and Arthritis Branch, Division of Chronic Diseases, Public Health Service, Washington, D.C.*

It is the responsibility of the dietitian and public health nutritionist to assist patients to apply in their daily lives the current scientific knowledge of nutrition and diet therapy. As their contribution to medical care, the dietitian and nutritionist should be expected to assess the patient's dietary needs, interpret these to the physician and other members of the health team, and implement this aspect of care with the patient.

It has recently been pointed out that

to meet the changing health needs of our changing population a new concept of patient care is developing. It envisions a wide spectrum of medical and health service facilities—coordinated on a community-wide basis for both in-patient and out-patient care. It is designed to provide continuity of care in line with the patient's need and current medical knowledge (1).

This suggests that if the dietitian or public health nutritionist is to move with this trend, each must widen her horizons to encompass the entire continuum of medical care. Each must define her responsibilities to the in-patient cared for in the hospital, nursing home, or rehabilitation center; to the ambulatory patient seen in the doctor's office, out-patient clinic, or health center; and to the patient cared for in his own home. The dietitian or public health nutritionist must deepen her background in the basic sciences, the science of nutrition and therapeutic dietetics to fully develop her role as a consultant to her professional colleagues. And she must sharpen her understanding of the behavioral sciences and skills in educational methodology to be an effective counselor to patients and their families. It is a challenge to the dietitian or nutritionist to clearly state her contribu-

141

tions to patient care and delineate her functions. She must interpret to administrators and fellow workers that the job of modifying patterns of eating to improve dietary practices or as a part of therapy demands not only knowledge and skills, but the time, patience, and the ability to work with each individual at his own pace. In Chapter 12 on "Interviewing the Patient," Margaret Mead pictures the scope of responsibility of the dietitian and nutritionist in changing food habits, and suggests the perceptiveness that must be cultivated to counsel patients effectively.

A constructive diet therapy program requires the interaction of the dietitian or nutritionist with the physician, nurse, and social worker, along with the most important member of the team, the patient. With the trend toward enlarging the skills applied in health care this involvement can be extended to include the psychiatrist, dentist, health educator, physical, occupational, and speech therapist, and others. Auxiliary workers, such as the aide in the hospital or homemaker in home care, also assume responsibilities related to diet and become part of the team. Shorter periods of hospitalization and the increasing use of nursing home and home care services put stress on planning for continuity of care between the hospital, nursing home, and the home. The dietitian, with other staff in the hospital and out-patient clinic, must coordinate her efforts with those of the public health nutritionist and related health workers in the community who provide services to patients in their homes. Without coordination the only result can be confusion and frustration for the patient and his family.

To mobilize all of the resources, coordinate the variety of efforts, and provide meaningful dietary counseling, it is necessary for the dietitian and nutritionist to use every available channel of communication. To fully meet her responsibilities in patient care the dietitian or nutritionist must be able to communicate easily with (1) the patient and his family, (2) her professional co-workers, and (3) the staff of other community agencies.

### COMMUNICATION WITH THE PATIENT

*Learning about the patient's food intake.*—Through the process of dietary counseling the dietitian or nutritionist seeks to guide the patient to make those changes in his eating pattern that are necessary to improve his health. Since it is difficult for most patients to change firmly-rooted food habits, it is imperative that changes not be suggested unless they are necessary. Those changes which are recommended should be consistent with the patient's age, cultural background, financial situation, religious observances, present living situation, daily routine, and individual food preferences. The dietitian or nutritionist takes a giant stride toward the successful practice of diet therapy by identifying and understanding the distinguishing characteristics and variety of needs displayed by each individual she sees.

The basic tool for learning about the patient and his diet is a diet history or a record of past eating patterns. A written record from the patient of his current food practices provides the means for the diet counselor to become acquainted with the patient, and for the patient to develop an awareness of his own food intake. The food record provides the basis for assessment of the patient's diet and for developing an appropriate plan to meet his food needs. The nutrient analysis of dietary practices with which the dietitian or nutritionist can provide the physician can help him interpret some of the laboratory and clinical findings. An assessment of the patient's food habits further serves as a guide to the physician in prescribing the most appropriate and acceptable diet for the patient. For the dietitian or nutritionist the record of past eating practices serves importantly as the starting point for counseling about diet.

The tool for obtaining dietary information should be designed by the dietitian or nutritionist in collaboration with the physician and other interested co-workers. Guiding considerations in developing the device should be (*a*) the kind and amount of dietary information required, how it is to be evaluated and used, (*b*) the characteristics of the patient population—educational level, degree of physical, mental, and emotional incapacity, whether the patient is being seen in the hospital, the out-patient clinic, the office, or the home, and (*c*) the characteristics of the staff using the tool—the amount of time they can devote to obtaining the dietary information and their skill in interviewing.

Two distinct methods of collecting food intake information have been identified. Both of these methods which have been used in research are also applicable to planning for the dietary aspects of patient care. One of these methods is based upon record of food intake or diary in which meal by meal notes are kept of all food eaten during a stated period of time. The other approach to the diet history is based upon a detailed verbal statement of food consumed during the recent past. This may be for the past day, or two days, or a description of the "usual" food pattern. (2)

The record of food intake should be kept by the patient or those who care for him either at home, in the hospital, or in the nursing home. The format for record keeping at home can be simple, including sufficient space to write down all food eaten at each meal and between meals in estimated or measured amounts, and to describe the method of preparation. Such a record has the advantage of showing the actual food eaten and the variations from day to day. In the hospital the food consumed should be accurately observed, assessed, and recorded as part of the medical record. Recognizing the importance of food on the patient's progress in the hospital, the Joint Commission on Accreditation of Hospitals now asks whether notes on the patient's food intake are being included in the medical record. (3) In using and interpreting the patient's food intake while he is in the hospital, it should be remembered that for many reasons the kind and amount of food the individual eats in the hospital may be different from what he eats at home.

A food record is also needed from patients in a nursing home, under home care, or for those who are being seen regularly in the office or out-patient clinic. For patients at home, the record usually covers a stated period of time, a minimum of three days being desirable. Obvious disadvantages of the food record kept by the patient are that he may omit items, describe amounts incorrectly, or he may make some changes in his habits during the period recorded. However, many patients find the discipline of keeping a food record helpful in modifying their eating habits and the changes they make can indicate their knowledge about diet. For patients at home who have writing or language difficulties, someone else in the home may be able to keep the record.

An interview is commonly used to "recall" food intake information, particularly in the out-patient clinic, office, or home. Obtaining a detailed diet history is a time-consuming procedure which cannot be hurried. When good rapport is achieved and the dietitian is relaxed and an educated listener, the conference provides many additional, useful insights into the abilities, attitudes, and personality of the patient. Frequently an outline or interview form is used to structure the discussion. However, in designing such a form, a conversational approach should be preserved. Open-ended statements such as, "Tell me what you usually eat for breakfast," are more productive than leading questions like, "Do you drink orange juice for breakfast?" Questions leading to a "Yes" or "No" reply should be used only after the patient has had an uninterrupted opportunity to describe his eating practices in his own words. The meal pattern can be identified by asking the respondent to recall all of the food eaten during the previous 24 to 48 hours, or by asking him to describe his "usual" meals and snacks. The risk in recalling the previous day is that the day cited may not be typical. On the other hand, if the individual has erratic ways of eating, the "usual" meals may be difficult for him to describe and his replies may be misleading. With perceptive use, a cross-check for both of these methods should be possible by determining the frequency with which a wide variety of individual food items are eaten. Desserts, sweets, soft drinks, and alcoholic beverages must be included on the check list along with a wide variety of the basic food items—milk, eggs, cheeses, meats, fats, breads, cereals, fruits, vegetables. Although the check list should be constructed to include all the foods most commonly used locally, the interviewer should be alert to any additional items eaten which may not be on the list. While asking about frequency of consumption of each specific food item, it also is helpful to ask the patient to indicate his like or dislike for it.

Other ways of obtaining information about eating patterns may be possible with persons who express themselves easily in writing. For example, a food preference questionnaire requires only a short form with questions stated simply and clearly so that patients can complete the form themselves with little or no assistance. Questions must be appropriately worded to elicit the desired information. To gain the patient's cooperation, the worker using the form should take a few minutes to explain the purpose and use of the questionnaire and to give instructions on the degree of detail expected in the responses. This approach has the advantage of taking less time for the dietitian who is unable to spend the longer period required for the detailed diet-history interview. Meanwhile the patient is free to give considered responses and to take the time he needs to write the answers to the questionnaire thoughtfully. The form should be given to the patient to complete at a time when he will not be distracted or under pressure. Upon its completion the form must be reviewed by the dietitian with the patient to give them an opportunity to discuss and amplify responses. Those patients who are unable or unwilling to complete the questionnaire should not be urged to use it. In fact, unwillingness may be a significant clue concerning attitudes toward diagnosis, dietary restriction, or the authority of those involved in the dietary treatment. For such patients the more personal approach to the dietary interview is preferable. The food preference questionnaire appears to be particularly useful for hospitalized patients, but it can be used with patients seen in the office, clinic, or at home.

*Learning about the patient's needs and problems.*—In addition to the information about the meal pattern, some additional questions must be asked to learn how the patient feels about the dietary changes to be recommended, and to determine his ability and motivation to change his food habits. For these purposes answers must be obtained to the following:

What does the patient know about his present health problem and about its dietary treatment?

What past experiences has this patient had with a diet prescribed by a physician?

What feelings does the patient have about his ability to change his present eating pattern or about the suggested dietary treatment?

What foods are particularly important to this individual and would be most difficult for him to do without?

What foods can he not eat because of allergy, intolerance, or dislike?

Where are meals and snacks usually eaten, and at what hours?

What kinds of meals or refreshments are part of the patient's usual business, social, or recreational activities?

Who prepares the patient's meals? If meals are prepared at home, what are the facilities for food storage and preparation? If meals are eaten away from home, such as in a restaurant or school lunch, what choices are available?

Does the patient eat alone or with others? If alone, does this limit his food choices and methods of preparation? If with others, how does this limit the kinds and amount of food available to him?

Is the individual or family budget adequate and will it cover any possible additional costs for the modified diet? If it is not adequate, are there any resources such as public assistance, food stamp plan, or commodities?

What physical, emotional, intellectual, or social incapacities does this patient
have that should be considered in giving him dietary guidance?

What kinds of educational programs and materials would be most suitable
for this patient and what other resources are available to him for additional or continuing dietary guidance?

For guidance in the actual preparation and design of tools to obtain a diet history, some of the pertinent references are listed at the
end of this chapter. It may also be helpful to learn about procedures
and forms used by other dietitians and public health nutritionists in
the geographical area.

*Assessing the patient's food intake.*—Having obtained the food intake information, an assessment or appraisal of the patient's dietary
needs and needs for counseling can be made. The early chapters of
this handbook provide the basic principles for evaluation of the
patient's food intake, using the requirements for a "normal diet"
or a diet modified for specific therapy as the criteria. When working
with the physician to develop procedures for the dietary assessment,
it should be decided whether an appraisal of the food intake by food
groups is appropriate, or a more detailed calculation of specific
nutrients is preferred. Calculations of nutrients should be viewed as
important indicators of the nutrient quality of the dietary pattern,
not as absolute values. A short method of calculation is generally
used in the clinical situation. In the near future the use of computers
for calculating nutrients may streamline the mechanical aspects of
dietary assessment (5).

In interpreting the information obtained, it should be made clear
that it is based on a dietary appraisal. A *nutrition history* and appraisal to describe nutritional status is a much more comprehensive
procedure including extensive laboratory and clinical observations in
addition to dietary studies and is beyond the scope of this handbook.

*Planning and implementing the patient's dietary care and counseling.*
—Using the background information from the food record and the
dietary assessment, the physician can prescribe the diet and the plan
for dietary care of the patient that can reflect the strengths of the
individual's own eating pattern. Thus, past eating habits can be
modified to meet therapeutic needs (4). Where drastic changes must
be made these changes should be explained, and the patient involved
in the decision about how best to handle them. For the in-patient,

the food served can demonstrate how dietary changes can be made and the selective menu or patient cafeteria used for teaching. In addition to discussions with the patient about his diet, individualized written plans should be provided. In preparing written materials and selecting supplementary printed teaching materials, the language skills and reading level of the patient and his family should be considered.

Group counseling or classes can supplement individual counseling for patients having a similar condition. Such classes have proved useful in motivating members in the group, and in helping them to share problems and their solutions. In addition, a larger patient audience can be reached when professional time is limited. Films, filmstrips, slides, and other audio-visual aids prepared on diabetes, heart disease, arthritis, weight control, and other subjects can be useful in presenting basic information to such groups. Programmed instruction also has been found to be an effective method to provide basic information to patients with diabetes. This is a new technique which has possibilities in other areas of health education. As new teaching tools become available, the dietitian and public health nutritionist should participate in testing their potentialities to develop more effective methods of patient education (6).

The dietary plan, once made and introduced, must be reviewed and adjusted periodically for the patient in the hospital or at home. Patients require continuing encouragement and support to continue to adhere to the modified dietary pattern. The record of food intake is needed for follow-up purposes to determine the patient's understanding of the diet and his ability to cope with the new way of eating. When the dietitian talks with the patient in the hospital or clinic, or the public health nurse or nutritionist sees him at home, some plan must be made to provide continuing dietary guidance. This might be offered either by the dietitian or nutritionist who initiates the counseling or by others with whom she coordinates her efforts.

### COMMUNICATION WITH PROFESSIONAL CO-WORKERS

*The medical record.*—To best serve the patient, the dietitian or nutritionist must coordinate her efforts with those of other health workers providing care. The medical record is the basic means of communication between professional staff within the hospital, nursing home, or out-patient clinic. Here will be found recorded information such as the patient's medical history, the physician's physical findings, diagnostic impressions, prognosis and orders, laboratory reports, height and weight, and progress notes. Social service reports usually include financial data, and some description of the patient's family, home situation, and occupation. This information may reveal some of the problems in daily living which the individual faces and which may hinder his adherence to a planned dietary routine. Reports and notes from any consultants, other staff, or from cooperating community agencies provide additional insights into the patient's over-all problems and needs.

As the first step in planning for the patient's dietary care program, it is essential to read the medical record carefully. Further, the dietitian or nutritionist should note in this record the findings of the dietary assessment, the dietary care plan, counseling provided to the patient, and any pertinent impressions of the patient's ability to cope with the recommended diet modification. She can thereby share her experiences with other staff members and record her contribution to patient care as part of the total picture.

*Conferences and ward rounds.*—Participation in ward rounds and conferences with other staff giving service to the patient can help fill in details not found in the record. The dietitian or nutritionist should particularly confer with the physician in the early stages of patient care so that the dietary appraisal can be available to him and plans can be made for appropriately individualized dietary care. Conferences should also be sought with other staff on behalf of any patient having a special problem which might be resolved by cooperative planning. Case conferences are often used in both inpatient facilities and in home care services for cooperative planning and evaluation of care to selected patients. The dietitian or nutritionist should seek the opportunity to participate in such conferences, since joint planning to meet patient needs can often pay dividends both in improved patient care and saving of professional time. Unrecognized dietary needs can be identified as can problems interfering with the patient's dietary adherence.

COMMUNICATION WITH STAFF OF OTHER COMMUNITY AGENCIES

*Knowing community resources.*—For effective coordination and cooperation between the in-patient facilities and other health and social agencies it is increasingly necessary for dietitians and public health nutritionists to be well informed about the many resources available in their communities, and the channels for referral. Since, at home, total responsibility for diet is placed upon the patient and his family, they frequently need diet counseling even when they have received considerable guidance in the hospital. At home the situation is constantly changing and new needs become apparent. Diet counseling for the patient at home may be available through the public health nursing agency, the public health nutritionist, a diet counseling service, or as a service of a coordinated home care program. Some patients may have no one at home to prepare meals, and if unable to do so themselves, can benefit from homemaker services or a home-delivered-meal service (7).

To provide for continuity of care, many communities have developed an information and referral service and/or an interagency referral system. These mechanisms provide formalized channels by which information about the patient and his family can be exchanged between agencies. The information and referral service lists services available in the community and helps families to locate the best ones to meet their needs.

*The interagency referral system.*—With an interagency referral system, a referral may be initiated by any member of the health team in the hospital or community who recognizes a need which can be met by another agency. A standard form is usually developed for the community by an interagency committee and is the basis for the referral system. The form is used to supply complete information about the patient including identifying data, reason for referral, diagnosis and prognosis, physician's orders and instructions. Space is provided for instructions and comments by hospital or clinic personnel (physician, nurse, medical social worker, dietitian, physical therapist, occupational therapist, and others) and by the public health nurse or other community workers. Included as attachments are copies of any written dietary plans given to the patient for home use. The form is initiated in the agency making the referral and directed through the appropriate channels to the agency providing the needed services. With this kind of referral system the dietitian and public health nutritionist have the opportunity to exchange information with all other workers offering service to the patient. Using this procedure each worker benefits from the experience each has with the patient, and can relate his own efforts to the total patient care plan. Moreover, the referral form serves as a permanent record of these services. It also serves as a way of measuring patient progress and identifying the contributions of the various services (8).

By using all these formal, established channels, as well as the informal channels of communication available to her, the dietitian and public health nutritionist can improve and extend services to patients and better fulfill her role on the health team.

## REFERENCES

1. WALSH, HELEN E. The changing nature of public health, J. Am. Dietet. A., **46**:93–95, 1965.
2. BECKER, BERYL G., BEEUWKES, ADELIA M., and INDEK, BERNARD B. Dietary intake methodologies. A review. Ann Arbor, Mich.: Office of Research Administration, November, 1960.
3. Hospital Dietitians: Do you chart? J. Am. Dietet. A., **44**:361, 1964.
4. STONE, DANIEL B. A rational approach to diet and diabetes, J. Am. Dietet. A., **46**:30–35, 1965.
5. THOMPSON, ETHEL M., and TUCKER, HENRY. Computers in dietary studies, J. Am. Dietet. A., **40**:308, 1962.
6. KAUFMAN, MILDRED. Programmed instruction materials on diabetes, J. Am. Dietet. A., **46**:36–38, 1965.
7. PIPER, GERALDINE M. Planning new community nutrition services, J. Am. Dietet. A., **44**:461, 1964.
8. NEW YORK STATE DEPARTMENT OF HEALTH. Interagency referral form and instructions for interagency referral form. Albany.

## ADDITIONAL SELECTED REFERENCES ON METHODS FOR OBTAINING FOOD INTAKE INFORMATION

ADELSON, S. F. Some problems in collecting dietary data from individuals, J. Am. Dietet. A., **36**:453, 1960.
ANDERSON, L., and BROWE, J. Nutrition and family service. Philadelphia: W. B. Saunders Company, 1960, chapter 7.
*BLECHA, E. E. Dietary study methods. IV. The dietary history for use in diet therapy, J. Am. Dietet. A., **27**:968–69, 1951.
*BURKE, B. S. The dietary history as a tool in research, J. Am. Dietet. A., **23**:1041–46, 1946.
HAYES, O. B., ABRAHAM, S., and CACERES, C. A. Computers in epidemiologic dietary studies, J. Am. Dietet. A., **44**:456, 1964.
HUNSCHER, H. A., and MACY, I. G. Dietary study methods. I. Uses and abuses of dietary study methods, J. Am. Dietet. A., **27**:558–63, 1951.
INTERDEPARTMENTAL COMMITTEE ON NUTRITION FOR NATIONAL DEFENSE. Manual for Nutrition Surveys, 2d edition, 1963.

* Includes forms being used.

*Rosenthal, H., Baker, P. C., and McVey, W. A. Stern's applied dietetics. Baltimore: The Williams and Wilkins Co., 1949, pp. 8–12, 35.

Trulson, Martha F. Assessment of dietary study methods. I. Comparison of methods for obtaining data for clinical work, J. Am. Dietet. A., 30:991, 1954.

*Turner, D. The estimation of the patient's home dietary intake, J. Am. Dietet. A., 16:875–81, 1940.

Young, C. M. Diet therapy—interviewing the patient, Am. J. Clin. Nutr., 8: 523, 1960.

———. The interview itself, J. Am. Dietet. A., 35:677–81, 1959.

Young, C. M., and Musgrave, K. Dietary study methods. II. Uses of dietary score cards, J. Am. Dietet. A., 27:745–48, 1951.

Young, C. M., and Trulson, M. Methodology for dietary surveys in epidemiological surveys. II. Strengths and weaknesses of existing methods, Am. J. Pub. H., 50:803, 1960.

# APPENDIXES

FOOD VALUES IN COMMON PORTIONS

The 1964 revision of *Nutritive Value of Foods* (U.S. Department of Agriculture, Home and Garden Bulletin No. 72) provides a compact table on food composition of nearly 500 food items commonly used in this country. Edible portions are indicated in both weights and measures thereby providing a quick and convenient unit for assessing the nutrient content of diets.

The values are based on data in *Composition of Foods—Raw, Processed, Prepared* (U.S. Department of Agriculture, Agriculture Handbook No. 8 [December, 1963]). Data on more than 2,500 food items appear in this handbook, which is prepared by the Agricultural Research Service of United States Department of Agriculture.

### NIACIN AND NIACIN EQUIVALENT

The term niacin, used in Table 36, is a less inclusive term than niacin equivalent used in Table 3. Nearly all foods contain some tryptophan, an amino acid found in protein, which the body can convert to niacin. Niacin equivalent is the composite of the niacin already in the food and that which may be formed from tryptophan. Among the better sources of tryptophan are milk, meats, eggs, legumes, and nuts.

The average diet in the United States, which contains a generous amount of protein, provides enough tryptophan to increase the niacin value by about a third.

## TABLE 36A

## YIELD OF COOKED MEAT PER POUND OF RAW MEAT

| Meat as Purchased | Meat after Cooking (less Drippings) | |
| --- | --- | --- |
| | Parts weighed | Approximate weight of cooked parts per pound of raw meat purchased |
| | | *Ounces* |
| Chops or steaks for broiling or frying: | | |
| With bone and relatively large amount of fat, such as pork or lamb chops; beef rib, sirloin, or porterhouse steaks. | Lean, bone, fat | 10–12 |
| | Lean and fat | 7–10 |
| | Lean only | 5–7 |
| Without bone and with very little fat, such as round of beef, veal steaks | Lean and fat | 12–13 |
| | Lean only | 9–12 |
| Ground meat for broiling or frying, such as hamburger, lamb, or pork patties | Patties | 9–13 |
| Roasts for oven cooking (no liquid added): | | |
| With bone and relatively large amount of fat, such as beef rib, loin, chuck; lamb shoulder, leg; pork, fresh or cured. | Lean, bone, fat | 10–12 |
| | Lean and fat | 8–10 |
| | Lean only | 6–9 |
| Without bone. | Lean and fat | 10–12 |
| | Lean only | 7–10 |
| Cuts for pot-roasting, simmering, braising, stewing: | | |
| With bone and relatively large amount of fat, such as beef chuck, pork shoulder | Lean, bone, fat | 10–11 |
| | Lean and fat | 8–9 |
| | Lean only | 6–8 |
| Without bone and with relatively small amount of fat, such as trimmed beef, veal | Lean with adhering fat | 9–11 |

# TABLE 36—NUTRITIVE VALUES OF THE EDIBLE PART OF FOODS

Reprinted from *Nutritive Value of Foods* (U.S. Department of Agriculture, Home and Garden Bulletin No. 72).

[Dashes show that no basis could be found for imputing a value although there was some reason to believe that a measurable amount of the constituent might be present]

| Food, Approximate Measure, and Weight (in Grams) | | Food Energy | Protein | Fat (Total Lipid) | Fatty acids | | | Carbohydrate | Calcium | Iron | Vitamin A Value | Thiamine | Riboflavin | Niacin | Ascorbic Acid |
| | | | | | Saturated (Total) | Unsaturated Oleic | Linoleic | | | | | | | | |
| | Grams | (Calories) | (Gm.) | (Gm.) | (Gm.) | (Gm.) | (Gm.) | (Gm.) | (Mg.) | (Mg.) | (I.U.) | (Mg.) | (Mg.) | (Mg.) | (Mg.) |
| **MILK, CREAM, CHEESE; RELATED PRODUCTS** | | | | | | | | | | | | | | | |
| Milk, cow's: | | | | | | | | | | | | | | | |
| Fluid, whole (3.5% fat). 1 cup | 244 | 160 | 9 | 9 | 5 | 3 | Trace | 12 | 288 | 0.1 | 350 | 0.08 | 0.42 | 0.1 | 2 |
| Fluid, nonfat (skim) 1 cup | 246 | 90 | 9 | Trace | -- | -- | -- | 13 | 298 | .1 | 10 | .10 | .44 | .2 | 2 |
| Buttermilk, cultured, from skim milk. 1 cup | 246 | 90 | 9 | Trace | -- | -- | -- | 13 | 298 | .1 | 10 | .09 | .44 | .2 | 2 |
| Evaporated, unsweetened, undiluted. 1 cup | 252 | 345 | 18 | 20 | 11 | 7 | 1 | 24 | 635 | .3 | 820 | .10 | .84 | .5 | 3 |
| Condensed, sweetened, undiluted. 1 cup | 306 | 980 | 25 | 27 | 15 | 9 | 1 | 166 | 802 | .3 | 1,090 | .23 | 1.17 | .5 | 3 |
| Dry, whole. 1 cup | 103 | 515 | 27 | 28 | 16 | 9 | 1 | 39 | 936 | .5 | 1,160 | .30 | 1.50 | .7 | 6 |
| Dry, nonfat, instant. 1 cup | 70 | 250 | 25 | Trace | -- | -- | -- | 36 | 905 | .4 | 20 | .24 | 1.25 | .6 | 5 |
| Milk, goat's: | | | | | | | | | | | | | | | |
| Fluid, whole. 1 cup | 244 | 165 | 8 | 10 | 6 | 2 | Trace | 11 | 315 | .2 | 390 | .10 | .27 | .7 | 2 |
| Cream: | | | | | | | | | | | | | | | |
| Half-and-half (cream and milk). 1 cup | 242 | 325 | 8 | 28 | 16 | 9 | 1 | 11 | 261 | .1 | 1,160 | .08 | .38 | .1 | 2 |
| 1 tablespoon | 15 | 20 | Trace | 2 | 1 | 1 | Trace | 1 | 16 | Trace | 70 | Trace | .02 | Trace | Trace |
| Light, coffee or table. 1 cup | 240 | 505 | 7 | 49 | 27 | 16 | 1 | 10 | 245 | .1 | 2,030 | .07 | .36 | .1 | 2 |
| 1 tablespoon | 15 | 30 | Trace | 3 | 2 | 1 | Trace | 1 | 15 | Trace | 130 | Trace | .02 | Trace | Trace |
| Whipping, unwhipped (volume about double when whipped): | | | | | | | | | | | | | | | |
| Light. 1 cup | 239 | 715 | 6 | 75 | 41 | 25 | 2 | 9 | 203 | .1 | 3,070 | .06 | .30 | .1 | 2 |
| 1 tablespoon | 15 | 45 | Trace | 5 | 3 | 2 | Trace | 1 | 13 | Trace | 190 | Trace | .02 | Trace | Trace |
| Heavy. 1 cup | 238 | 840 | 5 | 89 | 49 | 29 | 3 | 7 | 178 | .1 | 3,670 | .05 | .26 | .1 | 2 |
| 1 tablespoon | 15 | 55 | Trace | 6 | 3 | 2 | Trace | Trace | 11 | Trace | 230 | Trace | .02 | Trace | Trace |
| Cheese: | | | | | | | | | | | | | | | |
| Blue or Roquefort type. 1 ounce | 28 | 105 | 6 | 9 | 5 | 3 | Trace | 1 | 89 | .1 | 350 | .01 | .17 | .1 | 0 |
| Cheddar or American: | | | | | | | | | | | | | | | |
| Ungrated. 1 inch cube | 17 | 70 | 4 | 5 | 3 | 2 | Trace | Trace | 128 | .2 | 220 | Trace | .08 | Trace | 0 |
| Grated. 1 cup | 112 | 445 | 28 | 36 | 20 | 12 | 1 | 2 | 840 | 1.1 | 1,470 | .03 | .51 | .1 | 0 |
| 1 tablespoon | 7 | 30 | 2 | 2 | 1 | 1 | Trace | Trace | 52 | .1 | 90 | Trace | .03 | Trace | 0 |
| Cheddar, process. 1 ounce | 28 | 105 | 7 | 9 | 5 | 3 | Trace | 1 | 219 | .3 | 350 | Trace | .12 | Trace | 0 |
| Cheese foods, Cheddar. 1 ounce | 28 | 90 | 6 | 7 | 4 | 2 | Trace | 2 | 162 | .2 | 280 | .01 | .16 | Trace | 0 |

TABLE 36—*Continued*

| Food, Approximate Measure, and Weight (in Grams) | Food Energy (Calories) | Protein (Gm.) | Fat (Total Lipid) (Gm.) | Fatty acids Saturated (Total) (Gm.) | Fatty acids Unsaturated Oleic (Gm.) | Fatty acids Unsaturated Linoleic (Gm.) | Carbohydrate (Gm.) | Calcium (Mg.) | Iron (Mg.) | Vitamin A Value (I.U.) | Thiamine (Mg.) | Riboflavin (Mg.) | Niacin (Mg.) | Ascorbic Acid (Mg.) |
|---|---|---|---|---|---|---|---|---|---|---|---|---|---|---|
| **MILK, CREAM, CHEESE; RELATED PRODUCTS—Continued** | | | | | | | | | | | | | | |
| Cheese—Continued | | | | | | | | | | | | | | |
| Cottage cheese, from skim milk: | | | | | | | | | | | | | | |
| Creamed _____ 1 cup_____ 225 | 240 | 31 | 9 | 5 | 3 | Trace | 7 | 212 | 0.7 | 380 | 0.07 | 0.56 | 0.2 | 0 |
| 1 ounce_____ 28 | 30 | 4 | 1 | 1 | Trace | Trace | 1 | 27 | .1 | 50 | .01 | .07 | Trace | 0 |
| Uncreamed_____ 1 cup_____ 225 | 195 | 38 | 1 | Trace | Trace | Trace | 6 | 202 | .9 | 20 | .07 | .63 | .2 | 0 |
| 1 ounce_____ 28 | 25 | 5 | Trace | | | | 1 | 26 | .1 | Trace | .01 | .08 | Trace | 0 |
| Cream cheese_____ 1 ounce_____ 28 | 105 | 2 | 11 | 6 | 4 | Trace | 1 | 18 | .1 | 440 | Trace | .07 | Trace | 0 |
| 1 tablespoon_____ 15 | 55 | 1 | 6 | 3 | 2 | Trace | Trace | 9 | Trace | 230 | Trace | .04 | Trace | 0 |
| Swiss (domestic)_____ 1 ounce_____ 28 | 105 | 8 | 8 | 4 | 3 | Trace | 1 | 262 | .3 | 320 | Trace | .11 | Trace | 0 |
| Milk beverages: | | | | | | | | | | | | | | |
| Cocoa_____ 1 cup_____ 242 | 235 | 9 | 11 | 6 | 4 | Trace | 26 | 286 | .9 | 390 | .09 | .45 | .4 | 2 |
| Chocolate-flavored milk drink (made with skim milk)_____ 1 cup_____ 250 | 190 | 8 | 6 | 3 | 2 | Trace | 27 | 270 | .4 | 210 | .09 | .41 | .2 | 2 |
| Malted milk_____ 1 cup_____ 270 | 280 | 13 | 12 | | | | 32 | 364 | .8 | 670 | .17 | .56 | .2 | 2 |
| Milk desserts: | | | | | | | | | | | | | | |
| Cornstarch pudding, plain (blanc mange)._____ 1 cup_____ 248 | 275 | 9 | 10 | 5 | 3 | Trace | 39 | 290 | .1 | 390 | .07 | .40 | .1 | 2 |
| Custard, baked_____ 1 cup_____ 248 | 285 | 13 | 14 | 6 | 5 | 1 | 28 | 278 | 1.0 | 870 | .10 | .47 | .2 | 1 |
| Ice cream, plain, factory packed: | | | | | | | | | | | | | | |
| 1 slice or cut brick, ⅛ of quart brick._____ 71 | 145 | 3 | 9 | 5 | 3 | Trace | 15 | 87 | .1 | 370 | .03 | .13 | .1 | 1 |
| Container_____ 3½ fluid ounces._____ 62 | 130 | 2 | 8 | 4 | 3 | Trace | 13 | 76 | .1 | 320 | .03 | .12 | .1 | 1 |
| Container_____ 8 fluid ounces._____ 142 | 295 | 6 | 18 | 10 | 6 | 1 | 29 | 175 | .1 | 740 | .06 | .27 | .1 | 1 |
| Ice milk_____ 1 cup_____ 187 | 285 | 9 | 10 | 6 | 3 | Trace | 42 | 292 | .2 | 390 | .09 | .41 | .2 | 2 |
| Yoghurt, from partially skimmed milk._____ 1 cup_____ 246 | 120 | 8 | 4 | 2 | 1 | Trace | 13 | 295 | .1 | 170 | .09 | .43 | .2 | 2 |
| **EGGS** | | | | | | | | | | | | | | |
| Eggs, large, 24 ounces per dozen: | | | | | | | | | | | | | | |

## MEAT, POULTRY, FISH, SHELLFISH; RELATED PRODUCTS

| Food, approximate measure | Weight (g) | Food energy (cal.) | Protein (g) | Fat (g) | Saturated fat (g) | Oleic (g) | Linoleic (g) | Carbohydrate (g) | Calcium (mg) | Iron (mg) | Vitamin A (I.U.) | Thiamine (mg) | Riboflavin (mg) | Niacin (mg) | Ascorbic acid (mg) |
|---|---|---|---|---|---|---|---|---|---|---|---|---|---|---|---|
| Yolk of egg — 1 yolk | 17 | 60 | 3 | 5 | 2 | 2 | Trace | Trace | 24 | .9 | 580 | .04 | .07 | Trace | 0 |
| Cooked: | | | | | | | | | | | | | | | |
| Boiled, shell removed — 2 eggs | 100 | 160 | 13 | 12 | 4 | 5 | 1 | 1 | 54 | 2.3 | 1,180 | .09 | .28 | .1 | 0 |
| Scrambled, with milk and fat — 1 egg | 64 | 110 | 7 | 8 | 3 | 3 | Trace | 1 | 51 | 1.1 | 690 | .05 | .18 | Trace | 0 |
| Bacon, broiled or fried, crisp — 2 slices | 16 | 100 | 5 | 8 | 3 | 4 | 1 | 1 | 2 | .5 | 0 | .08 | .05 | .8 | ---- |
| Beef, trimmed to retail basis,[1] cooked: | | | | | | | | | | | | | | | |
| Cuts braised, simmered, or pot-roasted: | | | | | | | | | | | | | | | |
| Lean and fat — 3 ounces | 85 | 245 | 23 | 16 | 8 | 7 | Trace | 0 | 10 | 2.9 | 30 | .04 | .18 | 3.5 | ---- |
| Lean only — 2.5 ounces | 72 | 140 | 22 | 5 | 2 | 2 | Trace | 0 | 10 | 2.7 | 10 | .04 | .16 | 3.3 | ---- |
| Hamburger (ground beef), broiled: | | | | | | | | | | | | | | | |
| Lean — 3 ounces | 85 | 185 | 23 | 10 | 5 | 4 | Trace | 0 | 10 | 3.0 | 20 | .08 | .20 | 5.1 | ---- |
| Regular — 3 ounces | 85 | 245 | 21 | 17 | 8 | 8 | Trace | 0 | 9 | 2.7 | 30 | .07 | .18 | 4.6 | ---- |
| Roast, oven-cooked, no liquid added: | | | | | | | | | | | | | | | |
| Relatively fat, such as rib: | | | | | | | | | | | | | | | |
| Lean and fat — 3 ounces | 85 | 375 | 17 | 34 | 16 | 15 | 1 | 0 | 8 | 2.2 | 70 | .05 | .13 | 3.1 | ---- |
| Lean only — 1.8 ounces | 51 | 125 | 14 | 7 | 3 | 3 | Trace | 0 | 6 | 1.8 | 10 | .04 | .11 | 2.6 | ---- |
| Relatively lean, such as heel of round: | | | | | | | | | | | | | | | |
| Lean and fat — 3 ounces | 85 | 165 | 25 | 7 | 3 | 3 | 1 | 0 | 11 | 3.2 | 10 | .06 | .19 | 4.5 | ---- |
| Lean only — 2.7 ounces | 78 | 125 | 24 | 3 | 1 | 1 | Trace | 0 | 10 | 3.0 | Trace | .06 | .18 | 4.3 | ---- |
| Steak, broiled: | | | | | | | | | | | | | | | |
| Relatively fat, such as sirloin: | | | | | | | | | | | | | | | |
| Lean and fat — 3 ounces | 85 | 330 | 20 | 27 | 13 | 12 | 1 | 0 | 9 | 2.5 | 50 | .05 | .16 | 4.0 | ---- |
| Lean only — 2.0 ounces | 56 | 115 | 18 | 4 | 2 | 2 | Trace | 0 | 7 | 2.2 | 10 | .05 | .14 | 3.6 | ---- |
| Relatively lean, such as round: | | | | | | | | | | | | | | | |
| Lean and fat — 3 ounces | 85 | 220 | 24 | 13 | 6 | 6 | Trace | 0 | 10 | 3.0 | 20 | .07 | .19 | 4.8 | ---- |
| Lean only — 2.4 ounces | 68 | 130 | 21 | 4 | 2 | 2 | Trace | 0 | 9 | 2.5 | 10 | .06 | .16 | 4.1 | ---- |
| Beef, canned: | | | | | | | | | | | | | | | |
| Corned beef — 3 ounces | 85 | 185 | 22 | 10 | 5 | 4 | Trace | 0 | 17 | 3.7 | 20 | .01 | .20 | 2.9 | ---- |
| Corned beef hash — 3 ounces | 85 | 155 | 7 | 10 | 5 | 4 | Trace | 9 | 11 | 1.7 | ---- | .01 | .08 | 1.8 | ---- |
| Beef, dried or chipped — 2 ounces | 57 | 115 | 19 | 4 | 2 | 2 | Trace | 0 | 11 | 2.9 | ---- | .04 | .18 | 2.2 | ---- |
| Beef and vegetable stew — 1 cup | 235 | 210 | 15 | 10 | 5 | 4 | Trace | 15 | 28 | 2.8 | 2,310 | .13 | .17 | 4.4 | 15 |
| Beef potpie, baked: Individual pie, 4¼-inch diameter, weight before baking about 8 ounces — 1 pie | 227 | 560 | 23 | 33 | 9 | 20 | 2 | 43 | 32 | 4.1 | 1,860 | .25 | .27 | 4.5 | 7 |

[1] Outer layer of fat on the cut was removed to within approximately ½ inch of the lean. Deposits of fat within the cut were not removed.

TABLE 36—*Continued*

## MEAT, POULTRY, FISH, SHELLFISH; RELATED PRODUCTS—Continued

| Food, Approximate Measure, and Weight (in Grams) | | Food Energy | Protein | Fat (Total Lipid) | Fatty acids | | | Carbohydrate | Calcium | Iron | Vitamin A Value | Thiamine | Riboflavin | Niacin | Ascorbic Acid |
|---|---|---|---|---|---|---|---|---|---|---|---|---|---|---|---|
| | | | | | Saturated (Total) | Unsaturated Oleic | Unsaturated Linoleic | | | | | | | | |
| | *Grams* | (Calories) | (Gm.) | (Gm.) | (Gm.) | (Gm.) | (Gm.) | (Gm.) | (Mg.) | (Mg.) | (I.U.) | (Mg.) | (Mg.) | (Mg.) | (Mg.) |
| Chicken, cooked: | | | | | | | | | | | | | | | |
| Flesh only, broiled_____ 3 ounces_____ | 85 | 115 | 20 | 3 | 1 | 1 | 1 | 0 | 8 | 1.4 | 80 | 0.05 | 0.16 | 7.4 | ----- |
| Breast, fried, ½ breast: | | | | | | | | | | | | | | | |
| With bone_____ 3.3 ounces_____ | 94 | 155 | 25 | 5 | 1 | 2 | 1 | 1 | 9 | 1.3 | 70 | .04 | .17 | 11.2 | ----- |
| Flesh and skin only_____ 2.7 ounces_____ | 76 | 155 | 25 | 5 | 1 | 2 | 1 | 1 | 9 | 1.3 | 70 | .04 | .17 | 11.2 | ----- |
| Drumstick, fried: | | | | | | | | | | | | | | | |
| With bone_____ 2.1 ounces_____ | 59 | 90 | 12 | 4 | 1 | 2 | 1 | Trace | 6 | .9 | 50 | .03 | .15 | 2.7 | ----- |
| Flesh and skin only_____ 1.3 ounces_____ | 38 | 90 | 12 | 4 | 1 | 2 | 1 | Trace | 6 | .9 | 50 | .03 | .15 | 2.7 | ----- |
| Chicken, canned, boneless. 3 ounces_____ | 85 | 170 | 18 | 10 | 3 | 4 | 2 | 0 | 18 | 1.3 | 200 | .03 | .11 | 3.7 | 3 |
| Chicken potpie. *See* Poultry potpie. | | | | | | | | | | | | | | | |
| Chile con carne, canned: | | | | | | | | | | | | | | | |
| With beans_____ 1 cup_____ | 250 | 335 | 19 | 15 | 7 | 7 | Trace | 30 | 80 | 4.2 | 150 | .08 | .18 | 3.2 | ----- |
| Without beans_____ 1 cup_____ | 255 | 510 | 26 | 38 | 18 | 17 | 1 | 15 | 97 | 3.6 | 380 | .05 | .31 | 5.6 | ----- |
| Heart, beef, lean, braised_____ 3 ounces_____ | 85 | 160 | 27 | 5 | ----- | ----- | ----- | 1 | 5 | 5.0 | 20 | .21 | 1.04 | 6.5 | 1 |
| Lamb, trimmed to retail basis,[1] cooked: | | | | | | | | | | | | | | | |
| Chop, thick, with bone, 1 chop, broiled. 4.8 ounces. | 137 | 400 | 25 | 33 | 18 | 12 | 1 | 0 | 10 | 1.5 | ----- | .14 | .25 | 5.6 | ----- |
| Lean and fat_____ 4.0 ounces_____ | 112 | 400 | 25 | 33 | 18 | 12 | 1 | 0 | 10 | 1.5 | ----- | .14 | .25 | 5.6 | ----- |
| Lean only_____ 2.6 ounces_____ | 74 | 140 | 21 | 6 | 3 | 2 | Trace | 0 | 9 | 1.5 | ----- | .11 | .20 | 4.5 | ----- |
| Leg, roasted: | | | | | | | | | | | | | | | |
| Lean and fat_____ 3 ounces_____ | 85 | 235 | 22 | 16 | 9 | 6 | Trace | 0 | 9 | 1.4 | ----- | .13 | .23 | 4.7 | ----- |
| Lean only_____ 2.5 ounces_____ | 71 | 130 | 20 | 5 | 3 | 2 | Trace | 0 | 9 | 1.4 | ----- | .12 | .21 | 4.4 | ----- |
| Shoulder, roasted: | | | | | | | | | | | | | | | |
| Lean and fat_____ 3 ounces_____ | 85 | 285 | 18 | 23 | 13 | 8 | 1 | 0 | 9 | 1.0 | ----- | .11 | .20 | 4.0 | ----- |
| Lean only_____ 2.3 ounces_____ | 64 | 130 | 17 | 6 | 3 | 2 | Trace | 0 | 8 | 1.0 | ----- | .10 | .18 | 3.7 | ----- |
| Liver, beef, fried_____ 2 ounces_____ | 57 | 130 | 15 | 6 | ----- | ----- | ----- | 3 | 6 | 5.0 | 30,280 | .15 | 2.37 | 9.4 | 15 |
| Pork, cured, cooked: | | | | | | | | | | | | | | | |
| Ham, light cure, lean 3 ounces_____ | 85 | 245 | 18 | 19 | 7 | 8 | 2 | 0 | 8 | 2.2 | 0 | .40 | .16 | 3.1 | ----- |

| | | | | | | | | | | | | | | | | |
|---|---|---|---|---|---|---|---|---|---|---|---|---|---|---|---|---|
| Boiled ham, sliced | 2 ounces | 57 | 135 | 11 | 10 | 4 | 4 | 1 | 0 | 6 | 1.6 | 0 | .25 | .09 | 1.5 | ----- |
| Canned, spiced or unspiced. | 2 ounces | 57 | 165 | 8 | 14 | 5 | 6 | 1 | 1 | 5 | 1.2 | 0 | .18 | .12 | 1.6 | ----- |
| Pork, fresh, trimmed to retail basis,[1] cooked: | | | | | | | | | | | | | | | | |
| Chop, thick, with bone. | 1 chop, 3.5 ounces. | 98 | 260 | 16 | 21 | 8 | 9 | 2 | 0 | 8 | 2.2 | 0 | .63 | .18 | 3.8 | ----- |
| Lean and fat | 2.3 ounces | 66 | 260 | 16 | 21 | 8 | 9 | 2 | 0 | 8 | 2.2 | 0 | .63 | .18 | 3.8 | ----- |
| Lean only | 1.7 ounces | 48 | 130 | 15 | 7 | 2 | 3 | 1 | 0 | 7 | 1.9 | 0 | .54 | .16 | 3.3 | ----- |
| Roast, oven-cooked, no liquid added: | | | | | | | | | | | | | | | | |
| Lean and fat | 3 ounces | 85 | 310 | 21 | 24 | 9 | 10 | 2 | 0 | 9 | 2.7 | 0 | .78 | .22 | 4.7 | ----- |
| Lean only | 2.4 ounces | 68 | 175 | 20 | 10 | 3 | 4 | 1 | 0 | 9 | 2.6 | 0 | .73 | .21 | 4.4 | ----- |
| Cuts, simmered: | | | | | | | | | | | | | | | | |
| Lean and fat | 3 ounces | 85 | 320 | 20 | 26 | 9 | 11 | 2 | 0 | 8 | 2.5 | 0 | .46 | .21 | 4.1 | ----- |
| Lean only | 2.2 ounces | 63 | 135 | 18 | 6 | 2 | 3 | 1 | 0 | 8 | 2.3 | 0 | .42 | .19 | 3.7 | ----- |
| Poultry potpie (based on chicken potpie). Individual pie, 4¼-inch diameter, weigh before baking about ounces. | 1 pie | 227 | 535 | 23 | 31 | 10 | 15 | 3 | 42 | 68 | 3.0 | 3,020 | .25 | .26 | 4.1 | 5 |
| Sausage: | | | | | | | | | | | | | | | | |
| Bologna, slice, 4.1 by 0.1 inch. | 8 slices | 227 | 690 | 27 | 62 | | | | 2 | 16 | 4.1 | | .36 | .49 | 6.0 | ----- |
| Frankfurter, cooked | 1 frankfurter | 51 | 155 | 6 | 14 | | | | 1 | 3 | .8 | | .08 | .10 | 1.3 | ----- |
| Pork, links or patty, cooked. | 4 ounces | 113 | 540 | 21 | 50 | 18 | 21 | 5 | Trace | 8 | 2.7 | 0 | .89 | .39 | 4.2 | ----- |
| Tongue, beef, braised | 3 ounces | 85 | 210 | 18 | 14 | | | | Trace | 6 | 1.9 | | .04 | .25 | 3.0 | ----- |
| Turkey potpie. See Poultry potpie. | | | | | | | | | | | | | | | | |
| Veal, cooked: | | | | | | | | | | | | | | | | |
| Cutlet, without bone, broiled. | 3 ounces | 85 | 185 | 23 | 9 | 5 | 4 | Trace | 0 | 9 | 2.7 | | .06 | .21 | 4.6 | ----- |
| Roast, medium fat, medium done; lean and fat. | 3 ounces | 85 | 230 | 23 | 14 | 7 | 6 | Trace | 0 | 10 | 2.9 | | .11 | .26 | 6.6 | ----- |
| Fish and shellfish: | | | | | | | | | | | | | | | | |
| Bluefish, baked or broiled. | 3 ounces | 85 | 135 | 22 | 4 | | | | 0 | 25 | .6 | 40 | .09 | .08 | 1.6 | ----- |
| Clams: | | | | | | | | | | | | | | | | |
| Raw, meat only | 3 ounces | 85 | 65 | 11 | 1 | | | | 2 | 59 | 5.2 | 90 | .08 | .15 | 1.1 | 8 |
| Canned, solids and liquid. | 3 ounces | 85 | 45 | 7 | 1 | | | | 2 | 47 | 3.5 | | .01 | .09 | .9 | ----- |
| Crabmeat, canned | 3 ounces | 85 | 85 | 15 | 2 | | | | 1 | 38 | .7 | | .07 | .07 | 1.6 | ----- |
| Fish sticks, breaded, cooked, frozen; stick, 3.8 by 1.0 by 0.5 inch. | 10 sticks or 8-ounce package. | 227 | 400 | 38 | 20 | 5 | 4 | 10 | 15 | 25 | .9 | | .09 | .16 | 3.6 | ----- |

[1] Outer layer of fat on the cut was removed to within approximately ½ inch of the lean. Deposits of fat within the cut were not removed.

TABLE 36—Continued

| Food, Approximate Measure, and Weight (in Grams) | Food Energy | Protein | Fat (Total Lipid) | Fatty acids | | | Carbohydrate | Calcium | Iron | Vitamin A Value | Thiamine | Riboflavin | Niacin | Ascorbic Acid |
| | | | | Saturated (Total) | Unsaturated | | | | | | | | | |
| | | | | | Oleic | Linoleic | | | | | | | | |
| | (Calories) | (Gm.) | (Gm.) | (Gm.) | (Gm.) | (Gm.) | (Gm.) | (Mg.) | (Mg.) | (I.U.) | (Mg.) | (Mg.) | (Mg.) | (Mg.) |
| **MEAT, POULTRY, FISH, SHELLFISH; RELATED PRODUCTS**—Continued | | | | | | | | | | | | | | |
| Fish and shellfish—Continued | | | | | | | | | | | | | | |
| Haddock, fried_____ 3 ounces_____ _Grams_ 85 | 140 | 17 | 5 | 1 | 3 | | 5 | 34 | 1.0 | ----- | 0.03 | 0.06 | 2.7 | 2 |
| Mackerel: | | | | | | | | | | | | | | |
| Broiled, Atlantic_____ 3 ounces_____ 85 | 200 | 19 | 13 | ----- | | | 0 | 5 | 1.0 | 450 | .13 | .23 | 6.5 | ----- |
| Canned, Pacific, solids and liquid.[2] 3 ounces 85 | 155 | 18 | 9 | ----- | | | 0 | 221 | 1.9 | 20 | .02 | .28 | 7.4 | ----- |
| Ocean perch, breaded (egg and breadcrumbs), fried. 3 ounces_____ 85 | 195 | 16 | 11 | ----- | | | 6 | 28 | 1.1 | ----- | .08 | .09 | 1.5 | ----- |
| Oysters, meat only: Raw, 13–19 medium selects. 1 cup_____ 240 | 160 | 20 | 4 | ----- | | | 8 | 226 | 13.2 | 740 | .33 | .43 | 6.0 | ----- |
| Oyster stew, 1 part oysters to 3 parts milk by volume, 3–4 oysters. 1 cup_____ 230 | 200 | 11 | 12 | ----- | | | 11 | 269 | 3.3 | 640 | .13 | .41 | 1.6 | ----- |
| Salmon, pink, canned__ 3 ounces_____ 85 | 120 | 17 | 5 | 1 | 1 | Trace | 0 | [3]167 | .7 | 60 | .03 | .16 | 6.8 | ----- |
| Sardines, Atlantic, canned in oil, drained solids. 3 ounces_____ 85 | 175 | 20 | 9 | ----- | | | 0 | 372 | 2.5 | 190 | .02 | .17 | 4.6 | ----- |
| Shad, baked_____ 3 ounces_____ 85 | 170 | 20 | 10 | ----- | | | 0 | 20 | .5 | 20 | .11 | .22 | 7.3 | ----- |
| Shrimp, canned, meat only. 3 ounces_____ 85 | 100 | 21 | 1 | ----- | | | 1 | 98 | 2.6 | 50 | .01 | .03 | 1.5 | ----- |
| Swordfish, broiled with butter or margarine. 3 ounces_____ 85 | 150 | 24 | 5 | ----- | | | 0 | 23 | 1.1 | 1,750 | .03 | .04 | 9.3 | ----- |
| Tuna, canned in oil, drained solids. 3 ounces_____ 85 | 170 | 24 | 7 | ----- | | | 0 | 7 | 1.6 | 70 | .04 | .10 | 10.1 | ----- |
| **MATURE DRY BEANS AND PEAS, NUTS, PEANUTS; RELATED PRODUCTS** | | | | | | | | | | | | | | |

Beans, dry:

| Food | Measure | Weight (g) | | | | | | | | | | | | | | |
|---|---|---|---|---|---|---|---|---|---|---|---|---|---|---|---|---|
| Common varieties, such as Great Northern, navy, and others, canned: | | | | | | | | | | | | | | | | |
| Red | 1 cup | 256 | 230 | 15 | 1 | — | — | — | 42 | 74 | 4.6 | Trace | .13 | .10 | 1.5 | — |
| White, with tomato sauce: | | | | | | | | | | | | | | | | |
| With pork | 1 cup | 261 | 320 | 16 | 7 | 3 | 3 | 1 | 50 | 141 | 4.7 | 340 | .20 | .08 | 1.5 | 5 |
| Without pork | 1 cup | 261 | 310 | 16 | 1 | — | — | — | 60 | 177 | 5.2 | 160 | .18 | .09 | 1.5 | 5 |
| Lima, cooked | 1 cup | 192 | 260 | 16 | 1 | — | — | — | 48 | 56 | 5.6 | Trace | .26 | .12 | 1.3 | Trace |
| Brazil nuts | 1 cup | 140 | 915 | 20 | 94 | 19 | 45 | 24 | 15 | 260 | 4.8 | Trace | 1.34 | .17 | 2.2 | — |
| Cashew nuts, roasted | 1 cup | 135 | 760 | 23 | 62 | 10 | 43 | 4 | 40 | 51 | 5.1 | 140 | .58 | .33 | 2.4 | — |
| Coconut: | | | | | | | | | | | | | | | | |
| Fresh, shredded | 1 cup | 97 | 335 | 3 | 34 | 29 | 2 | Trace | 9 | 13 | 1.6 | 0 | .05 | .02 | .5 | 3 |
| Dried, shredded, sweetened | 1 cup | 62 | 340 | 2 | 24 | 21 | 2 | Trace | 33 | 10 | 1.2 | 0 | .02 | .02 | .2 | 0 |
| Cowpeas or blackeye peas, dry, cooked | 1 cup | 248 | 190 | 13 | 1 | — | — | — | 34 | 42 | 3.2 | 20 | .41 | .11 | 1.1 | Trace |
| Peanuts, roasted, salted: | | | | | | | | | | | | | | | | |
| Halves | 1 cup | 144 | 840 | 37 | 72 | 16 | 31 | 21 | 27 | 107 | 3.0 | — | .46 | .19 | 24.7 | 0 |
| Chopped | 1 tablespoon | 9 | 55 | 2 | 4 | 1 | 2 | 1 | 2 | 7 | .2 | — | .03 | .01 | 1.5 | 0 |
| Peanut butter | 1 tablespoon | 16 | 95 | 4 | 8 | 2 | 4 | 2 | 3 | 9 | .3 | — | .02 | .02 | 2.4 | 0 |
| Peas, split, dry, cooked | 1 cup | 250 | 290 | 20 | 1 | — | — | — | 52 | 28 | 4.2 | 100 | .37 | .22 | 2.2 | — |
| Pecans: | | | | | | | | | | | | | | | | |
| Halves | 1 cup | 108 | 740 | 10 | 77 | 5 | 48 | 15 | 16 | 79 | 2.6 | 140 | .93 | .14 | 1.0 | 2 |
| Chopped | 1 tablespoon | 7.5 | 50 | 1 | 5 | Trace | 3 | 1 | 1 | 5 | .2 | 10 | .06 | .01 | .1 | Trace |
| Walnuts, shelled: | | | | | | | | | | | | | | | | |
| Black or native, chopped | 1 cup | 126 | 790 | 26 | 75 | 4 | 26 | 36 | 19 | Trace | 7.6 | 380 | .28 | .14 | .9 | — |
| English or Persian: | | | | | | | | | | | | | | | | |
| Halves | 1 cup | 100 | 650 | 15 | 64 | 4 | 10 | 40 | 16 | 99 | 3.1 | 30 | .33 | .13 | .9 | 3 |
| Chopped | 1 tablespoon | 8 | 50 | 1 | 5 | Trace | 1 | 3 | 1 | 8 | .2 | Trace | .03 | .01 | .1 | Trace |
| **VEGETABLES AND VEGETABLE PRODUCTS** | | | | | | | | | | | | | | | | |
| Asparagus: | | | | | | | | | | | | | | | | |
| Cooked, cut spears | 1 cup | 175 | 35 | 4 | Trace | — | — | — | 6 | 37 | 1.0 | 1,580 | .27 | .32 | 2.4 | 46 |
| Canned spears, medium: | | | | | | | | | | | | | | | | |
| Green | 6 spears | 96 | 20 | 2 | Trace | — | — | — | 3 | 18 | 1.8 | 770 | .06 | .10 | .8 | 14 |
| Bleached | 6 spears | 96 | 20 | 2 | Trace | — | — | — | 4 | 15 | 1.0 | 80 | .05 | .06 | .7 | 14 |
| Beans: | | | | | | | | | | | | | | | | |
| Lima, immature, cooked | 1 cup | 160 | 180 | 12 | 1 | — | — | — | 32 | 75 | 4.0 | 450 | .29 | .16 | 2.0 | 28 |
| Snap, green: | | | | | | | | | | | | | | | | |
| Cooked: | | | | | | | | | | | | | | | | |
| In small amount of water, short time. | 1 cup | 125 | 30 | 2 | Trace | — | — | — | 7 | 62 | .8 | 680 | .08 | .11 | .6 | 16 |

² Vitamin values based on drained solids.

³ Based on total contents of can. If bones are discarded, value will be greatly reduced

TABLE 36—Continued

| Food, Approximate Measure, and Weight (in Grams) | | Food Energy | Protein | Fat (Total Lipid) | Fatty acids | | | Carbo-hydrate | Calcium | Iron | Vitamin A Value | Thiamine | Ribo-flavin | Niacin | Ascorbic Acid |
|---|---|---|---|---|---|---|---|---|---|---|---|---|---|---|---|
| | | | | | Saturated (Total) | Unsaturated Oleic | Linoleic | | | | | | | | |
| | Grams | (Calories) | (Gm.) | (Gm.) | (Gm.) | (Gm.) | (Gm.) | (Gm.) | (Mg.) | (Mg.) | (I.U.) | (Mg.) | (Mg.) | (Mg.) | (Mg.) |
| **VEGETABLES AND VEGETABLE PRODUCTS—Continued** | | | | | | | | | | | | | | | |
| Beans—Continued | | | | | | | | | | | | | | | |
| Snap, green—Continued | | | | | | | | | | | | | | | |
| Cooked—Continued | | | | | | | | | | | | | | | |
| In large amount of water, long time. 1 cup | 125 | 30 | 2 | Trace | | | | 7 | 62 | 0.8 | 680 | 0.07 | 0.10 | 0.4 | 13 |
| Canned: | | | | | | | | | | | | | | | |
| Solids and liquid 1 cup | 239 | 45 | 2 | Trace | | | | 10 | 81 | 2.9 | 690 | .08 | .10 | .7 | 9 |
| Strained or chopped (baby food). 1 ounce | 28 | 5 | Trace | Trace | | | | 1 | 9 | .3 | 110 | .01 | .02 | .1 | Trace |
| Bean sprouts. *See* Sprouts. | | | | | | | | | | | | | | | |
| Beets, cooked, diced 1 cup | 165 | 50 | 2 | Trace | | | | 12 | 23 | .8 | 40 | .04 | .07 | .5 | 11 |
| Broccoli spears, cooked 1 cup | 150 | 40 | 5 | Trace | | | | 7 | 132 | 1.2 | 3,750 | .14 | .29 | 1.2 | 135 |
| Brussels sprouts, cooked 1 cup | 130 | 45 | 5 | 1 | | | | 8 | 42 | 1.4 | 680 | .10 | .18 | 1.1 | 113 |
| Cabbage: | | | | | | | | | | | | | | | |
| Raw: | | | | | | | | | | | | | | | |
| Finely shredded 1 cup | 100 | 25 | 1 | Trace | | | | 5 | 49 | .4 | 130 | .05 | .05 | .3 | 47 |
| Coleslaw 1 cup | 120 | 120 | 1 | 9 | 2 | 2 | 5 | 9 | 52 | .5 | 180 | .06 | .06 | .3 | 35 |
| Cooked: | | | | | | | | | | | | | | | |
| In small amount of water, short time. 1 cup | 170 | 35 | 2 | Trace | | | | 7 | 75 | .5 | 220 | .07 | .07 | .5 | 56 |
| In large amount of water, long time. 1 cup | 170 | 30 | 2 | Trace | | | | 7 | 71 | .5 | 200 | .04 | .04 | .2 | 40 |
| Cabbage, celery or Chinese: | | | | | | | | | | | | | | | |
| Raw, leaves and stalk, 1-inch pieces. 1 cup | 100 | 15 | 1 | Trace | | | | 3 | 43 | .6 | 150 | .05 | .04 | .6 | 25 |
| Cabbage, spoon (or pakchoy), cooked. 1 cup | 150 | 20 | 2 | Trace | | | | 4 | 222 | .9 | 4,650 | .07 | .12 | 1.1 | 23 |
| Carrots: | | | | | | | | | | | | | | | |
| Raw: | | | | | | | | | | | | | | | |
| Whole, 5½ by 1 inch, 1 carrot (25 thin strips). | 50 | 20 | 1 | Trace | | | | 5 | 18 | .4 | 5,500 | .03 | .03 | .3 | 4 |

| | | | | | | | | | | | | | | | | |
|---|---|---|---|---|---|---|---|---|---|---|---|---|---|---|---|---|
| Cooked, diced | 1 cup | 145 | 45 | 1 | Trace | ------ | ------ | ------ | 10 | 48 | .9 | 15,220 | .08 | .07 | .7 | 9 |
| Canned, strained or chopped (baby food). | 1 ounce | 28 | 10 | Trace | Trace | ------ | ------ | ------ | 2 | 7 | .1 | 3,690 | .01 | .01 | .1 | 1 |
| Cauliflower, cooked, flowerbuds. | 1 cup | 120 | 25 | 3 | Trace | ------ | ------ | ------ | 5 | 25 | .8 | 70 | .11 | .10 | .7 | 66 |
| Celery, raw: Stalk, large outer, 8 by about 1½ inches, at root end. | 1 stalk | 40 | 5 | Trace | Trace | ------ | ------ | ------ | 2 | 16 | .1 | 100 | .01 | .01 | .1 | 4 |
| Pieces, diced | 1 cup | 100 | 15 | 1 | Trace | ------ | ------ | ------ | 4 | 39 | .3 | 240 | .03 | .03 | .3 | 9 |
| Collards, cooked | 1 cup | 190 | 55 | 5 | 1 | ------ | ------ | ------ | 9 | 289 | 1.1 | 10,260 | .27 | .37 | 2.4 | 87 |
| Corn, sweet: Cooked, ear 5 by 1¾ inches.[4] | 1 ear | 140 | 70 | 3 | 1 | ------ | ------ | ------ | 16 | 2 | .5 | [5]310 | .09 | .08 | 1.0 | 7 |
| Canned, solids and liquid. | 1 cup | 256 | 170 | 5 | 2 | ------ | ------ | ------ | 40 | 10 | 1.0 | [5]690 | .07 | .12 | 2.3 | 13 |
| Cowpeas, cooked, immature seeds. | 1 cup | 160 | 175 | 13 | 1 | ------ | ------ | ------ | 29 | 38 | 3.4 | 560 | .49 | .18 | 2.3 | 28 |
| Cucumbers, 10-ounce; 7½ by about 2 inches: Raw, pared. | 1 cucumber | 207 | 30 | 1 | Trace | ------ | ------ | ------ | 7 | 35 | .6 | Trace | .07 | .09 | .4 | 23 |
| Raw, pared, center slice ⅛-inch thick. | 6 slices | 50 | 5 | Trace | Trace | ------ | ------ | ------ | 2 | 8 | .2 | Trace | .02 | .02 | .1 | 6 |
| Dandelion greens, cooked. | 1 cup | 180 | 60 | 4 | 1 | ------ | ------ | ------ | 12 | 252 | 3.2 | 21,060 | .24 | .29 | ---- | 32 |
| Endive, curly (including escarole). | 2 ounces | 57 | 10 | 1 | Trace | ------ | ------ | ------ | 2 | 46 | 1.0 | 1,870 | .04 | .08 | .3 | 6 |
| Kale, leaves including stems, cooked. | 1 cup | 110 | 30 | 4 | 1 | ------ | ------ | ------ | 4 | 147 | 1.3 | 8,140 | ---- | ---- | ---- | 68 |
| Lettuce, raw: Butterhead, as Boston types; head, 4-inch diameter. | 1 head | 220 | 30 | 3 | Trace | ------ | ------ | ------ | 6 | 77 | 4.4 | 2,130 | .14 | .13 | .6 | 18 |
| Crisphead, as Iceberg; head, 4¾-inch diameter. | 1 head | 454 | 60 | 4 | Trace | ------ | ------ | ------ | 13 | 91 | 2.3 | 1,500 | .29 | .27 | 1.3 | 29 |
| Looseleaf, or bunching varieties, leaves. | 2 large | 50 | 10 | 1 | Trace | ------ | ------ | ------ | 2 | 34 | .7 | 950 | .03 | .04 | .2 | 9 |
| Mushrooms, canned, solids and liquid. | 1 cup | 244 | 40 | 5 | Trace | ------ | ------ | ------ | 6 | 15 | 1.2 | Trace | .04 | .60 | 4.8 | 4 |
| Mustard greens, cooked | 1 cup | 140 | 35 | 3 | 1 | ------ | ------ | ------ | 6 | 193 | 2.5 | 8,120 | .11 | .19 | .9 | 68 |
| Okra, cooked, pod 3 by ⅝ inch. | 8 pods | 85 | 25 | 2 | Trace | ------ | ------ | ------ | 5 | 78 | .4 | 420 | .11 | .15 | .8 | 17 |

[4] Measure and weight apply to entire vegetable or fruit including parts not usually eaten.

[5] Based on yellow varieties; white varieties contain only a trace of cryptoxanthin and carotenes, the pigments in corn that have biological activity.

TABLE 36—Continued

| Food, Approximate Measure, and Weight (in Grams) | | Food Energy | Pro-tein | Fat (Total Lipid) | Fatty acids | | | Carbo-hy-drate | Cal-cium | Iron | Vita-min A Value | Thia-mine | Ribo-flavin | Niacin | Ascor-bic Acid |
|---|---|---|---|---|---|---|---|---|---|---|---|---|---|---|---|
| | | | | | Satu-rated (Total) | Unsaturated Oleic | Unsaturated Linoleic | | | | | | | | |
| | | (Calo-ries) | (Gm.) | (Gm.) | (Gm.) | (Gm.) | (Gm.) | (Gm.) | (Mg.) | (Mg.) | (I.U.) | (Mg.) | (Mg.) | (Mg.) | (Mg.) |
| VEGETABLES AND VEGETABLE PRODUCTS—Continued | | | | | | | | | | | | | | | |
| Onions: | | | | | | | | | | | | | | | |
| Mature: | | | | | | | | | | | | | | | |
| Raw, onion 2½-inch diameter. | 1 onion — 110 *Grams* | 40 | 2 | Trace | | | | 10 | 30 | 0.6 | 40 | 0.04 | 0.04 | 0.2 | 11 |
| Cooked | 1 cup — 210 | 60 | 3 | Trace | | | | 14 | 50 | .8 | 80 | .06 | .06 | .4 | 14 |
| Young green, small, without tops. | 6 onions — 50 | 20 | 1 | Trace | | | | 5 | 20 | .3 | Trace | .02 | .02 | .2 | 12 |
| Parsley, raw, chopped | 1 tablespoon — 3.5 | 1 | Trace | Trace | | | | Trace | 7 | .2 | 300 | Trace | .01 | Trace | 6 |
| Parsnips, cooked | 1 cup — 155 | 100 | 2 | 1 | | | | 23 | 70 | .9 | 50 | .11 | .13 | .2 | 16 |
| Peas, green: | | | | | | | | | | | | | | | |
| Cooked | 1 cup — 160 | 115 | 9 | 1 | | | | 19 | 37 | 2.9 | 860 | .44 | .17 | 3.7 | 33 |
| Canned, solids and liquid. | 1 cup — 249 | 165 | 9 | 1 | | | | 31 | 50 | 4.2 | 1,120 | .23 | .13 | 2.2 | 22 |
| Canned, strained (baby food). | 1 ounce — 28 | 15 | 1 | Trace | | | | 3 | 3 | .4 | 140 | .02 | .02 | .4 | 3 |
| Peppers, hot, red, without seeds, dried (ground chili powder, added seasonings). | 1 tablespoon — 15 | 50 | 2 | 2 | | | | 8 | 40 | 2.3 | 9,750 | .03 | .17 | 1.3 | 2 |
| Peppers, sweet: | | | | | | | | | | | | | | | |
| Raw, medium, about 6 per pound: | | | | | | | | | | | | | | | |
| Green pod without stem and seeds. | 1 pod — 62 | 15 | 1 | Trace | | | | 3 | 6 | .4 | 260 | .05 | .05 | .3 | 79 |
| Red pod without stem and seeds. | 1 pod — 60 | 20 | 1 | Trace | | | | 4 | 8 | .4 | 2,670 | .05 | .05 | .3 | 122 |
| Canned, pimientos, | 1 pod — 38 | 10 | Trace | Trace | | | | 2 | 3 | .6 | 870 | .01 | .02 | .1 | 36 |

| Food | Measure | Weight (g) | Food energy | Protein (g) | Fat (g) | Saturated | Oleic | Linoleic | Carbohydrate (g) | Calcium (mg) | Iron (mg) | Vitamin A (I.U.) | Thiamine (mg) | Riboflavin (mg) | Niacin (mg) | Ascorbic acid (mg) |
|---|---|---|---|---|---|---|---|---|---|---|---|---|---|---|---|---|
| **Potatoes, medium (about 3 per pound raw):** | | | | | | | | | | | | | | | | |
| Baked, peeled after baking. | 1 potato | 99 | 90 | 3 | Trace | — | — | — | 21 | 9 | .7 | Trace | .10 | .04 | 1.7 | 20 |
| **Boiled:** | | | | | | | | | | | | | | | | |
| Peeled after boiling | 1 potato | 136 | 105 | 3 | Trace | — | — | — | 23 | 10 | .8 | Trace | .13 | .05 | 2.0 | 22 |
| Peeled before boiling | 1 potato | 122 | 80 | 2 | Trace | — | — | — | 18 | 7 | .6 | Trace | .11 | .04 | 1.4 | 20 |
| **French-fried, piece 2 by ½ by ½ inch:** | | | | | | | | | | | | | | | | |
| Cooked in deep fat | 10 pieces | 57 | 155 | 2 | 7 | 2 | 2 | 4 | 20 | 9 | .7 | Trace | .07 | .04 | 1.8 | 12 |
| Frozen, heated | 10 pieces | 57 | 125 | 2 | 5 | 1 | 1 | 2 | 19 | 5 | 1.0 | Trace | .08 | .01 | 1.5 | 12 |
| **Mashed:** | | | | | | | | | | | | | | | | |
| Milk added | 1 cup | 195 | 125 | 4 | 1 | — | — | — | 25 | 47 | .8 | 50 | .16 | .10 | 2.0 | 19 |
| Milk and butter added. | 1 cup | 195 | 185 | 4 | 8 | 4 | 3 | Trace | 24 | 47 | .8 | 330 | .16 | .10 | 1.9 | 18 |
| Potato chips, medium, 2-inch diameter. | 10 chips | 20 | 115 | 1 | 8 | 2 | 2 | 4 | 10 | 8 | .4 | Trace | .04 | .01 | 1.0 | 3 |
| Pumpkin, canned | 1 cup | 228 | 75 | 2 | 1 | — | — | — | 18 | 57 | .9 | 14,590 | .07 | .12 | 1.3 | 12 |
| Radishes, raw, small, without tops. | 4 radishes | 40 | 5 | Trace | Trace | — | — | — | 1 | 12 | .4 | Trace | .01 | .01 | .1 | 10 |
| Sauerkraut, canned, solids and liquid. | 1 cup | 235 | 45 | 2 | Trace | — | — | — | 9 | 85 | 1.2 | 120 | .07 | .09 | .4 | 33 |
| **Spinach:** | | | | | | | | | | | | | | | | |
| Cooked | 1 cup | 180 | 40 | 5 | 1 | — | — | — | 6 | 167 | 4.0 | 14,580 | .13 | .25 | 1.0 | 50 |
| Canned, drained solids. | 1 cup | 180 | 45 | 5 | 1 | — | — | — | 6 | 212 | 4.7 | 14,400 | .03 | .21 | .6 | 24 |
| Canned, strained or chopped (baby food). | 1 ounce | 28 | 10 | 1 | Trace | — | — | — | 2 | 18 | .2 | 1,420 | .01 | .04 | .1 | 2 |
| **Sprouts, raw:** | | | | | | | | | | | | | | | | |
| Mung bean | 1 cup | 90 | 30 | 3 | Trace | — | — | — | 6 | 17 | 1.2 | 20 | .12 | .12 | .7 | 17 |
| Soybean | 1 cup | 107 | 40 | 6 | 2 | — | — | — | 4 | 46 | .7 | 90 | .17 | .16 | .8 | 4 |
| **Squash:** | | | | | | | | | | | | | | | | |
| Cooked: | | | | | | | | | | | | | | | | |
| Summer, diced | 1 cup | 210 | 30 | 2 | Trace | — | — | — | 7 | 52 | .8 | 820 | .10 | .16 | 1.6 | 21 |
| Winter, baked, mashed. | 1 cup | 205 | 130 | 4 | 1 | — | — | — | 32 | 57 | 1.6 | 8,610 | .10 | .27 | 1.4 | 27 |
| Canned, winter, strained and chopped (baby food). | 1 ounce | 28 | 10 | Trace | Trace | — | — | — | 2 | 7 | .1 | 510 | .01 | .01 | .1 | 1 |

TABLE 36—Continued

| Food, Approximate Measure, and Weight (in Grams) | | Food Energy | Protein | Fat (Total Lipid) | Fatty acids | | | Carbohydrate | Calcium | Iron | Vitamin A Value | Thiamine | Riboflavin | Niacin | Ascorbic Acid |
|---|---|---|---|---|---|---|---|---|---|---|---|---|---|---|---|
| | | | | | Saturated (Total) | Unsaturated | | | | | | | | | |
| | | | | | | Oleic | Linoleic | | | | | | | | |
| | | (Calories) | (Gm.) | (Gm.) | (Gm.) | (Gm.) | (Gm.) | (Gm.) | (Mg.) | (Mg.) | (I.U.) | (Mg.) | (Mg.) | (Mg.) | (Mg.) |
| **VEGETABLES AND VEGETABLE PRODUCTS—Continued** | Grams | | | | | | | | | | | | | | |
| Sweetpotatoes: | | | | | | | | | | | | | | | |
| Cooked, medium, 5 by 2 inches, weight raw about 6 ounces: | | | | | | | | | | | | | | | |
| Baked, peeled after baking. 1 sweetpotato. | 110 | 155 | 2 | 1 | | | | 36 | 44 | 1.0 | 8,910 | 0.10 | 0.07 | 0.7 | 24 |
| Boiled, peeled after boiling. 1 sweetpotato. | 147 | 170 | 2 | 1 | | | | 39 | 47 | 1.0 | 11,610 | .13 | .09 | .9 | 25 |
| Candied, 3½ by 2¼ inches. 1 sweetpotato. | 175 | 295 | 2 | 6 | 2 | 3 | 1 | 60 | 65 | 1.6 | 11,030 | .10 | .08 | .8 | 17 |
| Canned, vacuum or solid pack. 1 cup. | 218 | 235 | 4 | Trace | | | | 54 | 54 | 1.7 | 17,000 | .10 | .10 | 1.4 | 30 |
| Tomatoes: | | | | | | | | | | | | | | | |
| Raw, medium, 2 by 2½ inches, about 3 per pound. 1 tomato. | 150 | 35 | 2 | Trace | | | | 7 | 20 | .8 | 1,350 | .10 | .06 | 1.0 | [6]34 |
| Canned. 1 cup. | 242 | 50 | 2 | Trace | | | | 10 | 15 | 1.2 | 2,180 | .13 | .07 | 1.7 | 40 |
| Tomato juice, canned. 1 cup. | 242 | 45 | 2 | Trace | | | | 10 | 17 | 2.2 | 1,940 | .13 | .07 | 1.8 | 39 |
| Tomato catsup. 1 tablespoon. | 17 | 15 | Trace | Trace | | | | 4 | 4 | .1 | 240 | .02 | .01 | .3 | 3 |
| Turnips, cooked, diced. 1 cup. | 155 | 35 | 1 | Trace | | | | 8 | 54 | .6 | Trace | .06 | .08 | .5 | 33 |
| Turnip greens: | | | | | | | | | | | | | | | |
| Cooked: | | | | | | | | | | | | | | | |
| In small amount of water, short time. 1 cup. | 145 | 30 | 3 | Trace | | | | 5 | 267 | 1.6 | 9,140 | .21 | .36 | .8 | 100 |
| In large amount of water, long time. 1 cup. | 145 | 25 | 3 | Trace | | | | 5 | 252 | 1.4 | 8,260 | .14 | .33 | .8 | 68 |
| Canned, solids and liquid. 1 cup. | 232 | 40 | 3 | 1 | | | | 7 | 232 | 3.7 | 10,900 | .04 | .21 | 1.4 | 44 |
| **FRUITS AND FRUIT PRODUCTS** | | | | | | | | | | | | | | | |
| Apples, raw, medium, 2½-inch diameter, about 3 per pound.[4] 1 apple. | 150 | 70 | Trace | Trace | | | | 18 | 8 | .4 | 50 | .04 | .02 | .1 | 3 |
| Apple brown betty. 1 cup. | 230 | 345 | 4 | 8 | 4 | 3 | Trace | 68 | 41 | 1.4 | 230 | .13 | .10 | .9 | 3 |

|  |  |  |  |  |  |  |  |  |  |  |  |  |  |  |  |  |
|---|---|---|---|---|---|---|---|---|---|---|---|---|---|---|---|---|
| Apple juice, ... canned. | 1 cup | 2.. | 120 | Trace | Trace |  |  |  |  | 15 | 1.3 | ------ | .01 | .04 | .2 | 2 |
| Applesauce, canned: |  |  |  |  |  |  |  |  |  |  |  |  |  |  |  |  |
| Sweetened | 1 cup | 254 | 230 | 1 | Trace |  |  |  | 60 | 10 | 1.3 | 100 | .05 | .03 | .1 | 3 |
| Unsweetened or artificially sweetened. | 1 cup | 239 | 100 | Trace | Trace |  |  |  | 26 | 10 | 1.2 | 100 | .04 | .02 | .1 | 2 |
| Applesauce and apricots, canned, strained or junior (baby food). | 1 ounce | 28 | 25 | Trace | Trace |  |  |  | 6 | 1 | .1 | 170 | Trace | Trace | Trace | 1 |
| Apricots: |  |  |  |  |  |  |  |  |  |  |  |  |  |  |  |  |
| Raw, about 12 per pound.[4] | 3 apricots | 114 | 55 | 1 | Trace |  |  |  | 14 | 18 | .5 | 2,890 | .03 | .04 | .7 | 10 |
| Canned in heavy sirup: |  |  |  |  |  |  |  |  |  |  |  |  |  |  |  |  |
| Halves and sirup | 1 cup | 259 | 220 | 2 | Trace |  |  |  | 57 | 28 | .8 | 4,510 | .05 | .06 | .9 | 10 |
| Halves (medium) and sirup. | 4 halves; 2 tablespoons sirup. | 122 | 105 | 1 | Trace |  |  |  | 27 | 13 | .4 | 2,120 | .02 | .03 | .4 | 5 |
| Dried: |  |  |  |  |  |  |  |  |  |  |  |  |  |  |  |  |
| Uncooked, 40 halves, small. | 1 cup | 150 | 390 | 8 | 1 |  |  |  | 100 | 100 | 8.2 | 16,350 | .02 | .23 | 4.9 | 19 |
| Cooked, unsweetened, fruit and liquid. | 1 cup | 285 | 240 | 5 | 1 |  |  |  | 62 | 63 | 5.1 | 8,550 | .01 | .13 | 2.8 | 8 |
| Apricot nectar, canned | 1 cup | 250 | 140 | 1 | Trace |  |  |  | 36 | 22 | .5 | 2,380 | .02 | .02 | .5 | 7 |
| Avocados, raw: |  |  |  |  |  |  |  |  |  |  |  |  |  |  |  |  |
| California varieties, mainly Fuerte: |  |  |  |  |  |  |  |  |  |  |  |  |  |  |  |  |
| 10-ounce avocado, about 3⅓ by 4¼ inches, peeled, pitted. | ½ avocado | 108 | 185 | 2 | 18 | 4 | 8 | 2 | 6 | 11 | .6 | 310 | .12 | .21 | 1.7 | 15 |
| ½-inch cubes | 1 cup | 152 | 260 | 3 | 26 | 5 | 12 | 3 | 9 | 15 | .9 | 440 | .16 | .30 | 2.4 | 21 |
| Florida varieties: |  |  |  |  |  |  |  |  |  |  |  |  |  |  |  |  |
| 13-ounce avocado, about 4 by 3 inches, peeled, pitted. | ½ avocado | 123 | 160 | 2 | 14 | 3 | 6 | 2 | 11 | 12 | .7 | 360 | .13 | .24 | 2.0 | 17 |
| ½-inch cubes | 1 cup | 152 | 195 | 2 | 17 | 3 | 8 | 2 | 13 | 15 | .9 | 440 | .16 | .30 | 2.4 | 21 |
| Bananas, raw, 6 by 1½ inches, about 3 per pound.[4] | 1 banana | 150 | 85 | 1 | Trace |  |  |  | 23 | 8 | .7 | 190 | .05 | .06 | .7 | 10 |
| Blackberries, raw | 1 cup | 144 | 85 | 2 | 1 |  |  |  | 19 | 46 | 1.3 | 290 | .05 | .06 | .5 | 30 |
| Blueberries, raw | 1 cup | 140 | 85 | 1 | 1 |  |  |  | 21 | 21 | 1.4 | 140 | .04 | .08 | .6 | 20 |
| Cantaloups, raw; medium, 5-inch diameter, about 1⅔ pounds.[4] | ½ melon | 385 | 60 | 1 | Trace |  |  |  | 14 | 27 | .8 | [7]6,540 | .08 | .06 | 1.2 | 63 |

[4] Measure and weight apply to entire vegetable or fruit including parts not usually eaten.

[6] Year-round average. Samples marketed from November through May average around 15 milligrams per 150-gram tomato; from June through October, around 39 milligrams.

[7] Value based on varieties with orange-colored flesh; for green-fleshed varieties value is about 540 I.U. per ½ melon.

TABLE 36—*Continued*

| Food, Approximate Measure, and Weight (In Grams) | Food Energy | Protein | Fat (Total Lipid) | Fatty acids Saturated (Total) | Fatty acids Unsaturated Oleic | Fatty acids Unsaturated Linoleic | Carbohydrate | Calcium | Iron | Vitamin A Value | Thiamine | Riboflavin | Niacin | Ascorbic Acid |
|---|---|---|---|---|---|---|---|---|---|---|---|---|---|---|
| | (Calories) | (Gm.) | (Gm.) | (Gm.) | (Gm.) | (Gm.) | (Gm.) | (Mg.) | (Mg.) | (I.U.) | (Mg.) | (Mg.) | (Mg.) | (Mg.) |
| **FRUITS AND FRUIT PRODUCTS—Con.** | | | | | | | | | | | | | | |
| Cherries: | | | | | | | | | | | | | | |
| Raw, sweet, with stems⁴ 1 cup _____ 130 *Grams* | 80 | 2 | Trace | | | | 20 | 26 | 0.5 | 130 | 0.06 | 0.07 | 0.5 | 12 |
| Canned, red, sour, pitted, 1 cup _____ 260 heavy sirup. | 230 | 2 | 1 | | | | 59 | 36 | .8 | 1,680 | .07 | .06 | .4 | 13 |
| Cranberry juice cocktail, 1 cup _____ 250 canned. | 160 | Trace | Trace | | | | 41 | 12 | .8 | Trace | .02 | .02 | .1 | (8) |
| Cranberry sauce, sweetened, canned, strained. 1 cup _____ 277 | 405 | Trace | 1 | | | | 104 | 17 | .6 | 40 | .03 | .03 | .1 | 5 |
| Dates, domestic, natural and dry, pitted, cut. 1 cup _____ 178 | 490 | 4 | 1 | | | | 130 | 105 | 5.3 | 90 | .16 | .17 | 3.9 | 0 |
| Figs: | | | | | | | | | | | | | | |
| Raw, small, 1½-inch diameter, about 12 per pound. 3 figs _____ 114 | 90 | 1 | Trace | | | | 23 | 40 | .7 | 90 | .07 | .06 | .5 | 2 |
| Dried, large, 2 by 1 inch. 1 fig _____ 21 | 60 | 1 | Trace | | | | 15 | 26 | .6 | 20 | .02 | .02 | .1 | 0 |
| Fruit cocktail, canned in heavy sirup, solids and liquid. 1 cup _____ 256 | 195 | 1 | 1 | | | | 50 | 23 | 1.0 | 360 | .04 | .03 | 1.1 | 5 |
| Grapefruit: | | | | | | | | | | | | | | |
| Raw, medium, 4¼-inch diameter, size 64: | | | | | | | | | | | | | | |
| White⁴ _____ ½ grapefruit_ 285 | 55 | 1 | Trace | | | | 14 | 22 | .6 | 10 | .05 | .02 | .2 | 52 |
| Pink or red⁴ _____ ½ grapefruit_ 285 | 60 | 1 | Trace | | | | 15 | 23 | .6 | 640 | .05 | .02 | .3 | 52 |
| Raw sections, white ____ 1 cup _____ 194 | 75 | 1 | Trace | | | | 20 | 31 | .8 | 20 | .07 | .03 | .3 | 72 |
| Canned, white: | | | | | | | | | | | | | | |
| Sirup pack, solids and liquid. 1 cup _____ 249 | 175 | 1 | Trace | | | | 44 | 32 | .7 | 20 | .07 | .04 | .5 | 75 |
| Water pack, solids and liquid. 1 cup _____ 240 | 70 | 1 | Trace | | | | 18 | 31 | .7 | 20 | .07 | .04 | .5 | 72 |
| Grapefruit juice: | | | | | | | | | | | | | | |
| Fresh _____ 1 cup _____ 246 | 95 | 1 | Trace | | | | 23 | 22 | .5 | (9) | .09 | .04 | .4 | 92 |
| Canned, white: | | | | | | | | | | | | | | |
| Unsweetened _____ 1 cup _____ 247 | 100 | 1 | Trace | | | | 24 | 20 | 1.0 | 20 | .07 | .04 | .4 | 84 |
| Sweetened _____ 1 cup _____ 250 | 130 | 1 | Trace | | | | | | | | | | | 79 |

| Food | Measure | | | | | | | | | | | | | | |
|---|---|---|---|---|---|---|---|---|---|---|---|---|---|---|---|
| **Frozen, concentrate, unsweetened:** | | | | | | | | | | | | | | | |
| Undiluted, can, 6 fluid ounces. | 1 can | 207 | ------ | 300 | 4 | 1 | ------ | 72 | 70 | .8 | 60 | .29 | .12 | 1.4 | 286 |
| Diluted with 3 parts water, by volume. | 1 cup | 247 | ------ | 100 | 1 | Trace | ------ | 24 | 25 | .2 | 20 | .10 | .04 | .5 | 96 |
| **Frozen, concentrate, sweetened:** | | | | | | | | | | | | | | | |
| Undiluted, can, 6 fluid ounces. | 1 can | 211 | ------ | 350 | 3 | 1 | ------ | 85 | 59 | .6 | 50 | .24 | .11 | 1.2 | 245 |
| Diluted with 3 parts water, by volume. | 1 cup | 249 | ------ | 115 | 1 | Trace | ------ | 28 | 20 | .2 | 20 | .08 | .03 | .4 | 82 |
| **Dehydrated:** | | | | | | | | | | | | | | | |
| Crystals, can, net weight 4 ounces. | 1 can | 114 | ------ | 430 | 5 | 1 | ------ | 103 | 99 | 1.1 | 90 | .41 | .18 | 2.0 | 399 |
| Prepared with water (1 pound yields about 1 gallon). | 1 cup | 247 | ------ | 100 | 1 | Trace | ------ | 24 | 22 | .2 | 20 | .10 | .05 | .5 | 92 |
| **Grapes, raw:** | | | | | | | | | | | | | | | |
| American type (slip skin), such as Concord, Delaware, Niagara, Catawba, and Scuppernong.[4] | 1 cup | 153 | ------ | 65 | 1 | 1 | ------ | 15 | 15 | .4 | 100 | .05 | .03 | .2 | 3 |
| European type (adherent skin), such as Malaga, Muscat, Thompson Seedless, Emperor, and Flame Tokay.[4] | 1 cup | 160 | ------ | 95 | 1 | Trace | ------ | 25 | 17 | .6 | 140 | .07 | .04 | .4 | 6 |
| Grape juice, bottled or canned. | 1 cup | 254 | ------ | 165 | 1 | Trace | ------ | 42 | 28 | .8 | ------ | .10 | .05 | .6 | Trace |
| Lemons, raw, medium, 2⅛-inch diameter, size 150.[4] | 1 lemon | 106 | ------ | 20 | 1 | Trace | ------ | 6 | 18 | .4 | 10 | .03 | .01 | .1 | 38 |
| **Lemon juice:** | | | | | | | | | | | | | | | |
| Fresh | 1 cup | 246 | ------ | 60 | 1 | Trace | ------ | 20 | 17 | .5 | 40 | .08 | .03 | .2 | 113 |
| | 1 tablespoon | 15 | ------ | 5 | Trace | Trace | ------ | 1 | 1 | Trace | Trace | Trace | Trace | Trace | 7 |
| Canned, unsweetened | 1 cup | 245 | ------ | 55 | 1 | Trace | ------ | 19 | 17 | .5 | 40 | .07 | .03 | .2 | 102 |
| **Lemonade concentrate, frozen, sweetened:** | | | | | | | | | | | | | | | |
| Undiluted, can, 6 fluid ounces. | 1 can | 220 | ------ | 430 | Trace | Trace | ------ | 112 | 9 | .4 | 40 | .05 | .06 | .7 | 66 |
| Diluted with 4⅓ parts water, by volume. | 1 cup | 248 | ------ | 110 | Trace | Trace | ------ | 28 | 2 | .1 | 10 | .01 | .01 | .2 | 17 |

[4] Measure and weight apply to entire vegetable or fruit including parts not usually eaten.

[8] About 5 milligrams per 8 fluid ounces is from cranberries. Ascorbic acid is usually added to approximately 100 milligrams per 8 fluid ounces.

[9] For white-fleshed varieties value is about 20 I.U. per cup; for red-fleshed varieties, 1,080 I.U. per cup.

TABLE 36—Continued

| Food, Approximate Measure, and Weight (in Grams) | Food Energy | Protein | Fat (Total Lipid) | Fatty acids Saturated (Total) | Fatty acids Unsaturated Oleic | Fatty acids Unsaturated Linoleic | Carbohydrate | Calcium | Iron | Vitamin A Value | Thiamine | Riboflavin | Niacin | Ascorbic Acid |
|---|---|---|---|---|---|---|---|---|---|---|---|---|---|---|
| | (Calories) | (Gm.) | (Gm.) | (Gm.) | (Gm.) | (Gm.) | (Gm.) | (Mg.) | (Mg.) | (I.U.) | (Mg.) | (Mg.) | (Mg.) | (Mg.) |
| FRUITS AND FRUIT PRODUCTS—Con. | | | | | | | | | | | | | | |
| Lime juice: | | | | | | | | | | | | | | |
| Fresh ------- 1 cup ------ *Grams* 246 | 65 | 1 | Trace | --- | --- | --- | 22 | 22 | 0.5 | 30 | 0.05 | 0.03 | 0.3 | 80 |
| Canned ------ 1 cup ------ 246 | 65 | 1 | Trace | --- | --- | --- | 22 | 22 | .5 | 30 | .05 | .03 | .3 | 52 |
| Limeade concentrate, frozen, sweetened: | | | | | | | | | | | | | | |
| Undiluted, can, 6 fluid ounces. 1 can ------ 218 | 410 | Trace | Trace | --- | --- | --- | 108 | 11 | .2 | Trace | .02 | .02 | .2 | 26 |
| Diluted with 4⅓ parts water, by volume. 1 cup ------ 248 | 105 | Trace | Trace | --- | --- | --- | 27 | 2 | Trace | Trace | Trace | Trace | Trace | 6 |
| Oranges, raw: | | | | | | | | | | | | | | |
| California, Navel (winter), 2⅝-inch diameter, size 88.4 1 orange ----- 180 | 60 | 2 | Trace | --- | --- | --- | 16 | 49 | .5 | 240 | .12 | .05 | .5 | 75 |
| Florida, all varieties, 3-inch diameter.4 1 orange ----- 210 | 75 | 1 | Trace | --- | --- | --- | 19 | 67 | .3 | 310 | .16 | .06 | .6 | 70 |
| Orange juice: | | | | | | | | | | | | | | |
| Fresh: | | | | | | | | | | | | | | |
| California, Valencia (summer). 1 cup ------ 249 | 115 | 2 | 1 | --- | --- | --- | 26 | 27 | .7 | 500 | .22 | .06 | .9 | 122 |
| Florida varieties: | | | | | | | | | | | | | | |
| Early and mid-season. 1 cup ------ 247 | 100 | 1 | Trace | --- | --- | --- | 23 | 25 | .5 | 490 | .22 | .06 | .9 | 127 |
| Late season, Valencia. 1 cup ------ 248 | 110 | 1 | Trace | --- | --- | --- | 26 | 25 | .5 | 500 | .22 | .06 | .9 | 92 |
| Canned, unsweetened--- 1 cup ------ 249 | 120 | 2 | Trace | --- | --- | --- | 28 | 25 | 1.0 | 500 | .17 | .05 | .6 | 100 |
| Frozen concentrate: | | | | | | | | | | | | | | |
| Undiluted, can, 6 fluid ounces. 1 can ------ 210 | 330 | 5 | Trace | --- | --- | --- | 80 | 69 | .8 | 1,490 | .63 | .10 | 2.4 | 332 |
| Diluted with 3 parts water, by volume. 1 cup ------ 248 | 110 | 2 | Trace | --- | --- | --- | 27 | 22 | .2 | 500 | .21 | .03 | .8 | 112 |
| Dehydrated: | | | | | | | | | | | | | | |
| Crystals, can, net weight 4 ounces. 1 can ------ 113 | 430 | 6 | 2 | --- | --- | --- | 100 | 95 | 1.9 | 1,900 | .76 | .24 | 3.3 | 406 |

| Food | Measure | Grams | Food energy (calories) | Protein (g) | Fat (g) | Saturated fatty acids (g) | Unsaturated Oleic (g) | Unsaturated Linoleic (g) | Carbohydrate (g) | Calcium (mg) | Iron (mg) | Vitamin A (I.U.) | Thiamine (mg) | Riboflavin (mg) | Niacin (mg) | Ascorbic acid (mg) |
|---|---|---|---|---|---|---|---|---|---|---|---|---|---|---|---|---|
| Prepared with water. 1 pound yields about 1 gallon. | 1 cup | 230 | | | | | | | | | | | | | | |
| Orange and grapefruit juice: Frozen concentrate: Undiluted, can, 6 fluid ounces. | 1 can | 209 | 325 | 4 | 1 | ---- | ---- | ---- | 78 | 61 | .8 | 790 | .47 | .06 | 2.3 | 301 |
| Diluted with 3 parts water, by volume. | 1 cup | 248 | 110 | 1 | Trace | ---- | ---- | ---- | 26 | 20 | .2 | 270 | .16 | .02 | .8 | 102 |
| Papayas, raw, ½-inch cubes. | 1 cup | 182 | 70 | 1 | Trace | ---- | ---- | ---- | 18 | 36 | .5 | 3,190 | .07 | .08 | .5 | 102 |
| Peaches: Raw: Whole, medium, 2-inch diameter, about 4 per pound.[4] | 1 peach | 114 | 35 | 1 | Trace | ---- | ---- | ---- | 10 | 9 | .5 | [10]1,320 | .02 | .05 | 1.0 | 7 |
| Sliced. | 1 cup | 168 | 65 | 1 | Trace | ---- | ---- | ---- | 16 | 15 | .8 | [10]2,230 | .03 | .08 | 1.6 | 12 |
| Canned, yellow-fleshed, solids and liquid: Sirup pack, heavy: Halves or slices | 1 cup | 257 | 200 | 1 | Trace | ---- | ---- | ---- | 52 | 10 | .8 | 1,100 | .02 | .06 | 1.4 | 7 |
| Halves (medium) and sirup. | 2 halves and 2 tablespoons sirup. | 117 | 90 | Trace | Trace | ---- | ---- | ---- | 24 | 5 | .4 | 500 | .01 | .03 | .7 | 3 |
| Water pack. | 1 cup | 245 | 75 | 1 | Trace | ---- | ---- | ---- | 20 | 10 | .7 | 1,100 | .02 | .06 | 1.4 | 7 |
| Strained or chopped (baby food). | 1 ounce | 28 | 25 | Trace | Trace | ---- | ---- | ---- | 6 | 2 | .1 | 140 | Trace | .01 | .2 | 1 |
| Dried: Uncooked | 1 cup | 160 | 420 | 5 | 1 | ---- | ---- | ---- | 109 | 77 | 9.6 | 6,240 | .02 | .31 | 8.5 | 28 |
| Cooked, unsweetened, 10-12 halves and 6 tablespoons liquid. | 1 cup | 270 | 220 | 3 | 1 | ---- | ---- | ---- | 58 | 41 | 5.1 | 3,290 | .01 | .15 | 4.2 | 6 |
| Frozen: Carton, 12 ounces, not thawed. | 1 carton | 340 | 300 | 1 | Trace | ---- | ---- | ---- | 77 | 14 | 1.7 | 2,210 | .03 | .14 | 2.4 | [11]135 |
| Can, 16 ounces, not thawed. | 1 can | 454 | 400 | 2 | Trace | ---- | ---- | ---- | 103 | 18 | 2.3 | 2,950 | .05 | .18 | 3.2 | [11]181 |
| Peach nectar, canned | 1 cup | 250 | 120 | Trace | Trace | ---- | ---- | ---- | 31 | 10 | .5 | 1,080 | .02 | .05 | 1.0 | 1 |
| Pears: Raw, 3 by 2½-inch diameter.[4] | 1 pear | 182 | 100 | 1 | 1 | ---- | ---- | ---- | 25 | 13 | .5 | 30 | .04 | .07 | .2 | 7 |

[4] Measure and weight apply to entire vegetable or fruit including parts not usually eaten.

[10] Based on yellow-fleshed varieties; for white-fleshed varieties value is about 50 I.U. per 114-gram peach and 80 I.U. per cup of sliced peaches.

[11] Average weighted in accordance with commercial freezing practices. For products without added ascorbic acid, value is about 37 milligrams per 12-ounce carton and 50 milligrams per 16-ounce can; for those with added ascorbic acid, 139 milligrams per 12 ounces and 186 milligrams per 16 ounces.

TABLE 36—*Continued*

| Food, Approximate Measure, and Weight (in Grams) | Food Energy | Protein | Fat (Total Lipid) | Fatty acids Saturated (Total) | Fatty acids Unsaturated Oleic | Fatty acids Unsaturated Linoleic | Carbohydrate | Calcium | Iron | Vitamin A Value | Thiamine | Riboflavin | Niacin | Ascorbic Acid |
|---|---|---|---|---|---|---|---|---|---|---|---|---|---|---|
| | (Calories) | (Gm.) | (Gm.) | (Gm.) | (Gm.) | (Gm.) | (Gm.) | (Mg.) | (Mg.) | (I.U.) | (Mg.) | (Mg.) | (Mg.) | (Mg.) |
| **FRUITS AND FRUIT PRODUCTS—Con.** | | | | | | | | | | | | | | |
| Pears—Continued | | | | | | | | | | | | | | |
| Canned, solids and liquid: | | | | | | | | | | | | | | |
| Sirup pack, heavy: | | | | | | | | | | | | | | |
| Halves or slices____ 1 cup_____ 255 | 195 | 1 | 1 | | | | 50 | 13 | 0.5 | Trace | 0.03 | 0.05 | 0.3 | 4 |
| Halves (medium) 2 halves and 2 table- spoons sirup. 117 | 90 | Trace | Trace | | | | 23 | 6 | .2 | Trace | .01 | .02 | .2 | 2 |
| Water pack_____ 1 cup_____ 243 | 80 | Trace | Trace | | | | 20 | 12 | .5 | Trace | .02 | .05 | .3 | 4 |
| Strained or chopped (baby food). 1 ounce____ 28 | 20 | Trace | Trace | | | | 5 | 2 | .1 | 10 | Trace | .01 | .1 | 1 |
| Pear nectar, canned____ 1 cup_____ 250 | 130 | 1 | Trace | | | | 33 | 8 | .2 | Trace | .01 | .05 | Trace | 1 |
| Persimmons, Japanese or kaki, raw, seedless, 2½-inch diameter.[4] 1 persimmon 125 | 75 | 1 | Trace | | | | 20 | 6 | .4 | 2,740 | .03 | .02 | .1 | 11 |
| Pineapple: | | | | | | | | | | | | | | |
| Raw, diced_____ 1 cup_____ 140 | 75 | 1 | Trace | | | | 19 | 24 | .7 | 100 | .12 | .04 | .3 | 24 |
| Canned, heavy sirup pack, solids and liquid: | | | | | | | | | | | | | | |
| Crushed_____ 1 cup_____ 260 | 195 | 1 | Trace | | | | 50 | 29 | .8 | 120 | .20 | .06 | .5 | 17 |
| Sliced, slices and juice. 2 small or 1 large and 2 table- spoons juice. 122 | 90 | Trace | Trace | | | | 24 | 13 | .4 | 50 | .09 | .03 | .2 | 8 |
| Pineapple juice, canned___ 1 cup_____ 249 | 135 | 1 | Trace | | | | 34 | 37 | .7 | 120 | .12 | .04 | .5 | 22 |
| Plums, all except prunes: | | | | | | | | | | | | | | |
| Raw, 2-inch diameter, about 2 ounces.[4] 1 plum_____ 60 | 25 | Trace | Trace | | | | 7 | 7 | .3 | 140 | .02 | .02 | .3 | 3 |
| Canned, sirup pack (Italian prunes): | | | | | | | | | | | | | | |
| Plums (with pits) 1 cup_____ 256 | 205 | 1 | Trace | | | | 53 | 22 | 2.2 | 2,970 | .05 | .05 | .9 | 4 |

| Food | Measure | Weight (grams) | Food energy | Protein | Fat | Saturated | Oleic | Linoleic | Carbohydrate | Calcium | Iron | Vitamin A | Thiamine | Riboflavin | Niacin | Ascorbic acid |
|---|---|---|---|---|---|---|---|---|---|---|---|---|---|---|---|---|
| Plums (without pits) and juice. | 3 plums and 2 tablespoons juice. | 122 | 100 | Trace | Trace | | | | 26 | 11 | 1.1 | 1,470 | .03 | .02 | .5 | 2 |
| Prunes, dried, "softenized", medium: | | | | | | | | | | | | | | | | |
| Uncooked [4] | 4 prunes | 32 | 70 | 1 | Trace | | | | 18 | 14 | 1.1 | 440 | .02 | .04 | .4 | 1 |
| Cooked, unsweetened, 17–18 prunes and ⅓ cup liquid.[4] | 1 cup | 270 | 295 | 2 | 1 | | | | 78 | 60 | 4.5 | 1,860 | .08 | .18 | 1.7 | 2 |
| Prunes with tapioca, canned, strained or junior (baby food). | 1 ounce | 28 | 25 | Trace | Trace | | | | 6 | 2 | .3 | 110 | .01 | .02 | .1 | 1 |
| Prune juice, canned | 1 cup | 256 | 200 | 1 | Trace | | | | 49 | 36 | 10.5 | --- | .02 | .03 | 1.1 | 4 |
| Raisins, dried | 1 cup | 160 | 460 | 4 | Trace | | | | 124 | 99 | 5.6 | 30 | .18 | .13 | .9 | 2 |
| Raspberries, red: | | | | | | | | | | | | | | | | |
| Raw | 1 cup | 123 | 70 | 1 | 1 | | | | 17 | 27 | 1.1 | 160 | .04 | .11 | 1.1 | 31 |
| Frozen, 10-ounce carton, not thawed. | 1 carton | 284 | 275 | 2 | 1 | | | | 70 | 37 | 1.7 | 200 | .06 | .17 | 1.7 | 59 |
| Rhubarb, cooked, sugar added. | 1 cup | 272 | 385 | 1 | Trace | | | | 98 | 212 | 1.6 | 220 | .06 | .15 | .7 | 17 |
| Strawberries: | | | | | | | | | | | | | | | | |
| Raw, capped | 1 cup | 149 | 55 | 1 | 1 | | | | 13 | 31 | 1.5 | 90 | .04 | .10 | 1.0 | 88 |
| Frozen, 10-ounce carton, not thawed. | 1 carton | 284 | 310 | 1 | 1 | | | | 79 | 40 | 2.0 | 90 | .06 | .17 | 1.5 | 150 |
| Frozen, 16-ounce can, not thawed. | 1 can | 454 | 495 | 2 | 1 | | | | 126 | 64 | 3.2 | 150 | .09 | .27 | 2.4 | 240 |
| Tangerines, raw, medium, 2½-inch diameter, about 4 per pound.[4] | 1 tangerine | 114 | 40 | 1 | Trace | | | | 10 | 34 | .3 | 350 | .05 | .02 | .1 | 26 |
| Tangerine juice: | | | | | | | | | | | | | | | | |
| Canned, unsweetened | 1 cup | 248 | 105 | 1 | Trace | | | | 25 | 45 | .5 | 1,040 | .14 | .04 | .3 | 56 |
| Frozen concentrate: Undiluted, can, 6 fluid ounces. | 1 can | 210 | 340 | 4 | 1 | | | | 80 | 130 | 1.5 | 3,070 | .43 | .12 | .9 | 202 |
| Diluted with 3 parts water, by volume. | 1 cup | 248 | 115 | 1 | Trace | | | | 27 | 45 | .5 | 1,020 | .14 | .04 | .3 | 67 |
| Watermelon, raw, wedge, 4 by 8 inches (1/16 of 10 by 16-inch melon, about 2 pounds with rind).[4] | 1 wedge | 925 | 115 | 2 | 1 | | | | 27 | 30 | 2.1 | 2,510 | .13 | .13 | .7 | 30 |

[4] Measure and weight apply to entire vegetable or fruit including parts not usually eaten.

TABLE 36—Continued

| Food, Approximate Measure, and Weight (In Grams) | | Food Energy | Protein | Fat (Total Lipid) | Fatty acids | | | Carbohydrate | Calcium | Iron | Vitamin A Value | Thiamine | Riboflavin | Niacin | Ascorbic Acid |
| | | | | | Saturated (Total) | Unsaturated | | | | | | | | | |
| | | | | | | Oleic | Linoleic | | | | | | | | |
| | | (Calories) | (Gm.) | (Gm.) | (Gm.) | (Gm.) | (Gm.) | (Gm.) | (Mg.) | (Mg.) | (I.U.) | (Mg.) | (Mg.) | (Mg.) | (Mg.) |
| | Grams | | | | | | | | | | | | | | |
| **GRAIN PRODUCTS** | | | | | | | | | | | | | | | |
| Barley, pearled, light, uncooked. 1 cup | 203 | 710 | 17 | 2 | Trace | 1 | 1 | 160 | 32 | 4.1 | 0 | 0.25 | 0.17 | 6.3 | 0 |
| Biscuits, baking powder with enriched flour, 2½-inch diameter. 1 biscuit | 38 | 140 | 3 | 6 | 2 | 3 | 1 | 17 | 46 | .6 | Trace | .08 | .08 | .7 | Trace |
| Bran flakes (40 percent bran) added thiamine. 1 ounce | 28 | 85 | 3 | 1 | | | | 23 | 20 | 1.2 | 0 | .11 | .05 | 1.7 | 0 |
| Breads: | | | | | | | | | | | | | | | |
| Boston brown bread, slice, 3 by ¾ inch. 1 slice | 48 | 100 | 3 | 1 | | | | 22 | 43 | .9 | 0 | .05 | .03 | .6 | 0 |
| Cracked-wheat bread: | | | | | | | | | | | | | | | |
| Loaf, 1-pound, 20 slices. 1 loaf | 454 | 1,190 | 39 | 10 | 2 | 5 | 2 | 236 | 399 | 5.0 | Trace | .53 | .42 | 5.8 | Trace |
| Slice. 1 slice | 23 | 60 | 2 | 1 | | | | 12 | 20 | .3 | Trace | .03 | .02 | .3 | Trace |
| French or vienna bread: | | | | | | | | | | | | | | | |
| Enriched, 1-pound loaf. 1 loaf | 454 | 1,315 | 41 | 14 | 3 | 8 | 2 | 251 | 195 | 10.0 | Trace | 1.26 | .98 | 11.3 | Trace |
| Unenriched, 1-pound loaf. 1 loaf | 454 | 1,315 | 41 | 14 | 3 | 8 | 2 | 251 | 195 | 3.2 | Trace | .39 | .39 | 3.6 | Trace |
| Italian bread: | | | | | | | | | | | | | | | |
| Enriched, 1-pound loaf. 1 loaf | 454 | 1,250 | 41 | 4 | Trace | 1 | 2 | 256 | 77 | 10.0 | 0 | 1.31 | .93 | 11.7 | 0 |
| Unenriched, 1-pound loaf. 1 loaf | 454 | 1,250 | 41 | 4 | Trace | 1 | 2 | 256 | 77 | 3.2 | 0 | .39 | .27 | 3.6 | 0 |
| Raisin bread: | | | | | | | | | | | | | | | |
| Loaf, 1-pound, 20 slices. 1 loaf | 454 | 1,190 | 30 | 13 | 3 | 8 | 2 | 243 | 322 | 5.9 | Trace | .24 | .42 | 3.0 | Trace |
| Slice. 1 slice | 23 | 60 | 2 | 1 | | | | 12 | 16 | .3 | Trace | .01 | .02 | .2 | Trace |
| Rye bread: | | | | | | | | | | | | | | | |
| American, light (1/3 rye, 2/3 wheat): Loaf, 1-pound, 20 slices. 1 loaf | 454 | 1,100 | 41 | 5 | | | | 236 | 340 | 7.3 | 0 | .81 | .33 | 6.4 | 0 |

| Food and approximate measure | | Grams | | | | | | | | | | | | | | |
|---|---|---|---|---|---|---|---|---|---|---|---|---|---|---|---|---|
| Pumpernickel, loaf, 1 pound. | 1 loaf | 454 | 1,115 | 41 | 5 | ---- | ---- | ---- | 241 | 381 | 10.9 | 0 | 1.05 | .63 | 5.4 | 0 |
| **White bread, enriched:** | | | | | | | | | | | | | | | | |
| 1 to 2 percent nonfat dry milk: | | | | | | | | | | | | | | | | |
| Loaf, 1-pound, 20 slices. | 1 loaf | 454 | 1,225 | 39 | 15 | 3 | 8 | 2 | 229 | 318 | 10.9 | Trace | 1.13 | .77 | 10.4 | Trace |
| Slice. | 1 slice | 23 | 60 | 2 | 1 | Trace | Trace | Trace | 12 | 16 | .6 | Trace | .06 | .04 | .5 | Trace |
| 3 to 4 percent nonfat dry milk:[12] | | | | | | | | | | | | | | | | |
| Loaf, 1-pound. | 1 loaf | 454 | 1,225 | 39 | 15 | 3 | 8 | 2 | 229 | 381 | 11.3 | Trace | 1.13 | .95 | 10.8 | Trace |
| Slice, 20 per loaf. | 1 slice | 23 | 60 | 2 | 1 | Trace | Trace | Trace | 12 | 19 | .6 | Trace | .06 | .05 | .6 | Trace |
| Slice, toasted. | 1 slice | 20 | 60 | 2 | 1 | Trace | Trace | Trace | 12 | 19 | .6 | Trace | .05 | .05 | .6 | Trace |
| Slice, 26 per loaf. | 1 slice | 17 | 45 | 1 | 1 | Trace | Trace | Trace | 9 | 14 | .4 | Trace | .04 | .04 | .4 | Trace |
| 5 to 6 percent nonfat dry milk: | | | | | | | | | | | | | | | | |
| Loaf, 1-pound, 20 slices. | 1 loaf | 454 | 1,245 | 41 | 17 | 4 | 10 | 2 | 228 | 435 | 11.3 | Trace | 1.22 | .91 | 11.0 | Trace |
| Slice. | 1 slice | 23 | 65 | 2 | 1 | Trace | Trace | Trace | 12 | 22 | .6 | Trace | .06 | .05 | .6 | Trace |
| **White bread, unenriched:** | | | | | | | | | | | | | | | | |
| 1 to 2 percent nonfat dry milk: | | | | | | | | | | | | | | | | |
| Loaf, 1-pound, 20 slices. | 1 loaf | 454 | 1,225 | 39 | 15 | 3 | 8 | 2 | 229 | 318 | 3.2 | Trace | .40 | .36 | 5.6 | Trace |
| Slice. | 1 slice | 23 | 60 | 2 | 1 | Trace | Trace | Trace | 12 | 16 | .2 | Trace | .02 | .02 | .3 | Trace |
| 3 to 4 percent nonfat dry milk:[12] | | | | | | | | | | | | | | | | |
| Loaf, 1-pound. | 1 loaf | 454 | 1,225 | 39 | 15 | 3 | 8 | 2 | 229 | 381 | 3.2 | Trace | .31 | .39 | 5.0 | Trace |
| Slice, 20 per loaf. | 1 slice | 23 | 60 | 2 | 1 | Trace | Trace | Trace | 12 | 19 | .2 | Trace | .02 | .02 | .3 | Trace |
| Slice, toasted. | 1 slice | 20 | 60 | 2 | 1 | Trace | Trace | Trace | 12 | 19 | .2 | Trace | .01 | .02 | .3 | Trace |
| Slice, 26 per loaf. | 1 slice | 17 | 45 | 1 | 1 | Trace | Trace | Trace | 9 | 14 | .1 | Trace | .01 | .01 | .2 | Trace |
| 5 to 6 percent nonfat dry milk: | | | | | | | | | | | | | | | | |
| Loaf, 1 pound, 20 slices. | 1 loaf | 454 | 1,245 | 41 | 17 | 4 | 10 | 2 | 228 | 435 | 3.2 | Trace | .32 | .59 | 4.1 | Trace |
| Slice. | 1 slice | 23 | 65 | 2 | 1 | Trace | Trace | Trace | 12 | 22 | .2 | Trace | .02 | .03 | .2 | Trace |
| Whole-wheat bread, made with 2 percent nonfat dry milk: | | | | | | | | | | | | | | | | |
| Loaf, 1-pound, 20 slices. | 1 loaf | 454 | 1,105 | 48 | 14 | 3 | 6 | 3 | 216 | 449 | 10.4 | Trace | 1.17 | .56 | 12.9 | Trace |
| Slice. | 1 slice | 23 | 55 | 2 | 1 | Trace | Trace | Trace | 11 | 23 | .5 | Trace | .06 | .03 | .7 | Trace |
| Slice, toasted. | 1 slice | 19 | 55 | 2 | 1 | Trace | Trace | Trace | 11 | 22 | .5 | Trace | .05 | .03 | .6 | Trace |
| Breadcrumbs, dry, grated. | 1 cup | 88 | 345 | 11 | 4 | 1 | 2 | 1 | 65 | 107 | 3.2 | Trace | .19 | .26 | 3.1 | Trace |
| **Cakes:[13]** | | | | | | | | | | | | | | | | |
| Angelfood cake; sector, 2-inch (1/12 of 8-inch-diameter cake). | 1 sector | 40 | 110 | 3 | Trace | ---- | ---- | ---- | 24 | 4 | .1 | 0 | Trace | .06 | .1 | 0 |

[12] When the amount of nonfat dry milk in commercial white bread is unknown, values for bread with 3 to 4 percent nonfat dry milk are suggested.

[13] Unenriched cake flour and vegetable cooking fat used unless otherwise specified.

TABLE 36—*Continued*

| Food, Approximate Measure, and Weight (In Grams) | | Food Energy | Protein | Fat (Total Lipid) | Fatty acids | | | Carbohydrate | Calcium | Iron | Vitamin A Value | Thiamine | Riboflavin | Niacin | Ascorbic Acid |
|---|---|---|---|---|---|---|---|---|---|---|---|---|---|---|---|
| | | | | | Saturated (Total) | Unsaturated | | | | | | | | | |
| | | | | | | Oleic | Linoleic | | | | | | | | |
| | *Grams* | (Calories) | (Gm.) | (Gm.) | (Gm.) | (Gm.) | (Gm.) | (Gm.) | (Mg.) | (Mg.) | (I.U.) | (Mg.) | (Mg.) | (Mg.) | (Mg.) |
| **GRAIN PRODUCTS—Continued** | | | | | | | | | | | | | | | |
| Cakes [13]—Continued | | | | | | | | | | | | | | | |
| Chocolate cake, chocolate icing; sector, 2-inch (1/16 of 10-inch-diameter layer cake). 1 sector | 120 | 445 | 5 | 20 | 8 | 10 | 1 | 67 | 84 | 1.2 | [14]190 | 0.03 | 0.12 | 0.3 | Trace |
| Fruitcake, dark (made with enriched flour); piece, 2 by 2 by ½ inch. 1 piece | 30 | 115 | 1 | 5 | 1 | 3 | 1 | 18 | 22 | .8 | [14]40 | .04 | .04 | .2 | Trace |
| Gingerbread (made with enriched flour); piece, 2 by 2 by 2 inches. 1 piece | 55 | 175 | 2 | 6 | 1 | 4 | Trace | 29 | 37 | 1.3 | 50 | .06 | .06 | .5 | 0 |
| Plain cake and cupcakes, without icing: | | | | | | | | | | | | | | | |
| Piece, 3 by 2 by 1½ inches. 1 piece | 55 | 200 | 2 | 8 | 2 | 5 | 1 | 31 | 35 | .2 | [14]90 | .01 | .05 | .1 | Trace |
| Cupcake, 2¾-inch diameter. 1 cupcake | 40 | 145 | 2 | 6 | 1 | 3 | Trace | 22 | 26 | .2 | [14]70 | .01 | .03 | .1 | Trace |
| Plain cake and cupcakes, with chocolate icing: | | | | | | | | | | | | | | | |
| Sector, 2-inch (1/16 of 10-inch-layer cake). 1 sector | 100 | 370 | 4 | 14 | 5 | 7 | 1 | 59 | 63 | .6 | [14]180 | .02 | .09 | .2 | Trace |
| Cupcake, 2¾-inch diameter. 1 cupcake | 50 | 185 | 2 | 7 | 2 | 4 | Trace | 30 | 32 | .3 | [14]90 | .01 | .04 | .1 | Trace |
| Poundcake, old-fashioned (equal weights flour, sugar, fat, eggs); slice, 2¾ by 3 by ⅝ inch. 1 slice | 30 | 140 | 2 | 9 | 2 | 5 | 1 | 14 | 6 | .2 | [14]80 | .01 | .03 | .1 | 0 |
| Sponge cake; sector, 2-inch (1/12 of 8-inch-diameter cake). 1 sector | 40 | 120 | 3 | 2 | 1 | 1 | Trace | 22 | 12 | .5 | 180 | .02 | .06 | .1 | Trace |
| Cookies: | | | | | | | | | | | | | | | |
| Plain and assorted, 1 cooky | 25 | 120 | 1 | 5 | ------ | ------ | ------ | 18 | 9 | .2 | 20 | .01 | .01 | .1 | Trace |

| Food, approximate measure, and weight | Measure | Grams | Food energy (Calories) | Protein (g) | Fat (g) | Saturated (g) | Oleic (g) | Linoleic (g) | Carbohydrate (g) | Calcium (mg) | Iron (mg) | Vitamin A (I.U.) | Thiamine (mg) | Riboflavin (mg) | Niacin (mg) | Ascorbic acid (mg) |
|---|---|---|---|---|---|---|---|---|---|---|---|---|---|---|---|---|
| Corn, rice and wheat flakes, mixed, added nutrients. | 1 ounce | 28 | 110 | 2 | Trace | | | | 24 | 11 | .5 | 0 | .11 | ---- | .9 | 0 |
| Corn flakes, added nutrients: | | | | | | | | | | | | | | | | |
| Plain | 1 ounce | 28 | 110 | 2 | Trace | | | | 24 | 5 | .4 | 0 | .12 | .02 | .6 | 0 |
| Sugar-covered | 1 ounce | 28 | 110 | 1 | Trace | | | | 26 | 3 | .3 | 0 | .12 | .01 | .5 | 0 |
| Corn grits, degermed, cooked: | | | | | | | | | | | | | | | | |
| Enriched | 1 cup | 242 | 120 | 3 | Trace | | | | 27 | 2 | [15].7 | [16]150 | [15].10 | [15].07 | [15]1.0 | 0 |
| Unenriched | 1 cup | 242 | 120 | 3 | Trace | | | | 27 | 2 | .2 | [16]150 | .05 | .02 | .5 | 0 |
| Cornmeal, white or yellow, dry: | | | | | | | | | | | | | | | | |
| Whole ground, unbolted | 1 cup | 118 | 420 | 11 | 5 | 1 | 2 | 2 | 87 | 24 | 2.8 | [16]600 | .45 | .13 | 2.4 | 0 |
| Degermed, enriched | 1 cup | 145 | 525 | 11 | 2 | Trace | 1 | 1 | 114 | 9 | [15]4.2 | [16]640 | [15].64 | [15].38 | [15]5.1 | 0 |
| Corn muffins, made with enriched degermed cornmeal and enriched flour; muffin, 2¾-inch diameter. | 1 muffin | 48 | 150 | 3 | 5 | 1 | 2 | 1 | 23 | 50 | .8 | [17]80 | .09 | .11 | .8 | Trace |
| Corn, puffed, presweetened, added nutrients. | 1 ounce | 28 | 110 | 1 | Trace | | | | 26 | 3 | .5 | 0 | .12 | .05 | .6 | 0 |
| Corn, shredded, added nutrients. | 1 ounce | 28 | 110 | 2 | Trace | | | | 25 | 1 | .7 | 0 | .12 | .05 | .6 | 0 |
| Crackers: | | | | | | | | | | | | | | | | |
| Graham, plain | 4 small or 2 medium | 14 | 55 | 1 | 1 | | | | 10 | 6 | .2 | 0 | .01 | .03 | .2 | 0 |
| Saltines, 2 inches square. | 2 crackers | 8 | 35 | 1 | 1 | | | | 6 | 2 | .1 | 0 | Trace | Trace | .1 | 0 |
| Soda: | | | | | | | | | | | | | | | | |
| Cracker, 2½ inches square. | 2 crackers | 11 | 50 | 1 | 1 | | | | 8 | 2 | .2 | 0 | Trace | Trace | .1 | 0 |
| Oyster crackers | 10 crackers | 10 | 45 | 1 | 1 | | | | 7 | 2 | .2 | 0 | Trace | Trace | .1 | 0 |
| Cracker meal | 1 tablespoon | 10 | 45 | 1 | Trace | | | | 7 | 2 | .1 | 0 | .01 | Trace | .1 | 0 |
| Doughnuts, cake type | 1 doughnut | 32 | 125 | 1 | 6 | 1 | 4 | 1 | 16 | 13 | [18].4 | 30 | [18].05 | [18].05 | [18].4 | Trace |
| Farina, regular, enriched, cooked. | 1 cup | 238 | 100 | 3 | Trace | | | | 21 | 10 | [15].7 | 0 | [15].11 | [15].07 | [15]1.0 | 0 |

13 Unenriched cake flour and vegetable cooking fat used unless otherwise specified.

14 If the fat used in the recipe is butter or fortified margarine, the vitamin A value for chocolate cake with chocolate icing will be 490 I.U. per 2-inch sector, item 360; 100 I.U. for fruitcake, item 361; for plain cake without icing, 300 I.U. per piece, item 363; 220 I.U. per cupcake, item 364; for plain cake with icing, 440 I.U. per 2-inch sector, item 365; 220 I.U. per cupcake, item 366; and 300 I.U. for poundcake, item 367.

15 Iron, thiamine, riboflavin, and niacin are based on the minimum levels of enrichment specified in standards of identity promulgated under the Federal Food, Drug, and Cosmetic Act.

16 Vitamin A value based on yellow product. White product contains only a trace.

17 Based on recipe using white cornmeal; if yellow cornmeal is used, the vitamin A value is 140 I.U. per muffin.

18 Based on product made with enriched flour. With unenriched flour, approximate values per doughnut are: Iron, 0.2 milligram; thiamine, 0.01 milligram; riboflavin, 0.01 milligram; niacin, 0.2 milligram.

# TABLE 36—Continued

| Food, Approximate Measure, and Weight (in Grams) | Food Energy | Protein | Fat (Total Lipid) | Fatty acids | | | Carbohydrate | Calcium | Iron | Vitamin A Value | Thiamine | Riboflavin | Niacin | Ascorbic Acid |
|---|---|---|---|---|---|---|---|---|---|---|---|---|---|---|
| | | | | Saturated (Total) | Unsaturated Oleic | Linoleic | | | | | | | | |
| | (Calories) | (Gm.) | (Gm.) | (Gm.) | (Gm.) | (Gm.) | (Gm.) | (Mg.) | (Mg.) | (I.U.) | (Mg.) | (Mg.) | (Mg.) | (Mg.) |
| **GRAIN PRODUCTS—Continued** | | | | | | | | | | | | | | |
| Macaroni, cooked: | | | | | | | | | | | | | | |
| Enriched: | | | | | | | | | | | | | | |
| Cooked, firm stage (8 to 10 minutes; undergoes additional cooking in a food mixture). 1 cup ___ _Grams_ 130 | 190 | 6 | 1 | | | | 39 | 14 | [15] 1.4 | 0 | [15] 0.23 | [15] 0.14 | [15] 1.9 | 0 |
| Cooked until tender __ 1 cup ___ 140 | 155 | 5 | 1 | | | | 32 | 11 | [15] 1.3 | 0 | [15] .19 | [15] .11 | [15] 1.5 | 0 |
| Unenriched: | | | | | | | | | | | | | | |
| Cooked, firm stage (8 to 10 minutes; undergoes additional cooking in a food mixture). 1 cup ___ 130 | 190 | 6 | 1 | | | | 39 | 14 | .6 | 0 | .02 | .02 | .5 | 0 |
| Cooked until tender __ 1 cup ___ 140 | 155 | 5 | 1 | | | | 32 | 11 | .6 | 0 | .02 | .02 | .4 | 0 |
| Macaroni (enriched) and cheese, baked. 1 cup ___ 220 | 470 | 18 | 24 | 11 | 10 | 1 | 44 | 398 | 2.0 | 950 | .22 | .44 | 2.0 | Trace |
| Muffins, with enriched white flour; muffin, 2¾-inch diameter. 1 muffin ___ 48 | 140 | 4 | 5 | 1 | 3 | Trace | 20 | 50 | .8 | 50 | .08 | .11 | .7 | Trace |
| Noodles (egg noodles), cooked: | | | | | | | | | | | | | | |
| Enriched _____ 1 cup ___ 160 | 200 | 7 | 2 | 1 | 1 | Trace | 37 | 16 | [15] 1.4 | 110 | [15] .23 | [15] .14 | [15] 1.8 | 0 |
| Unenriched _____ 1 cup ___ 160 | 200 | 7 | 2 | 1 | 1 | Trace | 37 | 16 | 1.0 | 110 | .04 | .03 | .7 | 0 |
| Oats (with or without corn) puffed, added nutrients. 1 ounce __ 28 | 115 | 3 | 2 | Trace | 1 | 1 | 21 | 50 | 1.3 | 0 | .28 | .05 | .5 | 0 |
| Oatmeal or rolled oats, regular or quick-cooking, cooked. 1 cup ___ 236 | 130 | 5 | 2 | Trace | 1 | 1 | 23 | 21 | 1.4 | 0 | .19 | .05 | .3 | 0 |
| Pancakes (griddlecakes), 4-inch diameter: | | | | | | | | | | | | | | |
| Wheat, enriched flour 1 cake ___ 27 | 60 | 2 | 2 | Trace | 1 | Trace | 9 | 27 | .4 | 30 | .05 | .06 | .3 | Trace |

| Food | Measure | Grams | Food energy (Calories) | Protein (g) | Fat (g) | Saturated (g) | Oleic (g) | Linoleic (g) | Carbohydrate (g) | Calcium (mg) | Iron (mg) | Vitamin A (I.U.) | Thiamine (mg) | Riboflavin (mg) | Niacin (mg) | Ascorbic acid (mg) |
|---|---|---|---|---|---|---|---|---|---|---|---|---|---|---|---|---|
| Buckwheat (buckwheat) pancake mix, made with egg and milk). | 1 cake | 27 | 55 | 2 | 2 | 1 | 1 | Trace | 6 | 59 | .4 | 60 | .03 | .04 | .2 | Trace |
| Piecrust, plain, baked: Enriched flour: | | | | | | | | | | | | | | | | |
|   Lower crust, 9-inch shell. | 1 crust | 135 | 675 | 8 | 45 | 10 | 29 | 3 | 59 | 19 | 2.3 | 0 | .27 | .19 | 2.4 | 0 |
|   Double crust, 9-inch pie. | 1 double crust | 270 | 1,350 | 16 | 90 | 21 | 58 | 7 | 118 | 38 | 4.6 | 0 | .55 | .39 | 4.9 | 0 |
| Unenriched flour: | | | | | | | | | | | | | | | | |
|   Lower crust, 9-inch shell. | 1 crust | 135 | 675 | 8 | 45 | 10 | 29 | 3 | 59 | 19 | .7 | 0 | .04 | .04 | .6 | 0 |
|   Double crust, 9-inch pie. | 1 double crust | 270 | 1,350 | 16 | 90 | 21 | 58 | 7 | 118 | 38 | 1.4 | 0 | .08 | .07 | 1.3 | 0 |
| Pies (piecrust made with unenriched flour); sector, 4-inch, 1/7 of 9-inch-diameter pie: | | | | | | | | | | | | | | | | |
|   Apple. | 1 sector | 135 | 345 | 3 | 15 | 4 | 9 | 1 | 51 | 11 | .4 | 40 | .03 | .02 | .5 | 1 |
|   Cherry. | 1 sector | 135 | 355 | 4 | 15 | 4 | 10 | 1 | 52 | 19 | .4 | 590 | .03 | .03 | .6 | 1 |
|   Custard. | 1 sector | 130 | 280 | 8 | 14 | 5 | 8 | 1 | 30 | 125 | .8 | 300 | .07 | .21 | .4 | 0 |
|   Lemon meringue. | 1 sector | 120 | 305 | 4 | 12 | 4 | 7 | 1 | 45 | 17 | .6 | 200 | .04 | .10 | .2 | 4 |
|   Mince. | 1 sector | 135 | 365 | 3 | 16 | 4 | 10 | 1 | 56 | 38 | 1.4 | Trace | .09 | .05 | .5 | 1 |
|   Pumpkin. | 1 sector | 130 | 275 | 5 | 15 | 5 | 7 | 1 | 32 | 66 | .6 | 3,210 | .04 | .13 | .6 | Trace |
| Pizza (cheese); 5½-inch sector; ⅛ of 14-inch-diameter pie. | 1 sector | 75 | 185 | 7 | 6 | 2 | 3 | Trace | 27 | 107 | .7 | 290 | .04 | .12 | .7 | 4 |
| Popcorn, popped, with added oil and salt. | 1 cup | 14 | 65 | 1 | 3 | 2 | Trace | | 8 | 1 | .3 | 0 | — | .01 | .2 | 0 |
| Pretzels, small stick. | 5 sticks | 5 | 20 | Trace | Trace | | | | 4 | 1 | 0 | 0 | Trace | Trace | Trace | 0 |
| Rice, white (fully milled or polished), enriched, cooked: | | | | | | | | | | | | | | | | |
|   Common commercial varieties, all types. | 1 cup | 168 | 185 | 3 | Trace | | | | 41 | 17 | [19] 1.5 | 0 | [19] .19 | [19] .01 | [19] 1.6 | 0 |
|   Long grain, parboiled. | 1 cup | 176 | 185 | 4 | Trace | | | | 41 | 33 | [19] 1.4 | 0 | [19] .19 | [19] .02 | [19] 2.0 | 0 |
| Rice, puffed, added nutrients (without salt). | 1 cup | 14 | 55 | 1 | Trace | | | | 13 | 3 | .3 | 0 | .06 | .01 | .6 | 0 |

[15] Iron, thiamine, riboflavin, and niacin are based on the minimum levels of enrichment specified in standards of identity promulgated under the Federal Food, Drug, and Cosmetic Act.

[19] Iron, thiamine, and niacin are based on the minimum levels of enrichment specified in standards of identity promulgated under the Federal Food, Drug, and Cosmetic Act. Riboflavin is based on unenriched rice. When the minimum level of enrichment for riboflavin specified in the standards of identity becomes effective the value will be 0.12 milligram per cup of parboiled rice and of white rice.

TABLE 36—Continued

| Food, Approximate Measure, and Weight (in Grams) | Food Energy | Protein | Fat (Total Lipid) | Fatty acids Saturated (Total) | Fatty acids Unsaturated Oleic | Fatty acids Unsaturated Linoleic | Carbohydrate | Calcium | Iron | Vitamin A Value | Thiamine | Riboflavin | Niacin | Ascorbic Acid |
|---|---|---|---|---|---|---|---|---|---|---|---|---|---|---|
| | (Calories) | (Gm.) | (Gm.) | (Gm.) | (Gm.) | (Gm.) | (Gm.) | (Mg.) | (Mg.) | (I.U.) | (Mg.) | (Mg.) | (Mg.) | (Mg.) |
| **GRAIN PRODUCTS—Continued** | | | | | | | | | | | | | | |
| Rice flakes, added nutrients. 1 cup — 30 *Grams* | 115 | 2 | Trace | | | | 26 | 9 | 0.5 | 0 | 0.10 | 0.02 | 1.6 | 0 |
| Rolls: | | | | | | | | | | | | | | |
| Plain, pan; 12 per 16 ounces: | | | | | | | | | | | | | | |
| Enriched — 1 roll — 38 | 115 | 3 | 2 | Trace | 1 | Trace | 20 | 28 | .7 | Trace | .11 | .07 | .8 | Trace |
| Unenriched — 1 roll — 38 | 115 | 3 | 2 | Trace | 1 | Trace | 20 | 28 | .3 | Trace | .02 | .03 | .3 | Trace |
| Hard, round; 12 per 22 ounces. 1 roll — 52 | 160 | 5 | 2 | Trace | 1 | Trace | 31 | 24 | .4 | Trace | .03 | .05 | .4 | Trace |
| Sweet, pan; 12 per 18 ounces. 1 roll — 43 | 135 | 4 | 4 | 1 | 2 | Trace | 21 | 37 | .3 | 30 | .03 | .06 | .4 | Trace |
| Rye wafers, whole-grain, 1⅞ by 3½ inches. 2 wafers — 13 | 45 | 2 | Trace | | | | 10 | 7 | .5 | 0 | .04 | .03 | .2 | 0 |
| Spaghetti: | | | | | | | | | | | | | | |
| Cooked, tender stage (14 to 20 minutes): | | | | | | | | | | | | | | |
| Enriched — 1 cup — 140 | 155 | 5 | 1 | | | | 32 | 11 | [15] 1.3 | 0 | [15] .19 | [15] .11 | [15] 1.5 | 0 |
| Unenriched — 1 cup — 140 | 155 | 5 | 1 | | | | 32 | 11 | .6 | 0 | .02 | .02 | .4 | 0 |
| Spaghetti with meat balls in tomato sauce (home recipe). 1 cup — 250 | 335 | 19 | 12 | 4 | 6 | 1 | 39 | 125 | 3.8 | 1,600 | .26 | .30 | 4.0 | 22 |
| Spaghetti in tomato sauce with cheese (home recipe). 1 cup — 250 | 260 | 9 | 9 | 2 | 5 | 1 | 37 | 80 | 2.2 | 1,080 | .24 | .18 | 2.4 | 14 |
| Waffles, with enriched flour, ½ by 4½ by 5½ inches. 1 waffle — 75 | 210 | 7 | 7 | 2 | 4 | 1 | 28 | 85 | 1.3 | 250 | .13 | .19 | 1.0 | Trace |
| Wheat, puffed: | | | | | | | | | | | | | | |
| With added nutrients (without salt). 1 ounce — 28 | 105 | 4 | Trace | | | | 22 | 8 | 1.2 | 0 | .15 | .07 | 2.2 | 0 |
| With added nutrients, with sugar and honey. 1 ounce — 28 | 105 | 2 | 1 | | | | 25 | 7 | .9 | 0 | .14 | .05 | 1.8 | 0 |

| | | | | | | | | | | | | | | | |
|---|---|---|---|---|---|---|---|---|---|---|---|---|---|---|---|---|
| Wheat, shredded, plain (long, round, or bite-size). | 1 ounce | 28 | 100 | 3 | 1 | --- | --- | --- | 23 | 12 | 1.0 | 0 | .06 | .03 | 1.2 | 0 |
| Wheat and malted barley flakes, with added nutrients. | 1 ounce | 28 | 110 | 2 | Trace | --- | --- | --- | 24 | 14 | .7 | 0 | .13 | .03 | 1.1 | 0 |
| Wheat flakes, with added nutrients. | 1 ounce | 28 | 100 | 3 | Trace | --- | --- | --- | 23 | 12 | 1.2 | 0 | .18 | .04 | 1.4 | 0 |
| Wheat flours: | | | | | | | | | | | | | | | | |
| Whole-wheat, from hard wheats, stirred. | 1 cup | 120 | 400 | 16 | 2 | Trace | 1 | 1 | 85 | 49 | 4.0 | 0 | .66 | .14 | 5.2 | 0 |
| All-purpose or family flour: | | | | | | | | | | | | | | | | |
| Enriched, sifted. | 1 cup | 110 | 400 | 12 | 1 | Trace | Trace | Trace | 84 | 18 | [15]3.2 | 0 | [15].48 | [15].29 | [15]3.8 | 0 |
| Unenriched, sifted. | 1 cup | 110 | 400 | 12 | 1 | Trace | Trace | Trace | 84 | 18 | .9 | 0 | .07 | .05 | 1.0 | 0 |
| Self-rising, enriched. | 1 cup | 110 | 385 | 10 | 1 | Trace | Trace | Trace | 82 | 292 | [15]3.2 | 0 | [15].49 | [15].29 | [15]3.9 | 0 |
| Cake or pastry flour, sifted. | 1 cup | 100 | 365 | 8 | 1 | Trace | Trace | Trace | 79 | 17 | .5 | 0 | .03 | .03 | .7 | 0 |
| Wheat germ, crude, commercially milled. | 1 cup | 68 | 245 | 18 | 7 | 2 | 4 | 2 | 32 | 49 | 6.4 | 0 | 1.36 | .46 | 2.9 | 0 |
| **FATS, OILS** | | | | | | | | | | | | | | | | |
| Butter, 4 sticks per pound: | | | | | | | | | | | | | | | | |
| Sticks, 2 | 1 cup | 227 | 1,625 | 1 | 184 | 101 | 61 | 6 | 1 | 45 | 0 | [20]7,500 | 0 | 0 | 0 | 0 |
| Stick, ⅛ | 1 tablespoon | 14 | 100 | Trace | 11 | 6 | 4 | Trace | Trace | 3 | 0 | [20]460 | 0 | 0 | 0 | 0 |
| Pat or square (64 per pound). | 1 pat | 7 | 50 | Trace | 6 | 3 | 2 | Trace | Trace | 1 | 0 | [20]230 | 0 | 0 | 0 | 0 |
| Fats, cooking: | | | | | | | | | | | | | | | | |
| Lard | 1 cup | 220 | 1,985 | 0 | 220 | 84 | 101 | 22 | 0 | 0 | 0 | 0 | --- | --- | --- | 0 |
| Lard | 1 tablespoon | 14 | 125 | 0 | 14 | 5 | 6 | 1 | 0 | 0 | 0 | 0 | --- | --- | --- | 0 |
| Vegetable fats | 1 cup | 200 | 1,770 | 0 | 200 | 46 | 130 | 14 | 0 | 0 | 0 | --- | --- | --- | --- | 0 |
| Vegetable fats | 1 tablespoon | 12.5 | 110 | 0 | 12 | 3 | 8 | 1 | 0 | 0 | 0 | --- | --- | --- | --- | 0 |
| Margarine, 4 sticks per pound: | | | | | | | | | | | | | | | | |
| Sticks, 2 | 1 cup | 227 | 1,635 | 1 | 184 | 37 | 105 | 33 | 1 | 45 | 0 | [21]7,500 | 0 | 0 | 0 | 0 |
| Stick, ⅛ | 1 tablespoon | 14 | 100 | Trace | 11 | 2 | 6 | 2 | Trace | 3 | 0 | [21]460 | 0 | 0 | 0 | 0 |
| Pat or square (64 per pound). | 1 pat | 7 | 50 | Trace | 6 | 1 | 3 | 1 | Trace | 1 | 0 | [21]230 | 0 | 0 | 0 | 0 |
| Oils, salad or cooking: | | | | | | | | | | | | | | | | |
| Corn | 1 tablespoon | 14 | 125 | 0 | 14 | 1 | 4 | 7 | 0 | 0 | 0 | 0 | 0 | 0 | 0 | 0 |
| Cottonseed | 1 tablespoon | 14 | 125 | 0 | 14 | 4 | 3 | 7 | 0 | 0 | 0 | 0 | 0 | 0 | 0 | 0 |
| Olive | 1 tablespoon | 14 | 125 | 0 | 14 | 2 | 11 | 1 | 0 | 0 | 0 | 0 | 0 | 0 | 0 | 0 |
| Soybean | 1 tablespoon | 14 | 125 | 0 | 14 | 2 | 3 | 7 | 0 | 0 | 0 | 0 | 0 | 0 | 0 | 0 |

[15] Iron, thiamine, riboflavin, and niacin are based on the minimum levels of enrichment specified in standards of identity promulgated under the Federal Food, Drug, and Cosmetic Act.

[20] Year-round average.

[21] Based on the average vitamin A content of fortified margarine. Federal specifications for fortified margarine require a minimum of 15,000 I.U. of vitamin A per pound.

## TABLE 36—Continued

| Food, Approximate Measure, and Weight (in Grams) | | | Food Energy | Protein | Fat (Total Lipid) | Fatty acids | | | Carbohydrate | Calcium | Iron | Vitamin A Value | Thiamine | Riboflavin | Niacin | Ascorbic Acid |
|---|---|---|---|---|---|---|---|---|---|---|---|---|---|---|---|---|
| | | | | | | Saturated (Total) | Unsaturated Oleic | Unsaturated Linoleic | | | | | | | | |
| | | Grams | (Calories) | (Gm.) | (Gm.) | (Gm.) | (Gm.) | (Gm.) | (Gm.) | (Mg.) | (Mg.) | (I.U.) | (Mg.) | (Mg.) | (Mg.) | (Mg.) |
| **FATS, OILS—Continued** | | | | | | | | | | | | | | | | |
| Salad dressings: | | | | | | | | | | | | | | | | |
| Blue cheese | 1 tablespoon | 16 | 80 | 1 | 8 | 2 | 2 | 4 | 1 | 13 | Trace | 30 | Trace | 0.02 | Trace | Trace |
| Commercial, mayonnaise type. | 1 tablespoon | 15 | 65 | Trace | 6 | 1 | 1 | 3 | 2 | 2 | Trace | 30 | Trace | Trace | Trace | Trace |
| French | 1 tablespoon | 15 | 60 | Trace | 6 | 1 | 1 | 3 | 3 | 2 | .1 | | .01 | .03 | Trace | --- |
| Home cooked, boiled | 1 tablespoon | 17 | 30 | 1 | 2 | 1 | 1 | Trace | 3 | 15 | .1 | 80 | .01 | .01 | Trace | Trace |
| Mayonnaise | 1 tablespoon | 15 | 110 | Trace | 12 | 2 | 3 | 6 | Trace | 3 | .1 | 40 | Trace | Trace | Trace | Trace |
| Thousand island | 1 tablespoon | 15 | 75 | Trace | 8 | 1 | 2 | 4 | 2 | 2 | .1 | 50 | Trace | Trace | Trace | Trace |
| **SUGARS, SWEETS** | | | | | | | | | | | | | | | | |
| Candy: | | | | | | | | | | | | | | | | |
| Caramels | 1 ounce | 28 | 115 | 1 | 3 | 2 | 1 | Trace | 22 | 42 | .4 | Trace | .01 | .05 | Trace | Trace |
| Chocolate, milk, plain | 1 ounce | 28 | 150 | 2 | 9 | 5 | 3 | Trace | 16 | 65 | .3 | 80 | .02 | .09 | .1 | Trace |
| Fudge, plain | 1 ounce | 28 | 115 | 1 | 3 | 2 | 1 | Trace | 21 | 22 | .3 | Trace | .01 | .03 | .1 | Trace |
| Hard candy | 1 ounce | 28 | 110 | 0 | Trace | --- | --- | --- | 28 | 6 | .5 | 0 | 0 | 0 | 0 | 0 |
| Marshmallows | 1 ounce | 28 | 90 | 1 | Trace | --- | --- | --- | 23 | 5 | .5 | 0 | 0 | Trace | Trace | 0 |
| Chocolate sirup, thin type | 1 tablespoon | 20 | 50 | Trace | Trace | Trace | Trace | Trace | 13 | 3 | .3 | 0 | Trace | .01 | .1 | 0 |
| Honey, strained or extracted. | 1 tablespoon | 21 | 65 | Trace | 0 | --- | --- | --- | 17 | 1 | .1 | 0 | Trace | .01 | .1 | Trace |
| Jams and preserves | 1 tablespoon | 20 | 55 | Trace | Trace | --- | --- | --- | 14 | 4 | .2 | Trace | Trace | .01 | Trace | Trace |
| Jellies | 1 tablespoon | 20 | 55 | Trace | Trace | --- | --- | --- | 14 | 4 | .3 | Trace | Trace | .01 | Trace | 1 |
| Molasses, cane: | | | | | | | | | | | | | | | | |
| Light (first extraction). | 1 tablespoon | 20 | 50 | --- | --- | --- | --- | --- | 13 | 33 | .9 | --- | .01 | .01 | Trace | Trace |
| Blackstrap (third extraction). | 1 tablespoon | 20 | 45 | --- | --- | --- | --- | --- | 11 | 137 | 3.2 | --- | .02 | .04 | .4 | --- |
| Sirup, table blends (chiefly corn, light and dark). | 1 tablespoon | 20 | 60 | 0 | 0 | --- | --- | --- | 15 | 9 | .8 | 0 | 0 | 0 | 0 | 0 |
| Sugars (cane or beet): | | | | | | | | | | | | | | | | |
| Granulated | 1 cup | 200 | 770 | 0 | 0 | --- | --- | --- | 199 | 0 | .2 | 0 | 0 | 0 | 0 | 0 |
| | 1 tablespoon | 12 | 45 | 0 | 0 | --- | --- | --- | 12 | 0 | Trace | 0 | 0 | 0 | 0 | 0 |
| Lump, 1⅛ by ¾ by ⅜ | 1 lump | 6 | 25 | 0 | 0 | --- | --- | --- | 6 | 0 | Trace | 0 | 0 | 0 | 0 | 0 |
| Powdered, stirred be- | 1 cup | 128 | 495 | 0 | 0 | --- | --- | --- | 127 | 0 | .1 | 0 | 0 | 0 | 0 | 0 |

## MISCELLANEOUS ITEMS

| Food | Measure | Grams | Calories | Protein (g) | Fat (g) | Saturated (g) | Oleic (g) | Linoleic (g) | Carbohydrate (g) | Calcium (mg) | Iron (mg) | Vitamin A (I.U.) | Thiamine (mg) | Riboflavin (mg) | Niacin (mg) | Ascorbic acid (mg) |
|---|---|---|---|---|---|---|---|---|---|---|---|---|---|---|---|---|
| *(continued from previous page)* | 1 tablespoon | 14 | 50 | 0 | 0 | 0 | | | 13 | 12 | .5 | 0 | Trace | Trace | Trace | 0 |
| Beer (average 3.6 percent alcohol by weight). | 1 cup | 240 | 100 | 1 | 0 | | | | 9 | 12 | Trace | 0 | .01 | .07 | 1.6 | 0 |
| Beverages, carbonated: | | | | | | | | | | | | | | | | |
| Cola type | 1 cup | 240 | 95 | 0 | 0 | | | | 24 | | | 0 | 0 | 0 | 0 | 0 |
| Ginger ale | 1 cup | 230 | 70 | 0 | 0 | | | | 18 | | | 0 | 0 | 0 | 0 | 0 |
| Bouillon cube, ⅝ inch | 1 cube | 4 | 5 | 1 | Trace | | | | Trace | | | | | | | |
| Chili powder. *See* Vegetables, peppers. | | | | | | | | | | | | | | | | |
| Chili sauce (mainly tomatoes). | 1 tablespoon | 17 | 20 | Trace | Trace | | | | 4 | 3 | .1 | 240 | .02 | .01 | .3 | 3 |
| Chocolate: | | | | | | | | | | | | | | | | |
| Bitter or baking | 1 ounce | 28 | 145 | 3 | 15 | 8 | 6 | Trace | 8 | 22 | 1.9 | 20 | .01 | .07 | .4 | 0 |
| Sweet | 1 ounce | 28 | 150 | 1 | 10 | 6 | 4 | Trace | 16 | 27 | .4 | Trace | .01 | .04 | .1 | 0 |
| Cider. *See* Fruits, apple juice. | | | | | | | | | | | | | | | | |
| Gelatin, dry: | | | | | | | | | | | | | | | | |
| Plain | 1 tablespoon | 10 | 35 | 9 | Trace | | | | 0 | | | | | | | |
| Dessert powder, 3-ounce package. | ½ cup | 85 | 315 | 8 | 0 | | | | 75 | | | | | | | |
| Gelatin dessert, ready-to-eat: | | | | | | | | | | | | | | | | |
| Plain | 1 cup | 239 | 140 | 4 | 0 | | | | 34 | | | | | | | |
| With fruit | 1 cup | 241 | 160 | 3 | Trace | | | | 40 | | | | | | | |
| Olives, pickled: | | | | | | | | | | | | | | | | |
| Green | 4 medium or 3 extra large or 2 giant. | 16 | 15 | Trace | 2 | Trace | 2 | Trace | Trace | 8 | .2 | 40 | | | | |
| Ripe: Mission | 3 small or 2 large. | 10 | 15 | Trace | 2 | Trace | 2 | Trace | Trace | 9 | .1 | 10 | | | | |
| Pickles, cucumber: | | | | | | | | | | | | | | | | |
| Dill, large, 4 by 1¾ inches. | 1 pickle | 135 | 15 | 1 | Trace | | | | 3 | 35 | 1.4 | 140 | Trace | .03 | Trace | 8 |
| Sweet, 2¾ by ¾ inches | 1 pickle | 20 | 30 | Trace | Trace | | | | 7 | 2 | .2 | 20 | Trace | Trace | Trace | 1 |
| Popcorn. *See* Grain products. | | | | | | | | | | | | | | | | |
| Sherbet, orange | 1 cup | 193 | 260 | 2 | 2 | | | | 59 | 31 | Trace | 110 | .02 | .06 | Trace | 4 |
| Soups, canned; ready-to-serve (prepared with equal volume of water): | | | | | | | | | | | | | | | | |
| Bean with pork | 1 cup | 250 | 170 | 8 | 6 | 1 | 2 | 2 | 22 | 62 | 2.2 | 650 | .14 | .07 | 1.0 | 2 |
| Beef noodle | 1 cup | 250 | 70 | 4 | 3 | 1 | 1 | 1 | 7 | 8 | 1.0 | 50 | .05 | .06 | 1.1 | Trace |
| Beef bouillon, broth, consomme. | 1 cup | 240 | 30 | 5 | 0 | | | | 3 | Trace | .5 | Trace | Trace | .02 | 1.2 | |

TABLE 36—Continued

| Food, Approximate Measure, and Weight (in Grams) | Food Energy (Calories) | Protein (Gm.) | Fat (Total Lipid) (Gm.) | Fatty acids Saturated (Total) (Gm.) | Fatty acids Unsaturated Oleic (Gm.) | Fatty acids Unsaturated Linoleic (Gm.) | Carbohydrate (Gm.) | Calcium (Mg.) | Iron (Mg.) | Vitamin A Value (I.U.) | Thiamine (Mg.) | Riboflavin (Mg.) | Niacin (Mg.) | Ascorbic Acid (Mg.) |
|---|---|---|---|---|---|---|---|---|---|---|---|---|---|---|
| MISCELLANEOUS ITEMS—Continued | | | | | | | | | | | | | | |
| Soups, canned; ready-to-serve—Con. | | | | | | | | | | | | | | |
| Chicken noodle 1 cup 250 | 65 | 4 | 2 | Trace | 1 | 1 | 8 | 10 | 0.5 | 50 | 0.02 | 0.02 | 0.8 | Trace |
| Clam chowder 1 cup 255 | 85 | 2 | 3 | ---- | 3 | 5 | 13 | 36 | 1.0 | 920 | .03 | .03 | 1.0 | ---- |
| Cream soup (mushroom) 1 cup 240 | 135 | 2 | 10 | 1 | | | 10 | 41 | .5 | 70 | .02 | .12 | .7 | Trace |
| Minestrone 1 cup 245 | 105 | 5 | 3 | ---- | | | 14 | 37 | 1.0 | 2,350 | .07 | .05 | 1.0 | 7 |
| Pea, green 1 cup 245 | 130 | 6 | 2 | 1 | 1 | Trace | 23 | 44 | 1.0 | 340 | .05 | .05 | 1.0 | ---- |
| Tomato 1 cup 245 | 90 | 2 | 2 | Trace | 1 | 1 | 16 | 15 | .7 | 1,000 | .06 | .05 | 1.1 | 12 |
| Vegetable with beef broth 1 cup 250 | 80 | 3 | 2 | ---- | | | 14 | 20 | .8 | 3,250 | .05 | .02 | 1.2 | ---- |
| Starch (cornstarch) 1 cup 128 | 465 | Trace | Trace | | | | 112 | 0 | 0 | 0 | 0 | 0 | 0 | 0 |
| 1 tablespoon 8 | 30 | Trace | Trace | | | | 7 | 0 | 0 | 0 | 0 | 0 | 0 | 0 |
| Tapioca, quick-cooking granulated, dry, stirred before measuring. 1 cup 152 | 535 | 1 | Trace | | | | 131 | 15 | .6 | 0 | 0 | 0 | 0 | 0 |
| 1 tablespoon 10 | 35 | Trace | Trace | | | | 9 | 1 | Trace | 0 | 0 | 0 | 0 | 0 |
| Vinegar 1 tablespoon 15 | 2 | 0 | | | | | 1 | 1 | .1 | | | | | |
| White sauce, medium 1 cup 265 | 430 | 10 | 33 | 18 | 11 | 1 | 23 | 305 | .5 | 1,220 | .12 | .44 | .6 | Trace |
| Yeast: | | | | | | | | | | | | | | |
| Baker's: | | | | | | | | | | | | | | |
| Compressed 1 ounce 28 | 25 | 3 | Trace | | | | 3 | 4 | 1.4 | Trace | .20 | .47 | 3.2 | Trace |
| Dry active 1 ounce 28 | 80 | 10 | Trace | | | | 11 | 12 | 4.6 | Trace | .66 | 1.53 | 10.4 | Trace |
| Brewer's, dry, debittered. 1 tablespoon 8 | 25 | 3 | Trace | | | | 3 | 17 | 1.4 | Trace | 1.25 | .34 | 3.0 | Trace |
| Yoghurt. See Milk, cream, cheese; related products. | | | | | | | | | | | | | | |

# APPENDIX 2

## DATA USED FOR CALCULATING ENERGY VALUES OF FOODS OR FOOD GROUPS BY THE ATWATER SYSTEM

### TABLE 37

| FOOD OR FOOD GROUP | PROTEIN | | | FAT | | | CARBOHYDRATE | | |
|---|---|---|---|---|---|---|---|---|---|
| | Coefficient of digestibility (Pct.) | Heat of combustion less 1.25* (Cal./gm.) | Factor to be applied to ingested nutrients (Cal./gm.) | Coefficient of digestibility (Pct.) | Heat of combustion (Cal./gm.) | Factor to be applied to ingested nutrients (Cal./gm.) | Coefficient of digestibility (Pct.) | Heat of combustion (Cal./gm.) | Factor to be applied to ingested nutrients (Cal./gm.) |
| **Eggs, Meat products, Milk products:** | | | | | | | | | |
| Eggs | 97 | 4.50 | 4.36 | 95 | 9.50 | 9.02 | 98 | 3.75 | 3.68 |
| Gelatin | 97 | 4.02 | 3.90 | 95 | 9.50 | 9.02 | 98 | 4.19 | 4.11 |
| Glycogen | | | | | | | | | † |
| Meat, fish | 97 | 4.40 | 4.27 | 95 | 9.50 | 9.02 | | | |
| Milk, milk products | 97 | 4.40 | 4.27 | 95 | 9.25 | 8.79 | 98 | 3.95 | 3.87 |
| **Fats, separated:** | | | | | | | | | |
| Butter | 97 | 4.40 | 4.27 | 95 | 9.25 | 8.79 | 98 | 3.95 | 3.87 |
| Other animal fats | | | | 95 | 9.50 | 9.02 | | | |
| Margarine, vegetable | | | | 95 | 9.30 | 8.84 | | | |
| Other vegetable fats and oils | 97 | 4.40 | 4.27 | 95 | 9.30 | 8.84 | | | |
| **Fruits:** | | | | | | | | | |
| All (except lemons, limes) | 85 | 3.95 | 3.36 | 90 | 9.30 | 8.37 | 90 | 4.00 | 3.60 |
| All fruit juice (except lemon, lime) unsweetened | 85 | 3.95 | 3.36 | 90 | 9.30 | 8.37 | 98‡ | 4.00 | 3.92‡ |
| Lemons, limes | 85 | 3.95 | 3.36 | 90 | 9.30 | 8.37 | 90‡ | 2.75 | 2.48‡ |
| Lemon juice, lime juice, unsweetened | 85 | 3.95 | 3.36 | 90 | 9.30 | 8.37 | 98 | 2.75 | 2.70 |
| **Grain products:** | | | | | | | | | |
| Barley, pearled | 78 | 4.55 | 3.55 | 90 | 9.30 | 8.37 | 94 | 4.20 | 3.95 |
| Buckwheat flour, dark | 74 | 4.55 | 3.37 | 90 | 9.30 | 8.37 | 90 | 4.20 | 3.78 |
| Buckwheat flour, light | 78 | 4.55 | 3.55 | 90 | 9.30 | 8.37 | 94 | 4.20 | 3.95 |
| Cornmeal, whole-ground | 60 | 4.55 | 2.73 | 90 | 9.30 | 8.37 | 96 | 4.20 | 4.03 |
| Cornmeal, degermed | 76 | 4.55 | 3.46 | 90 | 9.30 | 8.37 | 99 | 4.20 | 4.16 |
| Dextrin | | | | | | | 98 | 4.11 | 4.03 |
| Macaroni, spaghetti | 86 | 4.55 | 3.91 | 90 | 9.30 | 8.37 | 98 | 4.20 | 4.12 |
| Oatmeal, rolled oats | 76 | 4.55 | 3.46 | 90 | 9.30 | 8.37 | 98 | 4.20 | 4.12 |
| Rice, brown | 75 | 4.55 | 3.41 | 90 | 9.30 | 8.37 | 98 | 4.20 | 4.12 |
| Rice, white or polished | 84 | 4.55 | 3.82 | 90 | 9.30 | 8.37 | 99 | 4.20 | 4.16 |

* The correction, 1.25 calories, has been subtracted from the heat of combustion. This gives values applicable to grams of digested protein and is identical with Atwater's factors per gram of available protein.

† Carbohydrate factor, 3.87 for brain, heart, kidney, liver; 4.11 for tongue and shellfish.

‡ Unpublished revision made since 1955.

TABLE 37—Continued

| Food or Food Group | PROTEIN | | | FAT | | | CARBOHYDRATE | | |
|---|---|---|---|---|---|---|---|---|---|
| | Coefficient of digestibility (Pct.) | Heat of combustion less 1.25* (Cal./gm.) | Factor to be applied to ingested nutrients (Cal./gm.) | Coefficient of digestibility (Pct.) | Heat of combustion (Cal./gm.) | Factor to be applied to ingested nutrients (Cal./gm.) | Coefficient of digestibility (Pct.) | Heat of combustion (Cal./gm.) | Factor to be applied to ingested nutrients (Cal./gm.) |
| Rye flour, dark | 65 | 4.55 | 2.96 | 90 | 9.30 | 8.37 | 90 | 4.20 | 3.78 |
| Rye flour, whole-grain | 67 | 4.55 | 3.05 | 90 | 9.30 | 8.37 | 92 | 4.20 | 3.86 |
| Rye flour, medium | 71 | 4.55 | 3.23 | 90 | 9.30 | 8.37 | 95 | 4.20 | 3.99 |
| Rye flour, light | 75 | 4.55 | 3.41 | 90 | 9.30 | 8.37 | 97 | 4.20 | 4.07 |
| Sorghum (kaoliang), whole or nearly whole meal | 20 | 4.55 | .91 | 90 | 9.30 | 8.37 | 96 | 4.20 | 4.03 |
| Wheat, 97–100 per cent extraction | 79 | 4.55 | 3.59 | 90 | 9.30 | 8.37 | 90 | 4.20 | 3.78 |
| Wheat, 85–93 per cent extraction | 83 | 4.55 | 3.78 | 90 | 9.30 | 8.37 | 94 | 4.20 | 3.95 |
| Wheat, 70–74 per cent extraction | 89 | 4.55 | 4.05 | 90 | 9.30 | 8.37 | 98 | 4.20 | 4.12 |
| Wheat, flaked, puffed, rolled, shredded, whole meal | 79 | 4.55 | 3.59 | 90 | 9.30 | 8.37 | 90 | 4.20 | 3.78 |
| Wheat bran (100 per cent) | 40 | 4.55 | 1.82 | 90 | 9.30 | 8.37 | 56 | 4.20 | 2.35 |
| Other cereals, refined | 85 | 4.55 | 3.87 | 90 | 9.30 | 8.37 | 98 | 4.20 | 4.12 |
| Wild rice | 78 | 4.55 | 3.55 | 90 | 9.30 | 8.37 | 94 | 4.20 | 3.95 |
| Legumes, Nuts: | | | | | | | | | |
| Mature dry beans, cowpeas, peas, other legumes; nuts | 78 | 4.45 | 3.47 | 90 | 9.30 | 8.37 | 97 | 4.20 | 4.07 |
| Immature Lima beans, cowpeas, peas, other legumes | 78 | 4.45 | 3.47 | 90 | 9.30 | 8.37 | 97 | 4.20 | 4.07 |
| Soybeans, dry; soy flour, flakes, grits | 78 | 4.45 | 3.47 | 90 | 9.30 | 8.37 | 97 | 4.20 | 4.07 |
| Sugars: | | | | | | | | | |
| Cane or beet sugar (sucrose) | | | | | | | 98 | 3.95 | 3.87 |
| Glucose | | | | | | | 98 | 3.75 | 3.68 |
| Vegetables: | | | | | | | | | |
| Mushrooms | 70 | 3.75 | 2.62 | 90 | 9.30 | 8.37 | 85 | 4.10 | 3.48 |
| Potatoes and starchy roots | 74 | 3.75 | 2.78 | 90 | 9.30 | 8.37 | 96 | 4.20 | 4.03 |
| Other underground crops§ | 74 | 3.75 | 2.78 | 90 | 9.30 | 8.37 | 96 | 4.00 | 3.84 |
| Other vegetables | 65 | 3.75 | 2.44 | 90 | 9.30 | 8.37 | 85 | 4.20 | 3.57 |
| Miscellaneous foods: | | | | | | | | | |
| Alcohol‖ | | | | | | | | | |
| Chocolate, cocoa | 42 | 4.35 | 1.83 | 90 | 9.30 | 8.37 | 32 | 4.16 | 1.33 |
| Vinegar | | | | | | | 98 | 2.45 | 2.40 |
| Yeast | 80 | 3.75 | 3.00 | | | | 80 | 4.20 | 3.35 |

§ Vegetables such as beets, carrots, onions, parsnips, radishes.

‖ Coefficient of digestibility, 98 per cent; heat of combustion, 7.07 calories per gram; factor to apply to ingested alcohol, 6.93 calories per gram.

# APPENDIX 3

## Beverages—Alcoholic and Carbonated Non-alcoholic

*Alcoholic beverages.*—Food energy was calculated for alcoholic beverages as the total potential calories from any nutrients present (protein, fat, carbohydrate) plus those from alcohol. The factor 6.93 was applied to the alcoholic content by weight.

Dessert wines as classified in Table 38 include those containing more than 15 per cent alcohol (by volume), such as apple, muscatel, sherries, port, and tokay. Apertif wines and vermouths will also fall in this classification. Table wines to which the data in this table apply include those containing less than 15 per cent alcohol (by volume), such as barbera, burgundy, cabernet, chablis, champagnes, chianti, claret, Rhine wines, rosé, and sauternes. Cherry, peach, berry, and varietal wines usually fall in this class, although some may be high enough in alcohol content to be classified with dessert wines.

Within each group there is a rather wide range in total carbohydrate content. The carbohydrate is less in dry wines than in sweet wines.

## TABLE 38

### COMPOSITION OF BEVERAGES—ALCOHOLIC AND CARBONATED NON-ALCOHOLIC PER 100 GRAMS*

| | Food Energy | Protein | Carbo-hydrate | Calcium | Phosphorus | Iron | Thiamine | Riboflavin | Niacin |
|---|---|---|---|---|---|---|---|---|---|
| Beverages, alcoholic and carbonated non-alcoholic: | | | | | | | | | |
| Alcoholic: | | | | | | | | | |
| Beer, alcohol 4.5% by volume (3.6% by weight) | 42 | .3 | 3.8 | 5 | 30 | Trace | Trace | .03 | .6 |
| Gin, rum, vodka, whisky: | | | | | | | | | |
| 80-proof (33.4% alcohol by weight) | 231 | .... | Trace | | | | | | |
| 86-proof (36.0% alcohol by weight) | 249 | .... | Trace | | | | | | |
| 90-proof (37.9% alcohol by weight) | 263 | .... | Trace | | | | | | |
| 94-proof (39.7% alcohol by weight) | 275 | .... | Trace | | | | | | |
| 100-proof (42.5% alcohol by weight) | 295 | .... | Trace | | | | | | |
| Wines: | | | | | | | | | |
| Dessert, alcohol 18.8% by volume (15.3% by weight) | 137 | .1 | 7.7 | 8 | .... | .... | .01 | .02 | .2 |
| Table, alcohol 12.2% by volume (9.9% by weight) | 85 | .1 | 4.2 | 9 | 10 | .4 | Trace | .01 | .1 |
| Carbonated, non-alcoholic: | | | | | | | | | |
| Carbonated waters: | | | | | | | | | |
| Sweetened (quinine sodas) | 31 | .... | 8 | | | | | | |
| Unsweetened (club sodas) | .... | .... | .... | | | | | | |
| Cola type | 39 | .... | 10 | | | | | | |
| Cream sodas | 43 | .... | 11 | | | | | | |
| Fruit-flavored sodas (citrus, cherry, grape, strawberry, Tom Collins mixer, other) (10%–13% sugar) | 46 | .... | 12 | | | | | | |
| Ginger ale, pale dry and golden | 31 | .... | 8 | | | | | | |
| Root beer | 41 | .... | 10.5 | | | | | | |
| Special dietary drinks with artificial sweetener (less than 1 calorie per ounce) | .... | .... | .... | | | | | | |

* From *Composition of Foods—Raw, Processed, Prepared* (U.S. Department of Agriculture, Agriculture Handbook, No. 8 [December, 1963]).

# APPENDIX 4

## CHOLESTEROL CONTENT OF FOODS*

### TABLE 39

| ITEM | AMOUNT OF CHOLESTEROL IN: | | REFUSE FROM ITEM AS PURCHASED (Percent) |
|---|---|---|---|
| | 100 grams edible portion‡ (Mg.) | Edible portion of 1 pound as purchased (Mg.) | |
| Beef, raw: | | | |
| With bone† | 70 | 270 | 15 |
| Without bone† | 70 | 320 | 0 |
| Brains, raw | >2,000 | >9,000 | 0 |
| Butter | 250 | 1,135 | 0 |
| Cavier or fish roe | >300 | >1,300 | 0 |
| Cheese: | | | |
| Cheddar | 100 | 455 | 0 |
| Cottage, creamed | 15 | 70 | 0 |
| Cream | 120 | 545 | 0 |
| Other (25% to 30% fat) | 85 | 385 | 0 |
| Cheese spread | 65 | 295 | 0 |
| Chicken, flesh only, raw | 60 | .......... | 0 |
| Crab: | | | |
| In shell† | 125 | 270 | 52 |
| Meat only† | 125 | 565 | 0 |
| Egg, whole | 550 | 2,200 | 12 |
| Egg white | 0 | 0 | 0 |
| Egg yolk: | | | |
| Fresh | 1,500 | 6,800 | 0 |
| Frozen | 1,280 | 5,800 | 0 |
| Dried | 2,950 | 13,380 | 0 |
| Fish: | | | |
| Steak† | 70 | 265 | 16 |
| Fillet† | 70 | 320 | 0 |
| Heart, raw | 150 | 680 | 0 |
| Ice cream | 45 | 205 | 0 |
| Kidney, raw | 375 | 1,700 | 0 |
| Lamb, raw: | | | |
| With bone† | 70 | 265 | 16 |
| Without bone† | 70 | 320 | 0 |
| Lard and other animal fat | 95 | 430 | 0 |
| Liver, raw | 300 | 1,360 | 0 |
| Lobster: | | | |
| Whole† | 200 | 235 | 74 |
| Meat only† | 200 | 900 | 0 |
| Margarine: | | | |
| All vegetable fat | 0 | 0 | 0 |
| Two-thirds animal fat, one-third vegetable fat. | 65 | 295 | 0 |
| Milk: | | | |
| Fluid, whole | 11 | 50 | 0 |
| Dried, whole | 85 | 385 | 0 |
| Fluid, skim | 3 | 15 | 0 |

\* From *Composition of Foods—Raw, Processed, Prepared,* Department of Agriculture, Agriculture Handbook, No. 8 [December, 1963]).

† Designate items that have the same chemical composition for the edible portion but differ in the amount of refuse.

‡ Data apply to 100 grams of edible portion of the item, although it may be purchased with the refuse indicated and described or implied in the first column.

TABLE 39—*Continued*

| ITEM | AMOUNT OF CHOLESTEROL IN: | | REFUSE FROM ITEM AS PURCHASED (Percent) |
|---|---|---|---|
| | 100 grams edible portion‡ (Mg.) | Edible portion of 1 pound as purchased (Mg.) | |
| Mutton: | | | |
| With bone†................................ | 65 | 250 | 16 |
| Without bone†............................ | 65 | 295 | 0 |
| Oysters: | | | |
| In shell†.................................. | >200 | > 90 | 90 |
| Meat only†............................... | >200 | >900 | 0 |
| Pork: | | | |
| With bone†................................ | 70 | 260 | 18 |
| Without bone†............................ | 70 | 320 | 0 |
| Shrimp: | | | |
| In shell†.................................. | 125 | 390 | 31 |
| Flesh only†............................... | 125 | 565 | 0 |
| Sweetbreads (thymus)..................... | 250 | 1,135 | 0 |
| Veal: | | | |
| With bone†................................ | 90 | 320 | 21 |
| Without bone†............................ | 90 | 410 | 0 |

# APPENDIX 5

## Amino Acid Content of Foods

The following table is taken from a compilation prepared by M. L. Orr and B. K. Watt, as Home Economics Research Report No. 4 (1957), Household Economics Research Division, Institute of Home Economics, Agricultural Research Service, U.S. Department of Agriculture. The original report contains data on 18 amino acids in 202 food items. Only the average amounts of 8 "essential" amino acids, plus arginine and histidine, have been included in the following table. This table is useful when an average protein content may be assumed. When specific nitrogen or protein content of a food is known, reference may be made to the original publication.

## TABLE 40

### AMINO ACID CONTENT OF FOODS, 100 GM., EDIBLE PORTION

| Protein Content, and Nitrogen Conversion Factor | Tryptophan (Gm.) | Threonine (Gm.) | Isoleucine (Gm.) | Leucine (Gm.) | Lysine (Gm.) | Methionine (Gm.) | Cystine (Gm.) | Phenylalanine (Gm.) | Tyrosine (Gm.) | Valine (Gm.) | Arginine (Gm.) | Histidine (Gm.) |
|---|---|---|---|---|---|---|---|---|---|---|---|---|
| **MILK; MILK PRODUCTS** | | | | | | | | | | | | |
| *Milk (Protein, N×6.38):* | | | | | | | | | | | | |
| cow: | | | | | | | | | | | | |
|   fluid, whole and non-fat (3.5% protein) | 0.049 | 0.161 | 0.223 | 0.344 | 0.272 | 0.086 | 0.031 | 0.170 | 0.178 | 0.240 | 0.128 | 0.092 |
| canned: | | | | | | | | | | | | |
|   evaporated, unsweetened (7.0% protein) | 0.099 | 0.323 | 0.447 | 0.688 | 0.545 | 0.171 | 0.063 | 0.340 | 0.357 | 0.481 | 0.256 | 0.185 |
|   condensed, sweetened (8.1% protein) | 0.114 | 0.374 | 0.518 | 0.796 | 0.631 | 0.198 | 0.072 | 0.393 | 0.413 | 0.557 | 0.296 | 0.214 |
| dried: | | | | | | | | | | | | |
|   whole (25.8% protein) | 0.364 | 1.191 | 1.648 | 2.535 | 2.009 | 0.632 | 0.231 | 1.251 | 1.316 | 1.774 | 0.944 | 0.680 |
|   non-fat (35.6% protein) | 0.502 | 1.641 | 2.271 | 3.493 | 2.768 | 0.870 | 0.318 | 1.724 | 1.814 | 2.444 | 1.300 | 0.937 |
| goat (3.3% protein) | 0.039 | 0.217 | 0.087 | 0.278 | 0.312 | 0.065 | ..... | 0.121 | ..... | 0.139 | 0.174 | 0.068 |
| human (1.4% protein) | 0.023 | 0.062 | 0.075 | 0.124 | 0.090 | 0.028 | 0.027 | 0.060 | 0.071 | 0.086 | 0.055 | 0.030 |
| Indian buffalo (4.2% protein) | 0.059 | 0.212 | 0.204 | 0.420 | 0.331 | 0.112 | 0.058 | 0.177 | ..... | 0.255 | 0.136 | 0.086 |
| *Milk products:* | | | | | | | | | | | | |
| buttermilk (3.5% protein, N×6.38) | 0.038 | 0.165 | 0.219 | 0.348 | 0.291 | 0.082 | 0.032 | 0.186 | 0.137 | 0.262 | 0.168 | 0.099 |
| casein (100.0% protein, N×6.29) | 1.335 | 4.277 | 6.550 | 10.048 | 8.013 | 3.084 | 0.382 | 5.389 | 5.819 | 7.393 | 4.070 | 3.021 |
| cheese (protein, N×6.38): | | | | | | | | | | | | |
|   blue mold (21.5% protein) | 0.293 | 0.799 | 1.449 | 2.096 | 1.577 | 0.559 | 0.121 | 1.153 | 1.028 | 1.543 | 0.785 | 0.701 |
|   Camembert (17.5% protein) | 0.239 | 0.650 | 1.179 | 1.706 | 1.284 | 0.455 | 0.099 | 0.938 | 0.837 | 1.256 | 0.639 | 0.571 |
|   Cheddar (25.0% protein) | 0.341 | 0.929 | 1.685 | 2.437 | 1.834 | 0.650 | 0.141 | 1.340 | 1.195 | 1.794 | 0.913 | 0.815 |
|   Cheddar processed (23.2% protein) | 0.316 | 0.862 | 1.563 | 2.262 | 1.702 | 0.604 | 0.131 | 1.244 | 1.109 | 1.665 | 0.847 | 0.756 |
| cheese foods, Cheddar (20.5% protein) | 0.280 | 0.761 | 1.382 | 1.998 | 1.504 | 0.533 | 0.116 | 1.099 | 0.980 | 1.472 | 0.749 | 0.668 |
| cottage (17.0% protein) | 0.179 | 0.794 | 0.989 | 1.826 | 1.428 | 0.469 | 0.147 | 0.917 | 0.917 | 0.978 | 0.802 | 0.549 |

TABLE 40—*Continued*

| Protein Content, and Nitrogen Conversion Factor | Trypto-phan (Gm.) | Threo-nine (Gm.) | Iso-leucine (Gm.) | Leucine (Gm.) | Lysine (Gm.) | Methi-onine (Gm.) | Cystine (Gm.) | Phenyl-alanine (Gm.) | Tyro-sine (Gm.) | Valine (Gm.) | Argi-nine (Gm.) | Histi-dine (Gm.) |
|---|---|---|---|---|---|---|---|---|---|---|---|---|
| MILK PRODUCTS—*Continued* | | | | | | | | | | | | |
| cream cheese (9.0% protein) | 0.080 | 0.408 | 0.519 | 0.923 | 0.721 | 0.229 | 0.085 | 0.547 | 0.408 | 0.538 | 0.313 | 0.278 |
| Limburger (21.2% protein) | 0.289 | 0.788 | 1.429 | 2.067 | 1.555 | 0.552 | 0.120 | 1.136 | 1.014 | 1.522 | 0.774 | 0.691 |
| Parmesan (36.0% protein) | 0.491 | 1.337 | 2.426 | 3.510 | 2.641 | 0.937 | 0.203 | 1.930 | 1.721 | 2.584 | 1.315 | 1.174 |
| Swiss (27.5% protein) | 0.375 | 1.021 | 1.853 | 2.681 | 2.017 | 0.715 | 0.155 | 1.474 | 1.315 | 1.974 | 1.004 | 0.896 |
| Swiss processed (26.4% protein) | 0.360 | 0.981 | 1.779 | 2.574 | 1.937 | 0.687 | 0.149 | 1.415 | 1.262 | 1.895 | 0.964 | 0.861 |
| lactalbumin (100.0% protein, N× 6.49) | 2.203 | 5.239 | 6.209 | 12.342 | 9.060 | 2.250 | 3.405 | 4.360 | 3.806 | 5.686 | 3.498 | 1.911 |
| whey (Protein, N×6.49) | | | | | | | | | | | | |
| fluid (0.9% protein) | 0.010 | 0.048 | 0.052 | 0.074 | 0.055 | 0.013 | 0.018 | 0.023 | 0.009 | 0.045 | 0.017 | 0.011 |
| dried (12.7% protein) | 0.147 | 0.677 | 0.734 | 1.043 | 0.769 | 0.188 | 0.250 | 0.323 | 0.131 | 0.640 | 0.235 | 0.159 |
| EGGS, CHICKEN (Protein, N×6.25) | | | | | | | | | | | | |
| Fresh or stored: | | | | | | | | | | | | |
| whole (12.8% protein) | 0.211 | 0.637 | 0.850 | 1.126 | 0.819 | 0.401 | 0.299 | 0.739 | 0.551 | 0.950 | 0.840 | 0.307 |
| whites (10.8% protein) | 0.164 | 0.477 | 0.698 | 0.950 | 0.648 | 0.420 | 0.263 | 0.689 | 0.449 | 0.842 | 0.634 | 0.233 |
| yolks (16.3% protein) | 0.235 | 0.827 | 0.996 | 1.372 | 1.074 | 0.417 | 0.274 | 0.717 | 0.756 | 1.121 | 1.132 | 0.368 |
| Dried: | | | | | | | | | | | | |
| whole (46.8% protein) | 0.771 | 2.329 | 3.108 | 4.118 | 2.995 | 1.468 | 1.093 | 2.703 | 2.014 | 3.474 | 3.070 | 1.123 |
| whites (85.9% protein) | 1.306 | 3.793 | 5.553 | 7.559 | 5.154 | 3.340 | 2.089 | 5.484 | 3.573 | 6.693 | 5.044 | 1.855 |
| yolks (31.2% protein) | 0.449 | 1.582 | 1.907 | 2.626 | 2.057 | 0.799 | 0.524 | 1.373 | 1.448 | 2.147 | 2.167 | 0.704 |
| MEAT; POULTRY; FISH AND SHELL-FISH; THEIR PRODUCTS | | | | | | | | | | | | |
| *Meat* (Protein, N×6.25): | | | | | | | | | | | | |
| beef carcass or side: | | | | | | | | | | | | |
| thin (18.8% protein) | 0.220 | 0.830 | 0.984 | 1.540 | 1.642 | 0.466 | 0.238 | 0.773 | 0.638 | 1.044 | 1.212 | 0.653 |
| medium fat (17.5% protein) | 0.204 | 0.773 | 0.916 | 1.434 | 1.529 | 0.434 | 0.221 | 0.720 | 0.594 | 0.972 | 1.128 | 0.608 |
| fat (16.3% protein) | 0.190 | 0.720 | 0.853 | 1.335 | 1.424 | 0.404 | 0.206 | 0.670 | 0.553 | 0.905 | 1.051 | 0.566 |
| very fat (13.7% protein) | 0.160 | 0.605 | 0.717 | 1.122 | 1.197 | 0.340 | 0.173 | 0.563 | 0.465 | 0.761 | 0.883 | 0.476 |
| medium fat, trimmed to retail basis (18.2% protein) | 0.213 | 0.804 | 0.952 | 1.491 | 1.590 | 0.451 | 0.230 | 0.748 | 0.617 | 1.010 | 1.174 | 0.632 |

## TABLE 40—*Continued*

| Protein Content, and Nitrogen Conversion Factor | Trypto-phan (Gm.) | Threo-nine (Gm.) | Iso-leucine (Gm.) | Leucine (Gm.) | Lysine (Gm.) | Methi-onine (Gm.) | Cystine (Gm.) | Phenyl-alanine (Gm.) | Tyro-sine (Gm.) | Valine (Gm.) | Argi-nine (Gm.) | Histi-dine (Gm.) |
|---|---|---|---|---|---|---|---|---|---|---|---|---|
| MEAT; POULTRY; FISH—*Continued* | | | | | | | | | | | | |
| beef cuts, medium fat: | | | | | | | | | | | | |
| chuck (18.6% protein)......... | 0.217 | 0.821 | 0.973 | 1.524 | 1.625 | 0.461 | 0.235 | 0.765 | 0.631 | 1.033 | 1.199 | 0.646 |
| flank (19.9% protein)...... | 0.232 | 0.879 | 1.041 | 1.630 | 1.738 | 0.494 | 0.252 | 0.818 | 0.675 | 1.105 | 1.283 | 0.691 |
| hamburger (16.0% protein)..... | 0.187 | 0.707 | 0.837 | 1.311 | 1.308 | 0.397 | 0.202 | 0.658 | 0.543 | 0.888 | 1.032 | 0.556 |
| porterhouse (16.4% protein)..... | 0.192 | 0.724 | 0.858 | 1.343 | 1.433 | 0.407 | 0.207 | 0.674 | 0.556 | 0.911 | 1.057 | 0.569 |
| rib roast (17.4% protein)..... | 0.203 | 0.768 | 0.910 | 1.425 | 1.520 | 0.432 | 0.220 | 0.715 | 0.590 | 0.966 | 1.122 | 0.604 |
| round (19.5% protein)......... | 0.228 | 0.861 | 1.020 | 1.597 | 1.704 | 0.484 | 0.246 | 0.802 | 0.661 | 1.083 | 1.257 | 0.677 |
| rump (16.2% protein)...... | 0.189 | 0.715 | 0.848 | 1.327 | 1.415 | 0.402 | 0.205 | 0.666 | 0.550 | 0.899 | 1.045 | 0.562 |
| sirloin (17.3% protein)...... | 0.202 | 0.764 | 0.905 | 1.417 | 1.511 | 0.429 | 0.219 | 0.711 | 0.587 | 0.960 | 1.116 | 0.601 |
| beef, canned (25.0% protein)..... | 0.292 | 1.104 | 1.308 | 2.048 | 2.184 | 0.620 | 0.316 | 1.028 | 0.848 | 1.388 | 1.612 | 0.868 |
| beef, dried or chipped (34.3% protein)..... | 0.401 | 1.515 | 1.795 | 2.810 | 2.996 | 0.851 | 0.434 | 1.410 | 1.163 | 1.904 | 2.212 | 1.191 |
| lamb carcass or side: | | | | | | | | | | | | |
| thin (17.1% protein)...... | 0.222 | 0.782 | 0.886 | 1.324 | 1.384 | 0.410 | 0.224 | 0.695 | 0.594 | 0.843 | 1.114 | 0.476 |
| medium fat (15.7% protein)..... | 0.203 | 0.718 | 0.814 | 1.216 | 1.271 | 0.377 | 0.206 | 0.638 | 0.545 | 0.774 | 1.022 | 0.437 |
| fat (13.0% protein)..... | 0.168 | 0.595 | 0.674 | 1.007 | 1.052 | 0.312 | 0.171 | 0.528 | 0.451 | 0.641 | 0.847 | 0.362 |
| lamb cuts, medium fat: | | | | | | | | | | | | |
| leg (18.0% protein)...... | 0.233 | 0.824 | 0.933 | 1.394 | 1.457 | 0.432 | 0.236 | 0.732 | 0.625 | 0.887 | 1.172 | 0.501 |
| rib (14.9% protein)...... | 0.193 | 0.682 | 0.772 | 1.154 | 1.206 | 0.358 | 0.195 | 0.606 | 0.517 | 0.734 | 0.970 | 0.415 |
| shoulder (15.6% protein)..... | 0.202 | 0.714 | 0.809 | 1.208 | 1.263 | 0.374 | 0.205 | 0.634 | 0.542 | 0.769 | 1.016 | 0.434 |
| pork, packer's carcass or side: | | | | | | | | | | | | |
| thin (14.1% protein)...... | 0.183 | 0.654 | 0.724 | 1.038 | 1.157 | 0.352 | 0.165 | 0.555 | 0.503 | 0.733 | 0.864 | 0.487 |
| medium fat (11.9% protein)..... | 0.154 | 0.552 | 0.611 | 0.876 | 0.977 | 0.297 | 0.139 | 0.408 | 0.425 | 0.619 | 0.729 | 0.411 |
| fat (9.8% protein)..... | 0.127 | 0.455 | 0.503 | 0.721 | 0.804 | 0.245 | 0.114 | 0.386 | 0.350 | 0.510 | 0.601 | 0.339 |
| pork cuts, medium fat, fresh: | | | | | | | | | | | | |
| ham (15.2% protein)...... | 0.197 | 0.705 | 0.781 | 1.119 | 1.248 | 0.379 | 0.178 | 0.598 | 0.542 | 0.790 | 0.931 | 0.525 |
| loin (16.4% protein)...... | 0.213 | 0.761 | 0.842 | 1.207 | 1.346 | 0.409 | 0.192 | 0.646 | 0.585 | 0.853 | 1.005 | 0.567 |
| miscellaneous lean cuts (14.5% protein)...... | 0.188 | 0.673 | 0.745 | 1.067 | 1.190 | 0.362 | 0.169 | 0.571 | 0.517 | 0.754 | 0.889 | 0.501 |

TABLE 40—*Continued*

| Protein Content, and Nitrogen Conversion Factor | Trypto-phan (Gm.) | Threo-nine (Gm.) | Iso-leucine (Gm.) | Leucine (Gm.) | Lysine (Gm.) | Methi-onine (Gm.) | Cystine (Gm.) | Phenyl-alanine (Gm.) | Tyro-sine (Gm.) | Valine (Gm.) | Argi-nine (Gm.) | Histi-dine (Gm.) |
|---|---|---|---|---|---|---|---|---|---|---|---|---|
| MEAT; POULTRY; FISH—*Continued* | | | | | | | | | | | | |
| pork, cured: | | | | | | | | | | | | |
| bacon, medium fat (9.1% protein) | 0.095 | 0.306 | 0.399 | 0.728 | 0.587 | 0.141 | 0.106 | 0.434 | 0.234 | 0.434 | 0.622 | 0.246 |
| fat back or salt pork (3.9% protein) | 0.006 | 0.141 | 0.110 | 0.367 | 0.317 | 0.055 | 0.043 | 0.157 | 0.052 | 0.168 | 0.379 | 0.035 |
| ham (16.9% protein) | 0.162 | 0.692 | 0.841 | 1.306 | 1.420 | 0.411 | 0.273 | 0.646 | 0.652 | 0.879 | 1.068 | 0.544 |
| luncheon meat: | | | | | | | | | | | | |
| boiled ham (22.8% protein) | 0.219 | 0.934 | 1.135 | 1.762 | 1.915 | 0.554 | 0.368 | 0.872 | 0.879 | 1.186 | 1.441 | 0.733 |
| canned, spiced (14.9% protein) | 0.143 | 0.610 | 0.741 | 1.151 | 1.252 | 0.362 | 0.241 | 0.570 | 0.575 | 0.775 | 0.942 | 0.479 |
| rabbit, domesticated, flesh only (21.0% protein) | ........ | 1.021 | 1.082 | 1.636 | 1.818 | 0.541 | ........ | 0.793 | ........ | 1.021 | 1.176 | 0.474 |
| veal, carcass or side: | | | | | | | | | | | | |
| thin (19.7% protein) | 0.258 | 0.854 | 1.040 | 1.444 | 1.645 | 0.451 | 0.233 | 0.801 | 0.709 | 1.018 | 1.283 | 0.634 |
| medium fat (19.1% protein) | 0.251 | 0.828 | 1.008 | 1.400 | 1.595 | 0.437 | 0.226 | 0.776 | 0.688 | 0.987 | 1.244 | 0.614 |
| fat (18.5% protein) | 0.243 | 0.802 | 0.977 | 1.356 | 1.545 | 0.423 | 0.219 | 0.752 | 0.666 | 0.956 | 1.205 | 0.595 |
| veal cuts, medium fat: | | | | | | | | | | | | |
| round (19.5% protein) | 0.256 | 0.846 | 1.030 | 1.429 | 1.629 | 0.446 | 0.231 | 0.792 | 0.702 | 1.008 | 1.270 | 0.627 |
| shoulder (19.4% protein) | 0.255 | 0.841 | 1.024 | 1.422 | 1.620 | 0.444 | 0.230 | 0.788 | 0.698 | 1.003 | 1.263 | 0.624 |
| stew meat (18.3% protein) | 0.240 | 0.793 | 0.966 | 1.341 | 1.528 | 0.419 | 0.217 | 0.744 | 0.659 | 0.946 | 1.192 | 0.589 |
| *Poultry (Protein, N×6.25):* | | | | | | | | | | | | |
| chicken, flesh only: | | | | | | | | | | | | |
| broilers or fryers (20.6% protein) | 0.250 | 0.877 | 1.088 | 1.490 | 1.810 | 0.537 | 0.277 | 0.811 | 0.725 | 1.012 | 1.302 | 0.593 |
| hens (21.3% protein) | 0.259 | 0.907 | 1.125 | 1.540 | 1.871 | 0.556 | 0.286 | 0.838 | 0.750 | 1.046 | 1.346 | 0.613 |
| ducks, domesticated, flesh only (21.4% protein) | ........ | 0.935 | 1.109 | 1.657 | 1.842 | 0.531 | ........ | 0.842 | ........ | 1.027 | 1.301 | 0.486 |
| turkey, flesh only (24.0% protein) | ........ | 1.014 | 1.260 | 1.836 | 2.173 | 0.664 | 0.330 | 0.960 | ........ | 1.187 | 1.513 | 0.649 |

TABLE 40—Continued

| Protein Content, and Nitrogen Conversion Factor | Trypto-phan (Gm.) | Threo-nine (Gm.) | Iso-leucine (Gm.) | Leucine (Gm.) | Lysine (Gm.) | Methi-onine (Gm.) | Cystine (Gm.) | Phenyl-alanine (Gm.) | Tyro-sine (Gm.) | Valine (Gm.) | Argi-nine (Gm.) | Histi-dine (Gm.) |
|---|---|---|---|---|---|---|---|---|---|---|---|---|
| MEAT; POULTRY; FISH—*Continued* | | | | | | | | | | | | |
| *Fish and shellfish* (*Protein, N×6.25*): | | | | | | | | | | | | |
| bluefish (20.5% protein) | 0.203 | 0.889 | 1.040 | 1.548 | 1.797 | 0.597 | 0.276 | 0.761 | 0.554 | 1.092 | 1.155 | ...... |
| cod: | | | | | | | | | | | | |
|   fresh (16.5% protein) | 0.164 | 0.715 | 0.837 | 1.246 | 1.447 | 0.480 | 0.222 | 0.612 | 0.446 | 0.879 | 0.929 | ...... |
|   dried (81.8% protein) | 0.811 | 3.547 | 4.149 | 6.178 | 7.172 | 2.382 | 1.099 | 3.036 | 2.212 | 4.358 | 4.607 | ...... |
| croaker (17.8% protein) | 0.177 | 0.772 | 0.903 | 1.344 | 1.561 | 0.518 | 0.239 | 0.661 | 0.481 | 0.948 | 1.002 | ...... |
| eel (18.6% protein) | 0.185 | 0.806 | 0.943 | 1.405 | 1.631 | 0.542 | 0.250 | 0.690 | 0.503 | 0.991 | 1.048 | ...... |
| flounder (14.9% protein) | 0.148 | 0.646 | 0.756 | 1.125 | 1.306 | 0.434 | 0.200 | 0.553 | 0.403 | 0.794 | 0.839 | ...... |
| haddock (18.2% protein) | 0.181 | 0.789 | 0.923 | 1.374 | 1.596 | 0.530 | 0.245 | 0.676 | 0.492 | 0.970 | 1.025 | ...... |
| halibut (18.6% protein) | 0.185 | 0.806 | 0.943 | 1.495 | 1.631 | 0.542 | 0.250 | 0.690 | 0.503 | 0.991 | 1.048 | ...... |
| herring: | | | | | | | | | | | | |
|   Atlantic (18.3% protein) | 0.182 | 0.793 | 0.928 | 1.382 | 1.605 | 0.533 | 0.246 | 0.679 | 0.495 | 0.975 | 1.031 | ...... |
|   lake (18.5% protein) | 0.184 | 0.802 | 0.938 | 1.397 | 1.622 | 0.539 | 0.249 | 0.687 | 0.500 | 0.986 | 1.042 | ...... |
|   Pacific (16.6% protein) | 0.165 | 0.720 | 0.842 | 1.254 | 1.455 | 0.483 | 0.223 | 0.616 | 0.449 | 0.884 | 0.935 | ...... |
| mackerel: | | | | | | | | | | | | |
|   raw, common Atlantic (18.7% protein) | 0.186 | 0.811 | 0.948 | 1.412 | 1.640 | 0.545 | 0.251 | 0.694 | 0.506 | 0.996 | 1.053 | ...... |
|   canned, solids and liquid: | | | | | | | | | | | | |
|     Atlantic (19.3% protein) | 0.191 | 0.837 | 0.979 | 1.458 | 1.692 | 0.562 | 0.259 | 0.716 | 0.522 | 1.028 | 1.087 | ...... |
|     Pacific (21.1% protein) | 0.209 | 0.915 | 1.070 | 1.593 | 1.850 | 0.614 | 0.284 | 0.783 | 0.571 | 1.124 | 1.188 | ...... |
| salmon: | | | | | | | | | | | | |
|   raw, Pacific (Chinook or King) (17.4% protein) | 0.173 | 0.754 | 0.883 | 1.314 | 1.526 | 0.507 | 0.234 | 0.646 | 0.470 | 0.927 | 0.980 | ...... |
|   canned, solids and liquid (sockeye or red) (20.2% protein) | 0.200 | 0.876 | 1.025 | 1.526 | 1.771 | 0.588 | 0.271 | 0.750 | 0.546 | 1.076 | 1.138 | ...... |
| sardines, canned, solids and liquid: | | | | | | | | | | | | |
|   Atlantic type (21.1% protein) | 0.209 | 0.915 | 1.070 | 1.593 | 1.850 | 0.614 | 0.284 | 0.783 | 0.571 | 1.124 | 1.188 | ...... |
|   Pacific type (17.7% protein) | 0.176 | 0.767 | 0.898 | 1.337 | 1.552 | 0.515 | 0.238 | 0.657 | 0.479 | 0.943 | 0.997 | ...... |
| shrimp, canned, solids and liquid (18.7% protein) | 0.186 | 0.811 | 0.948 | 1.412 | 1.640 | 0.545 | 0.251 | 0.694 | 0.506 | 0.996 | 1.053 | ...... |

## TABLE 40—Continued

| Protein Content, and Nitrogen Conversion Factor | Trypto-phan (Gm.) | Threo-nine (Gm.) | Iso-leucine (Gm.) | Leucine (Gm.) | Lysine (Gm.) | Methi-onine (Gm.) | Cystine (Gm.) | Phenyl-alanine (Gm.) | Tyro-sine (Gm.) | Valine (Gm.) | Argi-nine (Gm.) | Histi-dine (Gm.) |
|---|---|---|---|---|---|---|---|---|---|---|---|---|
| **MEAT; POULTRY; FISH—***Continued* | | | | | | | | | | | | |
| *Products from meat, poultry, and fish (Protein, N×6.25):* | | | | | | | | | | | | |
| brains (10.4% protein) | 0.138 | 0.494 | 0.504 | 0.845 | 0.760 | 0.220 | 0.145 | 0.506 | 0.433 | 0.536 | 0.614 | 0.278 |
| chitterlings (8.6% protein) | 0.094 | 0.398 | 0.308 | 0.457 | 0.670 | 0.193 | 0.109 | 0.359 | 0.228 | 0.462 | 1.406 | 0.169 |
| fish flour (76.0% protein) | 0.754 | 4.378 | 4.232 | 6.189 | 7.381 | 2.019 | .... | 2.845 | .... | 3.916 | 5.204 | 1.289 |
| gelatin (85.6% protein, N×5.55) | 0.006 | 1.912 | 1.357 | 2.930 | 4.226 | 0.787 | 0.077 | 2.036 | 0.401 | 2.421 | 7.866 | 0.771 |
| gizzard, chicken (23.1% protein) | 0.207 | 1.072 | 1.094 | 1.689 | 1.567 | 0.554 | 0.218 | 0.968 | 0.680 | 1.116 | 1.741 | 0.480 |
| heart: | | | | | | | | | | | | |
| beef or pork (16.9% protein) | 0.219 | 0.776 | 0.857 | 1.509 | 1.387 | 0.403 | 0.168 | 0.765 | 0.627 | 0.973 | 1.068 | 0.433 |
| chicken (20.5% protein) | 0.266 | 0.941 | 1.040 | 1.830 | 1.683 | 0.489 | 0.203 | 0.928 | 0.761 | 1.181 | 1.296 | 0.525 |
| kidney: | | | | | | | | | | | | |
| beef (15.0% protein) | 0.221 | 0.665 | 0.730 | 1.301 | 1.087 | 0.307 | 0.182 | 0.706 | 0.557 | 0.876 | 0.934 | 0.377 |
| pork (16.3% protein) | 0.240 | 0.722 | 0.793 | 1.414 | 1.181 | 0.334 | 0.198 | 0.767 | 0.605 | 0.952 | 1.015 | 0.409 |
| sheep (16.6% protein) | 0.244 | 0.736 | 0.807 | 1.440 | 1.203 | 0.340 | 0.202 | 0.781 | 0.616 | 0.969 | 1.033 | 0.417 |
| liver: | | | | | | | | | | | | |
| beef or pork (19.7% protein) | 0.296 | 0.936 | 1.031 | 1.819 | 1.475 | 0.463 | 0.243 | 0.993 | 0.738 | 1.239 | 1.201 | 0.523 |
| calf (19.0% protein) | 0.286 | 0.903 | 0.994 | 1.754 | 1.423 | 0.447 | 0.234 | 0.958 | 0.711 | 1.195 | 1.158 | 0.505 |
| chicken (22.1% protein) | 0.332 | 1.050 | 1.156 | 2.040 | 1.655 | 0.520 | 0.272 | 1.114 | 0.827 | 1.390 | 1.347 | 0.587 |
| sheep or lamb (21.0% protein) | 0.316 | 0.998 | 1.099 | 1.939 | 1.572 | 0.494 | 0.259 | 1.058 | 0.786 | 1.320 | 1.280 | 0.558 |
| pancreas: | | | | | | | | | | | | |
| beef (13.5% protein) | 0.175 | 0.626 | 0.683 | 1.054 | 0.996 | 0.244 | .... | 0.562 | 0.590 | 0.724 | 0.771 | 0.266 |
| pork (14.5% protein) | 0.188 | 0.673 | 0.733 | 1.132 | 1.070 | 0.262 | .... | 0.603 | 0.633 | 0.777 | 0.828 | 0.285 |
| pork or beef, canned (14.3% protein) | 0.151 | 0.618 | 0.730 | 1.190 | 1.345 | 0.327 | 0.261 | 0.579 | 0.570 | 0.810 | 1.050 | 0.460 |
| potted meat (16.1% protein) | 0.149 | 0.662 | 0.641 | 1.203 | 1.061 | 0.361 | .... | 0.641 | .... | 0.943 | 1.002 | 0.322 |

TABLE 40—*Continued*

| Protein Content, and Nitrogen Conversion Factor | Tryptophan (Gm.) | Threonine (Gm.) | Isoleucine (Gm.) | Leucine (Gm.) | Lysine (Gm.) | Methionine (Gm.) | Cystine (Gm.) | Phenylalanine (Gm.) | Tyrosine (Gm.) | Valine (Gm.) | Arginine (Gm.) | Histidine (Gm.) |
|---|---|---|---|---|---|---|---|---|---|---|---|---|
| MEAT; POULTRY; FISH—*Continued* | | | | | | | | | | | | |
| sausage: | | | | | | | | | | | | |
| Bologna (14.8% protein) | 0.126 | 0.606 | 0.718 | 1.061 | 1.191 | 0.313 | 0.185 | 0.540 | 0.481 | 0.744 | 1.028 | 0.398 |
| Braunschweiger (15.4% protein) | 0.172 | 0.668 | 0.754 | 1.291 | 1.200 | 0.300 | 0.187 | 0.700 | 0.471 | 0.956 | 0.954 | 0.458 |
| frankfurters (14.2% protein) | 0.120 | 0.582 | 0.688 | 1.018 | 1.143 | 0.300 | 0.177 | 0.518 | 0.461 | 0.713 | 0.986 | 0.382 |
| head cheese (15.0% protein) | 0.079 | 0.418 | 0.509 | 0.946 | 0.907 | 0.250 | 0.209 | 0.569 | 0.569 | 0.617 | 1.075 | 0.278 |
| liverwurst (16.7% protein) | 0.187 | 0.724 | 0.818 | 1.400 | 1.301 | 0.347 | 0.203 | 0.759 | 0.510 | 1.037 | 1.034 | 0.497 |
| pork, links or bulk, raw (10.8% protein) | 0.092 | 0.442 | 0.524 | 0.774 | 0.869 | 0.228 | 0.135 | 0.394 | 0.351 | 0.543 | 0.750 | 0.290 |
| pork, bulk, canned (15.4% protein) | 0.131 | 0.631 | 0.747 | 1.104 | 1.239 | 0.325 | 0.192 | 0.562 | 0.500 | 0.774 | 1.069 | 0.414 |
| salami (23.9% protein) | 0.203 | 0.979 | 1.159 | 1.713 | 1.923 | 0.505 | 0.298 | 0.872 | 0.776 | 1.201 | 1.660 | 0.642 |
| Vienna sausage, canned (15.8% protein) | 0.134 | 0.647 | 0.766 | 1.133 | 1.272 | 0.334 | 0.197 | 0.576 | 0.513 | 0.794 | 1.097 | 0.425 |
| tongue: | | | | | | | | | | | | |
| beef (16.4% protein) | 0.197 | 0.708 | 0.792 | 1.286 | 1.364 | 0.357 | 0.207 | 0.661 | 0.548 | 0.840 | 1.065 | 0.412 |
| pork (16.8% protein) | 0.202 | 0.726 | 0.812 | 1.317 | 1.398 | 0.366 | 0.212 | 0.677 | 0.562 | 0.860 | 1.091 | 0.422 |
| veal and pork loaf, canned (17.2% protein) | 0.198 | 0.627 | 0.859 | 1.236 | 1.258 | 0.418 | 0.209 | 0.619 | 0.468 | 0.958 | 0.916 | 0.388 |
| LEGUMES (DRY SEED); COMMON NUTS; OTHER NUTS AND DRY SEEDS; THEIR PRODUCTS: | | | | | | | | | | | | |
| *Legume seeds and their products:* | | | | | | | | | | | | |
| beans (*Phaseolus vulgaris*) (N× 6.25): | | | | | | | | | | | | |
| pinto and red Mexican (23.0% protein) | 0.213 | 0.997 | 1.306 | 1.976 | 1.708 | 0.232 | 0.228 | 1.270 | 0.887 | 1.395 | 1.384 | 0.655 |
| red kidney: | | | | | | | | | | | | |
| raw (23.1% protein) | 0.214 | 1.002 | 1.312 | 1.985 | 1.715 | 0.233 | 0.229 | 1.275 | 0.891 | 1.401 | 1.390 | 0.658 |
| canned, solids and liquid (5.7% protein) | 0.053 | 0.247 | 0.324 | 0.490 | 0.423 | 0.057 | 0.057 | 0.315 | 0.220 | 0.346 | 0.343 | 0.162 |

TABLE 40—*Continued*

| Protein Content, and Nitrogen Conversion Factor | Trypto-phan (Gm.) | Threo-nine (Gm.) | Iso-leucine (Gm.) | Leucine (Gm.) | Lysine (Gm.) | Methi-onine (Gm.) | Cystine (Gm.) | Phenyl-alanine (Gm.) | Tyro-sine (Gm.) | Valine (Gm.) | Argi-nine (Gm.) | Histi-dine (Gm.) |
|---|---|---|---|---|---|---|---|---|---|---|---|---|
| LEGUMES; SEEDS; NUTS—*Continued* other common beans including navy, peabean, white marrow: | | | | | | | | | | | | |
| raw (21.4% protein) ........ | 0.199 | 0.928 | 1.216 | 1.839 | 1.589 | 0.216 | 0.212 | 1.181 | 0.825 | 1.298 | 1.287 | 0.609 |
| baked with pork, canned (5.8% protein) ........ | 0.057 | 0.274 | 0.291 | 0.486 | 0.354 | 0.059 | 0.018 | 0.333 | 0.165 | 0.312 | 0.251 | 0.186 |
| black gram, raw (23.6% protein, N×6.25) ........ | 0.242 | 0.801 | 1.390 | 2.062 | 1.510 | 0.332 | 0.287 | 1.242 | 0.551 | 1.450 | 1.552 | 0.559 |
| broadbeans, raw (25.4% protein, N×6.25) ........ | 0.236 | 0.829 | 1.593 | 2.211 | 1.426 | 0.106 | 0.179 | 1.057 | 0.687 | 1.276 | 1.780 | 0.748 |
| chickpeas (20.8% protein, N±6.25) | 0.170 | 0.739 | 1.195 | 1.538 | 1.434 | 0.276 | 0.296 | 1.012 | 0.692 | 1.025 | 1.551 | 0.559 |
| cowpeas (22.9% protein, N×6.25) .. | 0.220 | 0.901 | 1.110 | 1.715 | 1.491 | 0.352 | 0.297 | 1.198 | 0.678 | 1.293 | 1.473 | 0.692 |
| dolichos, twinflower (21.6% protein, N×6.25) | 0.221 | 0.836 | 1.448 | 1.707 | 1.700 | 0.294 | 0.480 | 1.486 | 0.560 | 1.286 | 1.230 | 0.650 |
| lentils, whole (25.0% protein, N× 6.25) | 0.216 | 0.896 | 1.316 | 1.760 | 1.528 | 0.180 | 0.204 | 1.104 | 0.664 | 1.360 | 1.908 | 0.548 |
| lima beans (20.7% protein, N×6.25) | 0.195 | 0.980 | 1.199 | 1.722 | 1.378 | 0.331 | 0.311 | 1.222 | 0.543 | 1.298 | 1.315 | 0.669 |
| lupine (32.3% protein, N×6.25) ... | ........ | 1.101 | 1.618 | 1.964 | 1.447 | 0.114 | ........ | 1.271 | ........ | 1.328 | 2.718 | 0.811 |
| moth beans (24.4% protein, N× 6.25) | 0.164 | ........ | 1.093 | 1.484 | 1.202 | 0.191 | 0.109 | 1.003 | 1.245 | 0.695 | ........ | 0.722 |
| mung beans (24.4% protein, 6.25) | 0.180 | 0.765 | 1.351 | 2.202 | 1.667 | 0.265 | 0.152 | 1.167 | 0.390 | 1.444 | 1.370 | 0.543 |
| peanuts (26.9% protein, N×5.46).. | 0.340 | 0.828 | 1.266 | 1.872 | 1.099 | 0.271 | 0.463 | 1.557 | 1.104 | 1.532 | 3.296 | 0.749 |
| peanut flour (51.2% protein, N× 5.46) | 0.647 | 1.575 | 2.410 | 3.563 | 2.091 | 0.516 | 0.881 | 2.963 | 2.100 | 2.916 | 6.273 | 1.425 |
| peanut butter (26.1% protein, N× 5.46) | 0.330 | 0.803 | 1.228 | 1.816 | 1.066 | 0.263 | 0.449 | 1.510 | 1.071 | 1.487 | 3.198 | 0.727 |

199

TABLE 40—Continued

| Protein Content, and Nitrogen Conversion Factor | Trypto-phan (Gm.) | Threo-nine (Gm.) | Iso-leucine (Gm.) | Leucine (Gm.) | Lysine (Gm.) | Methi-onine (Gm.) | Cystine (Gm.) | Phenyl-alanine (Gm.) | Tyro-sine (Gm.) | Valine (Gm.) | Argi-nine (Gm.) | Histi-dine (Gm.) |
|---|---|---|---|---|---|---|---|---|---|---|---|---|
| LEGUMES; SEEDS; NUTS—*Continued* | | | | | | | | | | | | |
| peas (*Pisum sativum*) (N×6.25): | | | | | | | | | | | | |
| entire seeds (23.8% protein) | 0.251 | 0.918 | 1.340 | 1.969 | 1.744 | 0.286 | 0.308 | 1.200 | 0.960 | 1.333 | 2.102 | 0.651 |
| split (24.5% protein) | 0.259 | 0.945 | 1.380 | 2.027 | 1.795 | 0.294 | 0.318 | 1.235 | 0.988 | 1.372 | 2.164 | 0.670 |
| pigeonpeas, without seed coat (21.9% protein, N×6.25) | 0.119 | 0.834 | 1.346 | 1.717 | 1.580 | 0.256 | 0.308 | 1.875 | 0.725 | 1.153 | 1.489 | 0.617 |
| soybeans, whole (34.9% protein, N×5.71) | 0.526 | 1.504 | 2.054 | 2.946 | 2.414 | 0.513 | 0.678 | 1.889 | 1.216 | 2.005 | 2.763 | 0.911 |
| soybean flour, flakes, and grits (protein, N×5.71): | | | | | | | | | | | | |
| low fat (44.7% protein) | 0.673 | 1.926 | 2.630 | 3.773 | 3.092 | 0.658 | 0.869 | 2.419 | 1.558 | 2.568 | 3.538 | 1.166 |
| medium fat (42.5% protein) | 0.640 | 1.831 | 2.501 | 3.588 | 2.940 | 0.625 | 0.826 | 2.300 | 1.481 | 2.441 | 3.364 | 1.109 |
| full fat (35.9% protein) | 0.541 | 1.547 | 2.112 | 3.030 | 2.483 | 0.528 | 0.698 | 1.943 | 1.251 | 2.062 | 2.842 | 0.937 |
| soybean curd (7.0% protein, N×5.71) | …… | …… | …… | …… | …… | 0.081 | 0.091 | …… | …… | …… | …… | …… |
| soybean milk (3.4% protein, N×5.71) | 0.051 | 0.176 | 0.175 | 0.395 | 0.269 | 0.054 | 0.071 | 0.195 | 0.193 | 0.186 | 0.302 | 0.121 |
| vetch (28.8% protein, N×6.25) | 0.203 | 0.899 | 2.198 | 2.290 | 1.898 | 0.346 | 0.336 | 1.014 | 0.369 | 1.442 | 2.249 | 0.659 |
| *Common nuts and their products:* | | | | | | | | | | | | |
| almonds (18.6 protein, N×5.18) | 0.176 | 0.610 | 0.873 | 1.454 | 0.582 | 0.259 | 0.377 | 1.146 | 0.618 | 1.124 | 2.729 | 0.517 |
| Brazil nuts (14.4% protein, N×5.46) | 0.187 | 0.422 | 0.593 | 1.129 | 0.443 | 0.941 | 0.504 | 0.617 | 0.483 | 0.823 | 2.247 | 0.367 |
| cashews (18.5% protein, N×5.30) | 0.471 | 0.737 | 1.222 | 1.522 | 0.792 | 0.353 | 0.527 | 0.946 | 0.712 | 1.592 | 2.098 | 0.415 |
| coconut (3.4% protein, N×5.30) | 0.033 | 0.129 | 0.180 | 0.269 | 0.152 | 0.071 | 0.062 | 0.174 | 0.101 | 0.212 | 0.486 | 0.069 |
| coconut meal (20.3% protein, N×5.30) | 0.199 | 0.770 | 1.076 | 1.605 | 0.908 | 0.421 | 0.372 | 1.038 | 0.605 | 1.268 | 2.899 | 0.414 |
| filberts (12.7% protein, N×5.30) | 0.211 | 0.415 | 0.853 | 0.939 | 0.417 | 0.139 | 0.165 | 0.537 | 0.434 | 0.934 | 2.171 | 0.288 |
| peanuts. *See* Legumes. | | | | | | | | | | | | |
| pecans (9.4% protein, N×5.30) | 0.138 | 0.389 | 0.553 | 0.773 | 0.435 | 0.153 | 0.216 | 0.564 | 0.316 | 0.525 | 1.185 | 0.273 |
| walnuts (English or Persian) (15.0% protein, N×5.30) | 0.175 | 0.589 | 0.767 | 1.228 | 0.441 | 0.306 | 0.320 | 0.767 | 0.583 | 0.974 | 2.287 | 0.405 |

TABLE 40—*Continued*

| Protein Content, and Nitrogen Conversion Factor | Trypto-phan (Gm.) | Threo-nine (Gm.) | Iso-leucine (Gm.) | Leucine (Gm.) | Lysine (Gm.) | Methi-onine (Gm.) | Cystine (Gm.) | Phenyl-alanine (Gm.) | Tyro-sine (Gm.) | Valine (Gm.) | Argi-nine (Gm.) | Histi-dine (Gm.) |
|---|---|---|---|---|---|---|---|---|---|---|---|---|
| LEGUMES; SEEDS; NUTS—*Continued* | | | | | | | | | | | | |
| *Other nuts and seeds and their products* | | | | | | | | | | | | |
| *(Protein N×5:30):* | | | | | | | | | | | | |
| acorns (10.4% protein) | 0.126 | 0.434 | 0.561 | 0.808 | 0.636 | 0.139 | 0.184 | 0.473 | ...... | 0.718 | 0.722 | 0.251 |
| amaranth (14.6% protein) | 0.149 | 0.832 | 0.882 | 1.209 | 1.074 | 0.372 | 0.521 | 1.141 | ...... | 0.849 | 1.747 | 0.441 |
| balsam pear seed meal (41.9% protein) | ...... | ...... | ...... | ...... | 1.265 | ...... | 0.142 | 2.609 | 0.617 | ...... | 5.914 | 0.917 |
| breadnut tree, Ramon (9.6% protein) | 0.261 | 0.373 | 0.543 | 1.041 | 0.418 | 0.056 | ...... | 0.453 | ...... | 0.927 | 0.884 | 0.147 |
| Chinese tallow tree-nut flour (57.6% protein) | 0.837 | 2.174 | 3.510 | 4.347 | 1.587 | 0.924 | 0.696 | 2.847 | 2.011 | 4.510 | 10.031 | 1.587 |
| chocolate tree, Nicaragua (38.5% protein) | 0.588 | 1.496 | 2.092 | 3.952 | 2.223 | 0.276 | ...... | 2.630 | ...... | 2.404 | 4.220 | 0.683 |
| cottonseed flour and meal (42.3% protein) | 0.591 | 1.764 | 1.884 | 2.945 | 2.139 | 0.686 | 0.814 | 2.610 | 1.365 | 2.458 | 5.603 | 1.325 |
| earpod tree, Guanacaste (34.1% protein) | 0.444 | 1.165 | 2.213 | 4.581 | 1.930 | 0.360 | ...... | 1.325 | ...... | 1.570 | 2.857 | 1.004 |
| lead tree (24.1% protein) | 0.191 | 0.828 | 1.651 | 1.787 | 1.164 | 0.055 | ...... | 0.855 | ...... | 0.864 | 2.410 | 0.564 |
| pumpkin seed (30.9% protein) | 0.560 | 0.933 | 1.737 | 2.437 | 1.411 | 0.577 | ...... | 1.749 | ...... | 1.679 | 4.810 | 0.711 |
| safflower seed meal (42.1% protein) | 0.675 | 1.462 | 1.914 | 2.740 | 1.525 | 0.731 | ...... | 2.605 | ...... | 2.446 | 4.623 | 0.985 |
| sesame: | | | | | | | | | | | | |
| seed (19.3% protein) | 0.331 | 0.707 | 0.951 | 1.679 | 0.583 | 0.637 | 0.495 | 1.457 | 0.951 | 0.885 | 1.992 | 0.441 |
| meal (33.4% protein) | 0.573 | 1.223 | 1.645 | 2.905 | 1.008 | 1.103 | 0.857 | 2.521 | 1.645 | 1.531 | 3.447 | 0.763 |
| sunflower: | | | | | | | | | | | | |
| kernel (23.0% protein) | 0.343 | 0.911 | 1.276 | 1.736 | 0.868 | 0.443 | 0.464 | 1.220 | 0.647 | 1.354 | 2.370 | 0.586 |
| meal (39.5% protein) | 0.589 | 1.565 | 2.191 | 2.981 | 1.491 | 0.760 | 0.797 | 2.094 | 1.110 | 2.325 | 4.069 | 1.006 |

TABLE 40—Continued

| Protein Content, and Nitrogen Conversion Factor | Trypto-phan (Gm.) | Threo-nine (Gm.) | Iso-leucine (Gm.) | Leucine (Gm.) | Lysine (Gm.) | Methi-onine (Gm.) | Cystine (Gm.) | Phenyl-alanine (Gm.) | Tyro-sine (Gm.) | Valine (Gm.) | Argi-nine (Gm.) | Histi-dine (Gm.) |
|---|---|---|---|---|---|---|---|---|---|---|---|---|
| **GRAINS AND THEIR PRODUCTS** | | | | | | | | | | | | |
| Barley (12.8% protein, N×5.83) | 0.160 | 0.433 | 0.545 | 0.889 | 0.433 | 0.184 | 0.257 | 0.661 | 0.466 | 0.643 | 0.659 | 0.239 |
| Bread, white (4% non-fat dry milk, flour basis) (8.5% protein, N×5.70) | 0.091 | 0.282 | 0.429 | 0.668 | 0.225 | 0.142 | 0.200 | 0.465 | 0.243 | 0.435 | 0.340 | 0.192 |
| Buckwheat flour: | | | | | | | | | | | | |
| dark (11.7% protein, N×6.25) | 0.165 | 0.461 | 0.440 | 0.683 | 0.687 | 0.206 | 0.228 | 0.442 | 0.240 | 0.607 | 0.930 | 0.256 |
| light (6.4% protein, N×6.25) | 0.090 | 0.252 | 0.241 | 0.374 | 0.376 | 0.113 | 0.125 | 0.242 | 0.131 | 0.332 | 0.509 | 0.140 |
| Cañihua (14.7% protein, N×6.25) | 0.118 | 0.706 | 1.000 | 0.851 | 0.882 | 0.263 | 0.162 | 0.529 | 0.294 | 0.677 | 1.162 | 0.367 |
| Cereal combinations: | | | | | | | | | | | | |
| corn and soy grits (18.0% protein, N×6.25) | 0.161 | 0.792 | 0.841 | 1.656 | 0.772 | 0.271 | 0.311 | 0.832 | 0.562 | 1.054 | 0.982 | 0.472 |
| infant food, precooked, mixed cereals with non-fat dry milk and yeast (19.4% protein, N×6.25) | 0.118 | | | | 0.273 | 0.310 | 0.137 | 0.543 | 0.447 | | 0.447 | 0.233 |
| oat-corn-rye mixture, puffed (14.5% protein, N×5.83) | 0.172 | 0.545 | 0.841 | 1.368 | 0.343 | 0.388 | 0.234 | 0.933 | 0.622 | 0.900 | 0.776 | 0.326 |
| Corn, field (10.0% protein, N×6.25) | 0.061 | 0.398 | 0.462 | 1.296 | 0.288 | 0.186 | 0.130 | 0.454 | 0.611 | 0.510 | 0.352 | 0.206 |
| Corn flour (7.8% protein, N×6.25) | 0.047 | 0.311 | 0.361 | 1.011 | 0.225 | 0.145 | 0.101 | 0.354 | 0.477 | 0.398 | 0.275 | 0.161 |
| Corn grits (8.7% protein, N×6.25) | 0.053 | 0.347 | 0.402 | 1.128 | 0.251 | 0.161 | 0.113 | 0.395 | 0.532 | 0.444 | 0.306 | 0.180 |
| Cornmeal: | | | | | | | | | | | | |
| whole ground (9.2% protein, N×6.25) | 0.056 | 0.367 | 0.425 | 1.192 | 0.265 | 0.171 | 0.119 | 0.418 | 0.562 | 0.470 | 0.324 | 0.190 |
| de-germed (7.9% protein, N×6.25) | 0.048 | 0.315 | 0.365 | 1.024 | 0.228 | 0.147 | 0.102 | 0.359 | 0.483 | 0.403 | 0.278 | 0.163 |
| Corn products: | | | | | | | | | | | | |
| flakes (8.1% protein, N×6.25) | 0.052 | 0.275 | 0.306 | 1.047 | 0.154 | 0.135 | 0.152 | 0.354 | 0.283 | 0.386 | 0.231 | 0.226 |
| germ (14.5% protein, N×6.25) | 0.144 | 0.622 | 0.578 | 1.030 | 0.791 | 0.232 | 0.130 | 0.483 | 0.343 | 0.789 | 1.134 | 0.464 |
| gluten (10.0% protein, N×6.25) | 0.059 | 0.344 | 0.443 | 1.563 | 0.179 | 0.282 | 0.141 | 0.558 | 0.582 | 0.512 | 0.322 | 0.200 |
| hominy (8.7% protein, N×6.25) | 0.084 | 0.316 | 0.349 | 0.810 | 0.358 | 0.099 | | 0.333 | 0.331 | 0.398 | 0.444 | 0.203 |
| masa (2.8% protein, N×6.25) | 0.010 | | | | 0.103 | 0.108 | 0.030 | | | | | |
| pozol (5.9% protein, N×6.25) | 0.042 | 0.336 | 0.304 | 0.591 | 0.234 | 0.087 | 0.087 | 0.254 | | 0.267 | 0.197 | 0.122 |
| tortilla (5.8% protein, N×6.25) | 0.031 | 0.235 | 0.345 | 0.939 | 0.145 | 0.111 | | 0.252 | | 0.304 | 0.223 | 0.128 |
| zein (16.1% protein, N×6.25) | 0.010 | 0.495 | 0.822 | 3.184 | | 0.281 | 0.162 | 1.664 | 0.981 | 0.654 | 0.286 | 0.216 |
| Job's tears (13.8% protein, N×5.83) | 0.066 | 0.620 | 1.065 | 3.506 | 0.362 | 0.459 | 0.265 | 0.703 | | | 0.518 | 0.317 |

TABLE 40—*Continued*

| Protein Content, and Nitrogen Conversion Factor | Trypto-phan (Gm.) | Threo-nine (Gm.) | Iso-leucine (Gm.) | Leucine (Gm.) | Lysine (Gm.) | Methi-onine (Gm.) | Cystine (Gm.) | Phenyl-alanine (Gm.) | Tyro-sine (Gm.) | Valine (Gm.) | Argi-nine (Gm.) | Histi-dine (Gm.) |
|---|---|---|---|---|---|---|---|---|---|---|---|---|
| **GRAINS AND PRODUCTS—*Continued*** | | | | | | | | | | | | |
| Millets: | | | | | | | | | | | | |
| foxtail millet (9.7% protein, N×5.83) | 0.103 | 0.323 | 0.790 | 1.737 | 0.218 | 0.291 | ..... | 0.697 | ..... | 0.717 | 0.374 | 0.218 |
| little millet (7.2% protein, N×5.83) | 0.047 | 0.262 | 0.517 | 0.841 | 0.138 | 0.178 | ..... | 0.370 | ..... | 0.471 | 0.363 | 0.147 |
| pearl millet (11.4% protein, N×5.83) | 0.248 | 0.456 | 0.635 | 1.746 | 0.383 | 0.270 | 0.152 | 0.506 | ..... | 0.682 | 0.524 | 0.240 |
| ragimillet (6.2% protein, N×5.83) | 0.085 | 0.270 | 0.398 | 0.620 | 0.202 | 0.270 | 0.187 | 0.263 | ..... | 0.473 | 0.100 | 0.079 |
| Oatmeal and rolled oats (14.2% protein, N×5.83) | 0.183 | 0.470 | 0.733 | 1.065 | 0.521 | 0.209 | 0.309 | 0.758 | 0.524 | 0.845 | 0.935 | 0.261 |
| Quinoa (11.0% protein, N×6.25) | 0.120 | 0.523 | 0.722 | 0.781 | 0.729 | 0.278 | 0.107 | 0.394 | 0.253 | 0.447 | 0.820 | 0.297 |
| Rice: | | | | | | | | | | | | |
| brown (7.5% protein, N×5.95) | 0.081 | 0.294 | 0.352 | 0.646 | 0.296 | 0.135 | 0.102 | 0.377 | 0.343 | 0.524 | 0.432 | 0.126 |
| white and converted (7.6% protein, N×5.95) | 0.082 | 0.298 | 0.356 | 0.655 | 0.300 | 0.137 | 0.103 | 0.382 | 0.347 | 0.531 | 0.438 | 0.128 |
| Rice products: | | | | | | | | | | | | |
| flakes or puffed (5.9% protein, N×5.95) | 0.046 | ..... | ..... | ..... | 0.056 | ..... | 0.044 | 0.286 | 0.124 | ..... | 0.137 | 0.137 |
| germ (14.2% protein, N×5.95) | 0.270 | 2.177 | 0.630 | 0.838 | 1.707 | 0.420 | 0.169 | 0.750 | 0.929 | 0.938 | 1.559 | 0.430 |
| Rye (12.1% protein, N×5.83) | 0.137 | 0.448 | 0.515 | 0.813 | 0.494 | 0.191 | 0.241 | 0.571 | 0.390 | 0.631 | 0.591 | 0.276 |
| Rye flour: | | | | | | | | | | | | |
| light (9.4% protein, N×5.83) | 0.106 | 0.348 | 0.400 | 0.632 | 0.384 | 0.148 | 0.187 | 0.443 | 0.303 | 0.490 | 0.459 | 0.214 |
| medium (11.4% protein, N×5.83) | 0.129 | 0.422 | 0.485 | 0.766 | 0.465 | 0.180 | 0.227 | 0.538 | 0.368 | 0.594 | 0.557 | 0.260 |
| Sorghum (11.0% protein, N×6.25) | 0.123 | 0.394 | 0.598 | 1.707 | 0.299 | 0.190 | 0.183 | 0.547 | 0.303 | 0.628 | 0.417 | 0.211 |
| Teosinte (22.0% protein, N×6.25) | 0.049 | ..... | ..... | ..... | 0.348 | 0.496 | ..... | ..... | ..... | ..... | ..... | ..... |
| Wheat, whole grain: | | | | | | | | | | | | |
| hard red spring (14.0% protein, N×5.83) | 0.173 | 0.403 | 0.607 | 0.939 | 0.384 | 0.214 | 0.307 | 0.691 | 0.523 | 0.648 | 0.670 | 0.286 |
| hard red winter (12.3% protein, N×5.83) | 0.152 | 0.354 | 0.534 | 0.825 | 0.338 | 0.188 | 0.270 | 0.608 | 0.460 | 0.570 | 0.589 | 0.251 |
| soft red winter (10.2% protein, N×5.83) | 0.126 | 0.294 | 0.443 | 0.684 | 0.280 | 0.156 | 0.224 | 0.504 | 0.382 | 0.472 | 0.488 | 0.208 |
| white (9.4% protein, N×5.83) | 0.116 | 0.271 | 0.408 | 0.630 | 0.258 | 0.143 | 0.206 | 0.464 | 0.351 | 0.435 | 0.450 | 0.192 |
| durum (12.7% protein, N×5.83) | 0.157 | 0.366 | 0.551 | 0.852 | 0.348 | 0.194 | 0.279 | 0.627 | 0.475 | 0.588 | 0.608 | 0.259 |

TABLE 40—Continued

| Protein Content, and Nitrogen Conversion Factor | Trypto-phan (Gm.) | Threo-nine (Gm.) | Iso-leucine (Gm.) | Leucine (Gm.) | Lysine (Gm.) | Methi-onine (Gm.) | Cystine (Gm.) | Phenyl-alanine (Gm.) | Tyro-sine (Gm.) | Valine (Gm.) | Argi-nine (Gm.) | Histi-dine (Gm.) |
|---|---|---|---|---|---|---|---|---|---|---|---|---|
| **GRAINS AND PRODUCTS—Continued** | | | | | | | | | | | | |
| Wheat flour: | | | | | | | | | | | | |
| whole grain (13.3% protein, N×5.83) | 0.164 | 0.383 | 0.577 | 0.892 | 0.365 | 0.203 | 0.292 | 0.657 | 0.497 | 0.616 | 0.636 | 0.271 |
| intermediate extraction (12.0% protein, N×5.70) | ...... | 0.392 | 0.619 | 0.924 | 0.356 | 0.198 | 0.320 | 0.732 | 0.335 | 0.583 | 0.549 | 0.286 |
| white (10.5% protein, N×5.70) | 0.129 | 0.302 | 0.483 | 0.809 | 0.239 | 0.138 | 0.210 | 0.577 | 0.359 | 0.453 | 0.406 | 0.210 |
| Wheat products: | | | | | | | | | | | | |
| bran (12.0% protein, N×6.31) | 0.196 | 0.342 | 0.485 | 0.717 | 0.491 | 0.145 | 0.270 | 0.434 | 0.259 | 0.552 | 0.742 | 0.280 |
| burghul (12.4% protein, N×5.83) | 0.070 | ...... | ...... | ...... | 0.430 | 0.300 | 0.319 | ...... | ...... | ...... | ...... | ...... |
| farina (10.9% protein, N×5.70) | 0.124 | ...... | 0.496 | 0.891 | 0.199 | 0.143 | 0.184 | 0.579 | 0.447 | ...... | 0.424 | 0.268 |
| flakes (10.8% protein, N×5.70) | 0.121 | 0.356 | ...... | ...... | 0.360 | 0.127 | 0.191 | 0.478 | 0.311 | 0.572 | 0.559 | 0.231 |
| germ (25.2% protein, N×5.80) | 0.265 | 1.343 | 1.177 | 1.708 | 1.534 | 0.404 | 0.287 | 0.908 | 0.882 | 1.364 | 1.825 | 0.687 |
| gluten, commercial (80.0% protein, N×5.70) | 0.856 | 2.119 | 3.677 | 5.993 | 1.530 | 1.389 | 1.726 | 4.351 | 2.596 | 3.789 | 3.481 | 1.825 |
| gluten flour (41.4% protein, N×5.70) | 0.443 | 1.097 | 1.903 | 3.101 | 0.792 | 0.719 | 0.893 | 2.252 | 1.344 | 1.961 | 1.801 | 0.944 |
| macaroni or, spaghetti (12.8% protein, N×5.70) | 0.150 | 0.499 | 0.642 | 0.849 | 0.413 | 0.193 | 0.243 | 0.669 | 0.422 | 0.728 | 0.582 | 0.303 |
| noodles, containing egg solids (12.6% protein, N×5.70) | 0.133 | 0.533 | 0.621 | 0.834 | 0.411 | 0.212 | 0.245 | 0.610 | 0.312 | 0.745 | 0.621 | 0.301 |
| Shredded Wheat (10.1% protein, N×5.83) | 0.085 | 0.495 | 0.449 | 0.684 | 0.331 | 0.139 | 0.204 | 0.481 | 0.236 | 0.577 | 0.523 | 0.236 |
| whole wheat with added germ (12.8% protein, N×5.83) | 0.136 | ...... | ...... | ...... | 0.466 | ...... | 0.246 | 0.755 | 0.481 | ...... | 0.742 | 0.371 |
| **FRUITS (Protein, N×6.25)** | | | | | | | | | | | | |
| Abiu (1.7% protein) | 0.028 | ...... | ...... | ...... | 0.085 | 0.013 | ...... | ...... | ...... | ...... | ...... | ...... |
| Avocados (1.3% protein) | 0.014 | ...... | ...... | ...... | 0.074 | 0.012 | ...... | ...... | ...... | ...... | ...... | ...... |
| Bananas ripe | | | | | | | | | | | | |
| common (1.2% protein) | 0.018 | ...... | ...... | ...... | 0.055 | 0.011 | ...... | ...... | ...... | ...... | ...... | ...... |
| dwarf (1.2% protein) | 0.012 | ...... | ...... | ...... | 0.049 | 0.004 | ...... | ...... | 0.031 | ...... | ...... | ...... |
| Dates (2.2% protein) | 0.061 | 0.061 | 0.074 | 0.077 | 0.065 | 0.027 | ...... | 0.063 | ...... | 0.094 | 0.049 | 0.049 |

TABLE 40—*Continued*

| Protein Content, and Nitrogen Conversion Factor | Trypto-phan (Gm.) | Threo-nine (Gm.) | Iso-leucine (Gm.) | Leucine (Gm.) | Lysine (Gm.) | Methi-onine (Gm.) | Cystine (Gm.) | Phenyl-alanine (Gm.) | Tyro-sine (Gm.) | Valine (Gm.) | Argi-nine (Gm.) | Histi-dine (Gm.) |
|---|---|---|---|---|---|---|---|---|---|---|---|---|
| **FRUITS—*Continued*** | | | | | | | | | | | | |
| Grapefruit (0.5% protein) | 0.001 | ... | ... | ... | 0.006 | 0.000 | | | | | | |
| Guavas, common (1.0% protein) | 0.010 | ... | ... | ... | 0.030 | 0.010 | | | | | | |
| Limes (0.8% protein) | 0.003 | ... | ... | ... | 0.015 | 0.002 | | | | | | |
| Mamey (0.5% protein) | 0.006 | ... | ... | ... | 0.040 | 0.007 | | | | | | |
| Mangos (0.7% protein) | 0.014 | ... | ... | ... | 0.093 | 0.008 | | | | | | |
| Muskmelons (0.6% protein) | 0.001 | ... | ... | ... | 0.015 | 0.002 | | | | | | |
| Oranges, sweet (0.9% protein) | 0.003 | ... | ... | ... | 0.024 | 0.003 | | | | | | |
| Orange juice (0.8% protein) | 0.003 | ... | ... | ... | 0.021 | 0.002 | | | | | | |
| Oranges, mandarin including tangerines (0.8% protein) | 0.005 | ... | ... | ... | 0.028 | 0.004 | | | | | | |
| Papayas (0.6% protein) | 0.012 | ... | ... | ... | 0.038 | 0.002 | | | | | | |
| Pineapple (0.4% protein) | 0.005 | ... | ... | ... | 0.009 | 0.001 | | | | | | |
| Plantain or baking banana (1.1% protein) | 0.010 | 0.027 | 0.056 | 0.059 | 0.050 | 0.005 | 0.016 | 0.049 | ... | 0.065 | 0.045 | |
| Soursop (1.0% protein) | 0.011 | ... | ... | ... | 0.060 | 0.007 | ... | ... | ... | ... | ... | |
| Sugarapple (1.8% protein) | 0.009 | ... | ... | ... | 0.071 | 0.008 | | | | | | |
| **VEGETABLES** | | | | | | | | | | | | |
| *Immature seeds (Protein, N×6.25):* | | | | | | | | | | | | |
| corn, sweet, white or yellow: | | | | | | | | | | | | |
|   raw (3.7% protein) | 0.023 | 0.151 | 0.137 | 0.407 | 0.137 | 0.072 | 0.062 | 0.207 | 0.124 | 0.231 | 0.174 | 0.095 |
|   canned, solids and liquid (2.0% protein) | 0.012 | 0.082 | 0.074 | 0.220 | 0.074 | 0.039 | 0.033 | 0.112 | 0.067 | 0.125 | 0.094 | 0.052 |
| cowpeas (9.4% protein) | 0.099 | 0.353 | 0.465 | 0.653 | 0.617 | 0.131 | ... | 0.523 | ... | 0.513 | 0.615 | 0.310 |
| lima beans: | | | | | | | | | | | | |
|   raw (7.5% protein) | 0.097 | 0.338 | 0.460 | 0.605 | 0.474 | 0.080 | 0.083 | 0.389 | 0.259 | 0.485 | 0.454 | 0.247 |
|   canned, solids and liquid (3.8% protein) | 0.049 | 0.171 | 0.233 | 0.306 | 0.240 | 0.041 | 0.042 | 0.197 | 0.131 | 0.246 | 0.230 | 0.125 |
| peas: | | | | | | | | | | | | |
|   raw (6.7% protein) | 0.056 | 0.245 | 0.308 | 0.418 | 0.316 | 0.054 | 0.073 | 0.257 | 0.163 | 0.274 | 0.595 | 0.109 |
|   canned, solids and liquid (3.4% protein) | 0.028 | 0.125 | 0.156 | 0.212 | 0.160 | 0.027 | 0.037 | 0.131 | 0.083 | 0.139 | 0.302 | 0.055 |

TABLE 40—Continued

| Protein Content, and Nitrogen Conversion Factor | Tryptophan (Gm.) | Threonine (Gm.) | Isoleucine (Gm.) | Leucine (Gm.) | Lysine (Gm.) | Methionine (Gm.) | Cystine (Gm.) | Phenylalanine (Gm.) | Tyrosine (Gm.) | Valine (Gm.) | Arginine (Gm.) | Histidine (Gm.) |
|---|---|---|---|---|---|---|---|---|---|---|---|---|
| VEGETABLES—Continued | | | | | | | | | | | | |
| *Leafy vegetables, raw (Protein, N× 6.25):* | | | | | | | | | | | | |
| amaranth (3.5% protein) | 0.038 | 0.056 | 0.164 | 0.206 | 0.141 | 0.025 | 0.024 | 0.096 | 0.105 | 0.136 | 0.134 | 0.069 |
| beet greens (2.0% protein) | 0.024 | 0.076 | 0.084 | 0.129 | 0.108 | 0.034 | ..... | 0.116 | ..... | 0.101 | 0.083 | 0.026 |
| Brussels sprouts (4.4% protein) | 0.044 | 0.153 | 0.186 | 0.194 | 0.197 | 0.046 | ..... | 0.148 | ..... | 0.193 | 0.279 | 0.106 |
| cabbage (1.4% protein) | 0.011 | 0.039 | 0.040 | 0.057 | 0.066 | 0.013 | 0.028 | 0.030 | 0.030 | 0.043 | 0.105 | 0.025 |
| chard (1.4% protein) | 0.014 | 0.058 | 0.060 | 0.076 | 0.055 | 0.004 | ..... | 0.046 | ..... | 0.055 | 0.035 | 0.018 |
| chicory (1.6% protein) | 0.024 | ..... | ..... | ..... | 0.052 | 0.016 | 0.006 | ..... | 0.040 | ..... | ..... | 0.024 |
| collards (3.9% protein) | 0.055 | 0.114 | 0.121 | 0.218 | 0.202 | 0.046 | 0.059 | 0.124 | 0.151 | 0.195 | 0.258 | 0.087 |
| kale (3.9% protein) | 0.042 | 0.139 | 0.133 | 0.252 | 0.121 | 0.035 | 0.036 | 0.158 | ..... | 0.184 | 0.202 | 0.062 |
| lettuce (1.2% protein) | 0.012 | ..... | ..... | ..... | 0.070 | 0.004 | ..... | ..... | ..... | ..... | ..... | ..... |
| mustard greens (2.3% protein) | 0.037 | 0.060 | 0.075 | 0.062 | 0.111 | 0.024 | 0.035 | 0.074 | 0.121 | 0.108 | 0.167 | 0.041 |
| parsley, curly garden (2.5% protein) | 0.050 | ..... | ..... | ..... | 0.160 | 0.012 | ..... | ..... | ..... | ..... | ..... | ..... |
| spinach (2.3% protein) | 0.037 | 0.102 | 0.107 | 0.176 | 0.142 | 0.039 | 0.046 | 0.099 | 0.073 | 0.126 | 0.116 | 0.049 |
| turnip greens (2.9% protein) | 0.045 | 0.125 | 0.107 | 0.207 | 0.129 | 0.052 | 0.045 | 0.146 | 0.105 | 0.149 | 0.167 | 0.051 |
| watercress (1.7% protein) | 0.028 | 0.084 | 0.076 | 0.131 | 0.091 | 0.010 | ..... | 0.062 | 0.036 | 0.084 | 0.053 | 0.034 |
| *Starchy roots and tubers (Protein, N× 6.25):* | | | | | | | | | | | | |
| *Apio arracacia* (1.2% protein) | 0.008 | ..... | ..... | ..... | 0.042 | 0.003 | | | | | | |
| cassava: | | | | | | | | | | | | |
| flour (1.6% protein) | 0.021 | 0.044 | 0.045 | 0.066 | 0.066 | 0.010 | 0.018 | 0.045 | 0.030 | 0.049 | 0.159 | 0.025 |
| root (1.1% protein) | 0.014 | 0.030 | 0.031 | 0.045 | 0.045 | 0.007 | 0.012 | 0.031 | 0.021 | 0.033 | 0.110 | 0.017 |
| potatoes: | | | | | | | | | | | | |
| raw (2.0% protein) | 0.021 | 0.079 | 0.088 | 0.100 | 0.107 | 0.025 | 0.019 | 0.088 | 0.036 | 0.107 | 0.099 | 0.029 |
| canned, solids and liquid (1.7% protein) | 0.018 | 0.067 | 0.075 | 0.085 | 0.091 | 0.021 | 0.016 | 0.075 | 0.030 | 0.091 | 0.084 | 0.024 |
| flour (7.1% protein) | 0.076 | 0.279 | 0.311 | 0.353 | 0.378 | 0.089 | 0.068 | 0.314 | 0.127 | 0.379 | 0.350 | 0.102 |

TABLE 40—*Continued*

| Protein Content, and Nitrogen Conversion Factor | Trypto-phan (Gm.) | Threo-nine (Gm.) | Iso-leucine (Gm.) | Leucine (Gm.) | Lysine (Gm.) | Methi-onine (Gm.) | Cystine (Gm.) | Phenyl-alanine (Gm.) | Tyro-sine (Gm.) | Valine (Gm.) | Argi-nine (Gm.) | Histi-dine (Gm.) |
|---|---|---|---|---|---|---|---|---|---|---|---|---|
| VEGETABLES—*Continued* | | | | | | | | | | | | |
| sweet potatoes (*Ipomaea batatas*): | | | | | | | | | | | | |
| raw (1.8% protein) | 0.031 | 0.085 | 0.087 | 0.103 | 0.085 | 0.033 | 0.029 | 0.100 | 0.081 | 0.135 | 0.094 | 0.036 |
| dehydrated (5.0% protein) | 0.087 | 0.235 | 0.241 | 0.286 | 0.236 | 0.093 | 0.080 | 0.278 | 0.225 | 0.374 | 0.261 | 0.099 |
| taro (1.0% protein) | 0.035 | 0.089 | 0.099 | 0.169 | 0.110 | 0.021 | …… | 0.099 | …… | 0.114 | 0.118 | 0.032 |
| yam (*Dioscorea* spp.) (2.1% protein) | 0.035 | …… | …… | …… | 0.110 | 0.034 | …… | …… | …… | …… | …… | …… |
| *Yautia malanga* (1.7% protein) | 0.023 | …… | …… | …… | 0.067 | 0.016 | …… | …… | …… | …… | …… | …… |
| *Other vegetables* (Protein, N×6.25): | | | | | | | | | | | | |
| asparagus: | | | | | | | | | | | | |
| raw (2.2% protein) | 0.027 | 0.066 | 0.080 | 0.096 | 0.103 | 0.032 | …… | 0.069 | …… | 0.106 | 0.123 | 0.036 |
| canned, solids and liquid (1.9% protein) | 0.023 | 0.057 | 0.069 | 0.083 | 0.089 | 0.027 | …… | 0.060 | …… | 0.092 | 0.106 | 0.031 |
| beans, snap: | | | | | | | | | | | | |
| raw (2.4% protein) | 0.033 | 0.091 | 0.109 | 0.139 | 0.126 | 0.035 | 0.024 | 0.057 | 0.050 | 0.115 | 0.101 | 0.045 |
| canned, solids and liquid (1.0% protein) | 0.014 | 0.038 | 0.045 | 0.058 | 0.052 | 0.014 | 0.010 | 0.024 | 0.021 | 0.048 | 0.042 | 0.019 |
| beets: | | | | | | | | | | | | |
| raw (1.6% protein) | 0.014 | 0.034 | 0.051 | 0.055 | 0.086 | 0.006 | …… | 0.027 | …… | 0.049 | 0.028 | 0.022 |
| canned, solids and liquid (0.9% protein) | 0.008 | 0.019 | 0.029 | 0.031 | 0.048 | 0.003 | …… | 0.015 | …… | 0.028 | 0.016 | 0.012 |
| broccoli (3.3% protein) | 0.037 | 0.122 | 0.126 | 0.163 | 0.147 | 0.050 | …… | 0.119 | …… | 0.170 | 0.192 | 0.063 |
| carrots: | | | | | | | | | | | | |
| raw (1.2% protein) | 0.010 | 0.043 | 0.046 | 0.065 | 0.052 | 0.010 | 0.029 | 0.042 | 0.020 | 0.056 | 0.041 | 0.017 |
| canned, solids and liquid (0.5% protein) | 0.004 | 0.018 | 0.019 | 0.027 | 0.022 | 0.004 | 0.012 | 0.018 | 0.008 | 0.023 | 0.017 | 0.007 |
| cauliflower (2.4% protein) | 0.033 | 0.102 | 0.104 | 0.162 | 0.134 | 0.047 | …… | 0.075 | 0.034 | 0.144 | 0.110 | 0.048 |
| celery (1.3% protein) | 0.012 | …… | …… | …… | 0.021 | 0.015 | 0.006 | …… | 0.016 | …… | …… | …… |
| chayote (0.6% protein) | 0.008 | …… | …… | …… | 0.038 | 0.001 | …… | …… | …… | …… | …… | …… |
| cowpeas, yardlong, immature pod (3.4% protein) | 0.034 | …… | …… | …… | 0.203 | 0.021 | …… | …… | …… | …… | …… | …… |
| cucumbers (0.7% protein) | 0.005 | 0.019 | 0.022 | 0.030 | 0.031 | 0.007 | …… | 0.016 | …… | 0.024 | 0.053 | 0.001 |
| cushaw (1.5% protein) | 0.014 | …… | …… | …… | 0.044 | 0.008 | …… | …… | …… | …… | …… | …… |
| eggplant (1.1% protein) | 0.010 | 0.038 | 0.056 | 0.068 | 0.030 | 0.006 | …… | 0.048 | …… | 0.065 | 0.037 | 0.019 |
| mallow (3.7% protein) | 0.144 | 0.155 | …… | 0.259 | 0.155 | 0.030 | …… | 0.166 | …… | 0.181 | 0.189 | 0.063 |

# TABLE 40—Continued

| Protein Content, and Nitrogen Conversion Factor | Trypto-phan (Gm.) | Threo-nine (Gm.) | Iso-leucine (Gm.) | Leucine (Gm.) | Lysine (Gm.) | Methi-onine (Gm.) | Cystine (Gm.) | Phenyl-alanine (Gm.) | Tyro-sine (Gm.) | Valine (Gm.) | Argi-nine (Gm.) | Histi-dine (Gm.) |
|---|---|---|---|---|---|---|---|---|---|---|---|---|
| VEGETABLES—Continued | | | | | | | | | | | | |
| mushrooms: | | | | | | | | | | | | |
| (Agaricus campestris)* | 0.006 | | 0.532 | 0.281 | | 0.167 | | | | 0.378 | 0.235 | |
| (Lactarius spp.)† | 0.006 | 0.156 | 0.201 | 0.139 | 0.088 | 0.021 | | 0.018 | | 0.116 | 0.021 | 0.027 |
| okra (1.8% protein) | 0.018 | 0.066 | 0.069 | 0.101 | 0.076 | 0.022 | 0.017 | 0.065 | 0.079 | 0.091 | 0.093 | 0.030 |
| onions, mature (1.4% protein) | 0.021 | 0.022 | 0.021 | 0.037 | 0.064 | 0.013 | | 0.039 | 0.046 | 0.031 | 0.180 | 0.014 |
| peppers (1.2% protein) | 0.009 | 0.050 | 0.046 | 0.046 | 0.051 | 0.016 | | 0.055 | | 0.033 | 0.024 | 0.014 |
| prickly pears (1.1% protein) | 0.009 | 0.053 | 0.044 | 0.057 | 0.044 | 0.008 | | 0.059 | | 0.041 | 0.032 | 0.016 |
| pumpkin (1.2% protein) | 0.016 | 0.028 | 0.044 | 0.063 | 0.058 | 0.011 | | 0.032 | | 0.045 | 0.043 | 0.019 |
| radishes (1.2% protein) | 0.005 | 0.059 | | | 0.034 | 0.002 | | | 0.016 | 0.030 | | |
| seepweed (2.6% protein) | 0.027 | 0.089 | 0.113 | 0.152 | 0.089 | 0.013 | | 0.116 | | 0.091 | 0.062 | 0.036 |
| soybean sprouts (6.2% protein) | | 0.159 | 0.225 | 0.265 | 0.211 | 0.045 | | 0.186 | | 0.225 | 0.225 | 0.133 |
| squash, summer (0.6% protein) | 0.005 | 0.014 | 0.019 | 0.027 | 0.023 | 0.008 | | 0.016 | | 0.022 | 0.027 | 0.009 |
| tomatoes and cherry tomatoes (1.0% protein) | 0.009 | 0.033 | 0.029 | 0.041 | 0.042 | 0.007 | | 0.028 | 0.014 | 0.028 | 0.029 | 0.015 |
| turnips (1.1% protein) | | | 0.020 | | 0.057 | 0.012 | | 0.020 | 0.029 | | | |
| waxgourd, Chinese (0.4% protein) | 0.002 | | | | 0.009 | 0.003 | | | | | | |
| MISCELLANEOUS FOOD ITEMS | | | | | | | | | | | | |
| Vegetable patty or steak (principally wheat protein) (15% protein, N× 5.70) | 0.142 | 0.411 | 0.884 | 1.079 | 0.321 | 0.253 | | 0.811 | | 0.705 | 0.597 | 0.321 |
| Yeast: | | | | | | | | | | | | |
| baker's, compressed‡ (N×6.25) | 0.122 | 0.655 | 0.655 | 1.151 | 0.914 | 0.248 | 0.120 | 0.607 | 0.580 | 0.840 | 0.536 | 0.353 |
| brewer's, dried§ (N×6.25) | 0.710 | 2.353 | 2.398 | 3.226 | 3.300 | 0.836 | 0.548 | 1.902 | 1.902 | 2.723 | 2.250 | 1.251 |
| primary, dried: | | | | | | | | | | | | |
| (Saccharomyces cerevisiae)§ (N×6.25) | 0.636 | 2.353 | 2.708 | 3.300 | 3.337 | 0.851 | 0.444 | 1.813 | 2.472 | 2.553 | 1.931 | 1.103 |
| (Torulopsis utilis)§ (N×6.25) | 0.636 | 2.331 | 3.323 | 3.797 | 3.648 | 0.710 | 0.422 | 2.361 | 2.464 | 2.901 | 3.337 | 1.251 |

*Total nitrogen is 0.58%. This is equivalent to 2.4% protein on the basis that two-thirds of the nitrogen is protein nitrogen. If total nitrogen is used for the calculation, the protein content is 3.6%.

†Total nitrogen is 0.69%. This is equivalent to 2.9% protein on the basis that two-thirds of the nitrogen is protein nitrogen. If total nitrogen is used for the calculation, the protein content is 4.3%.

‡Total nitrogen is 2.1%. This is equivalent to 10.6% protein on the basis that four-fifths of the nitrogen is protein nitrogen. If total nitrogen is used for the calculation, the protein content is 13.1%.

§Total nitrogen is 7.4%. This is equivalent to 36.9% protein on the basis that four-fifths of the nitrogen is protein nitrogen. If total nitrogen is used for the calculation, the protein content is 46.1%.

# APPENDIX 6

## Sodium and Potassium Content of Foods, 100 Grams Edible Portion[1]

### TABLE 41

| Food and description | Sodium (Mg.) | Potassium (Mg.) |
|---|---|---|
| Almonds: | | |
| Dried................................................ | 4 | 773 |
| Roasted and salted............................. | 198 | 773 |
| Apples: | | |
| Raw, pared........................................ | 1 | 110 |
| Frozen, sliced, sweetened......................... | 14 | 68 |
| Apple Brown Betty ............................... | 153 | 100 |
| Apple butter........................................ | 2 | 252 |
| Apple juice, canned or bottled....................... | 1 | 101 |
| Applesauce, canned, sweetened...................... | 2 | 65 |
| Apricots: | | |
| Raw................................................ | 1 | 281 |
| Canned, syrup pack, light........................... | 1 | 239 |
| Dried, sulfured, cooked, fruit, and liquid............. | 8 | 318 |
| Apricot nectar, canned (approx. 40% fruit)............. | Trace | 151 |
| Asparagus: | | |
| Cooked spears, boiled, drained.................... | 1 | 183 |
| Canned spears, green: | | |
| Regular pack, solids and liquid................... | 236[2] | 166 |
| Special dietary pack (low-sodium), solids and liquids. | 3 | 166 |
| Frozen: | | |
| Cuts and tips, cooked, boiled, drained............. | 1 | 220 |
| Spears, cooked, boiled, drained................... | 1 | 238 |
| Avocados, raw, all commercial varieties............... | 4 | 604 |
| Bacon, cured, cooked, broiled or fried, drained.......... | 1,021 | 236 |
| Bacon, Canadian, cooked, broiled or fried, drained....... | 2,555 | 432 |
| Baking powders: | | |
| Home use: | | |
| Straight phosphate............................. | 8,220 | 170 |
| Special low-sodium preparations................... | 6 | 10,948 |
| Bananas, raw, common.............................. | 1 | 370 |
| Barbecue sauce...................................... | 815 | 174 |
| Bass, black sea, raw................................ | 68 | 256 |
| Beans, common, mature seeds, dry: | | |
| White: | | |
| Cooked........................................ | 7 | 416 |
| Canned, solids and liquid, with pork and tomato sauce | 463 | 210 |
| Red, cooked....................................... | 3 | 340 |
| Beans, Lima: | | |
| Immature seeds: | | |
| Cooked, boiled, drained........................ | 1 | 422 |
| Canned: | | |
| Regular pack, solids and liquid.................. | 236[2] | 222 |
| Special dietary pack (low-sodium), solids and liquid | 4 | 222 |
| Frozen, thin-seeded types, commonly called baby Limas, cooked, boiled, drained.................. | 129 | 394 |
| Mature seeds, dry, cooked........................... | 2 | 612 |

1. Numbers in parentheses denote values imputed—usually from another form of the food or from a similar food. Dashes denote lack of reliable data for a constituent believed to be present in measurable amount. Values are selected from *Composition of Foods—Raw, Processed, Prepared* (U.S. Department of Agriculture, Agriculture Handbook No. 8 [December, 1963]).

2. Estimated average based on addition of salt in the amount of 0.6 percent of the finished product.

TABLE 41—*Continued*

| Food and description | Sodium (Mg.) | Potassium (Mg.) |
|---|---|---|
| Beans, mung, sprouted seeds, cooked, boiled, drained.... | 4 | 156 |
| Beans, snap: | | |
| Green: | | |
| Cooked, boiled, drained......................... | 4 | 151 |
| Canned: | | |
| Regular pack, solids and liquid.................. | 236[2] | 95 |
| Special dietary pack (low sodium), solids and liquid. | 2 | 95 |
| Frozen, cut, cooked, boiled, drained .............. | 1 | 152 |
| Yellow or wax: | | |
| Cooked, boiled, drained......................... | 3 | 151 |
| Canned: | | |
| Regular pack, solids and liquid.................. | 236[2] | 95 |
| Special dietary pack (low-sodium), solids and liquid. | 2 | 95 |
| Frozen, cut, cooked, boiled, drained............... | 1 | 164 |
| Beans and frankfurters, canned...................... | 539 | 262 |
| Beef: | | |
| Retail cuts, trimmed to retail level: | | |
| Round......................................... | 60 | 370 |
| Rump..:....................................... | 60 | 370 |
| Hamburger, regular ground, cooked............... | 47 | 450 |
| Beef and vegetable stew, canned..................... | 411 | 174 |
| Beef, corned, boneless: | | |
| Cooked, medium-fat............................. | 1,740 | 150 |
| Canned corned-beef hash (with potato).............. | 540 | 200 |
| Beef, dried, cooked, creamed........................ | 716 | 153 |
| Beef potpie, commercial, frozen, unheated.............. | 366 | 93 |
| Beets, common, red: | | |
| Canned: | | |
| Regular pack, solids and liquid................... | 236[2] | 167 |
| Special dietary pack (low-sodium), solids and liquid.. | 46 | 167 |
| Beet greens, common, cooked, boiled, drained.......... | 76 | 332 |
| Beverages, alcoholic: | | |
| Beer, alcohol 4.5% by volume (3.6% by weight) ...... | 7 | 25 |
| Gin, rum, vodka, whisky: | | |
| 80-proof (33.4% alcohol by weight)............... | 1 | 2 |
| 86-proof (36.0% alcohol by weight)............... | 1 | 2 |
| 90-proof (37.9% alcohol by weight)............... | 1 | 2 |
| 94-proof (39.7% alcohol by weight)............... | 1 | 2 |
| 100-proof (42.5% alcohol by weight)............... | 1 | 2 |
| Wines: | | |
| Dessert, alcohol 18.8% by volume (15.3% by weight) | 4 | 75 |
| Table, alcohol 12.2% by volume (9.9% by weight)... | 5 | 92 |
| Biscuits, baking powder, made with enriched flour....... | 626 | 117 |
| Biscuit dough, commercial, frozen.................... | 910 | 86 |
| Biscuit mix, with enriched flour, and biscuits baked from mix: | | |
| Mix, dry form.................................... | 1,300 | 80 |
| Biscuits, made with milk......................... | 973 | 116 |
| Blackberries, including dewberries, boysenberries, and youngberries, raw ................................. | 1 | 170 |
| Blackberries, canned, solids and liquid: | | |
| Water pack, with or without artificial sweetener....... | 1 | 115 |
| Syrup pack, heavy.............................. | 1 | 109 |
| Blueberries: | | |
| Raw........................................... | 1 | 81 |
| Frozen, not thawed, sweetened..................... | 1 | 66 |
| Bluefish, cooked: | | |
| Baked or broiled................................. | 104 | .......... |
| Fried.......................................... | 146 | .......... |

TABLE 41—*Continued*

| Food and description | Sodium (Mg.) | Potassium (Mg.) |
|---|---|---|
| Boston brown bread | 251 | 292 |
| Bouillon cubes or powder | 24,000 | 100 |
| Boysenberries, frozen, not thawed, sweetened | 1 | 105 |
| Bran, added sugar and malt extract | 1,060 | 1,070 |
| Bran flakes (40% bran), added thiamine | 925 | . . . . . . . . . . . |
| Bran flakes with raisins, added thiamine | 800 | . . . . . . . . . . . |
| Brazil nuts | 1 | 715 |
| Breads: | | |
|   Cracked-wheat | 529 | 134 |
|   French or Vienna, enriched | 580 | 90 |
|   Italian, enriched | 585 | 74 |
|   Raisin | 365 | 233 |
|   Rye, American (⅓ rye, ⅔ clear flour) | 557 | 145 |
|   White, enriched, made with 3%–4% non-fat dry milk | 507 | 105 |
|   Whole-wheat, made with 2% non-fat dry milk | 527 | 273 |
| Bread crumbs, dry, grated | 736 | 152 |
| Bread stuffing mix and stuffings prepared from mix: | | |
|   Mix, dry form | 1,331 | 172 |
| Broccoli: | | |
|   Cooked spears, boiled, drained | 10 | 267 |
|   Frozen, spears, cooked, boiled, drained | 12 | 220 |
| Brussels sprouts, frozen, cooked, boiled, drained | 14 | 295 |
| Buffalo fish, raw | 52 | 293 |
| Bulgur (parboiled wheat): | | |
|   Canned, made from hard red winter wheat: | | |
|     Unseasoned[3] | 599 | 87 |
|     Seasoned[4] | 460 | 112 |
| Butter[5] | 987 | 23 |
| Buttermilk, fluid, cultured (made from skim milk) | 130 | 140 |
| Cabbage: | | |
|   Common varieties (Danish, domestic, and pointed types): | | |
|     Raw | 20 | 233 |
|     Cooked, boiled until tender, drained, shredded, cooked in small amount of water | 14 | 163 |
|   Red, raw | 26 | 268 |
| Cabbage, Chinese (also called celery cabbage or petsai) | 23 | 253 |
| Cakes: | | |
|   Baked from home recipes: | | |
|     Angelfood | 283 | 88 |
|     Fruitcake, made with enriched flour, dark | 158 | 496 |
|     Gingerbread, made with enriched flour | 237 | 454 |
|     Plain cake or cupcake, without icing | 300 | 79 |
|     Pound, modified | 178 | 78 |
|   Frozen, commercial, devil's food, with chocolate icing | 420 | 119 |
| Candy: | | |
|   Caramels, plain or chocolate | 226 | 192 |
|   Chocolate, sweet | 33 | 269 |
|   Chocolate-coated, chocolate fudge | 228 | 193 |
|   Gum drops, starch jelly pieces | 35 | 5 |
|   Hard | 32 | 4 |
|   Marshmallows | 39 | 6 |
|   Peanut bars | 10 | 448 |
| Carp, raw | 50 | 286 |

3. Processed, partially debranned, whole-kernel wheat with salt added.

4. Processed, partially debranned, whole-kernel wheat with chicken fat, chicken stock base, dehydrated onion flakes, salt, monosodium glutamate, and herbs.

5. Values apply to salted butter. Unsalted butter contains less than 10 mg. of either sodium or potassium per 100 grams. Value for vitamin A is the year-round average.

TABLE 41—*Continued*

| Food and description | Sodium (Mg.) | Potassium (Mg.) |
|---|---|---|
| Carrots: | | |
|   Raw | 47 | 341 |
|   Canned: | | |
|     Regular pack, solids and liquid | 236[2] | 120 |
|     Special dietary pack (low-sodium), solids and liquid | 39 | 120 |
| Cashew nuts | 15[6] | 464 |
| Catfish, freshwater, raw | 60 | 330 |
| Cauliflower: | | |
|   Cooked, boiled, drained | 9 | 206 |
|   Frozen, cooked, boiled, drained | 10 | 207 |
| Caviar, sturgeon, granular | 2,200 | 180 |
| Celery, all, including green and yellow varieties: | | |
|   Raw | 126 | 341 |
|   Cooked, boiled, drained | 88 | 239 |
| Chard, Swiss, cooked, boiled, drained | 86 | 321 |
| Cheese straws | 721 | 63 |
| Cheeses: | | |
|   Natural cheeses: | | |
|     Cheddar (domestic type, commonly called American) | 700 | 82 |
|     Cottage (large or small curd): | | |
|       Creamed | 229 | 85 |
|       Uncreamed | 290 | 72 |
|     Cream | 250 | 74 |
|     Parmesan | 734 | 149 |
|     Swiss (domestic) | 710 | 104 |
|   Pasteurized process cheese, American | 1,136[7] | 80 |
|   Pasteurized process cheese spread, American | 1,625[7] | 240 |
| Cherries: | | |
|   Raw, sweet | 2 | 191 |
|   Canned: | | |
|     Sour, red, solids and liquid, water pack | 2 | 130 |
|     Sweet, solids and liquid, syrup pack, light | 1 | 128 |
|   Frozen, not thawed, sweetened | 2 | 130 |
| Chicken: | | |
|   All classes: | | |
|     Light meat without skin, cooked, roasted | 64 | 411 |
|     Dark meat without skin, cooked, roasted | 86 | 321 |
| Chicken potpie, commercial, frozen, unheated | 411 | 153 |
| Chicory, Witloof (also called French or Belgian endive), bleached head (forced), raw | 7 | 182 |
| Chili con carne, canned, with beans | 531 | 233 |
| Chocolate, bitter or baking | 4 | 830 |
| Chocolate syrup, fudge type | 89 | 284 |
| Chop suey, with meat, canned | 551 | 138 |
| Chow mein, chicken (without noodles), canned | 290 | 167 |
| Citron, candied | 290 | 120 |
| Clams, raw: | | |
|   Soft, meat only | 36 | 235 |
|   Hard or round, meat only | 205 | 311 |
| Clams, canned, including hard, soft, razor, and unspecified: | | |
|   Solids and liquid | ......... | 140 |

6. Applies to unsalted nuts. For salted nuts, value is approximately 200 mg. per 100 grams.

7. Values for phosphorus and sodium are based on use of 1.5 per cent anhydrous disodium phosphate as the emulsifying agent. If emulsifying agent does not contain either phosphorus or sodium, the content of these two nutrients in milligrams per 100 grams is as follows:

| | P | Na |
|---|---|---|
| American process cheese | 444 | 650 |
| Swiss process cheese | 540 | 681 |
| American cheese food | 427 | .... |
| American cheese spread | 548 | 1,139 |

TABLE 41—*Continued*

| Food and description | Sodium (Mg.) | Potassium (Mg.) |
|---|---|---|
| Cocoa and chocolate-flavored beverage powders: | | |
| Cocoa powder with non-fat dry milk............... | 525 | 800 |
| Mix for hot chocolate............................ | 382 | 605 |
| Cocoa, dry powder: | | |
| High-fat or breakfast: | | |
| Plain..................................... | 6 | 1,522 |
| Processed with alkali...................... | 717 | 651 |
| Coconut cream (liquid expressed from grated coconut meat) | 4 | 324 |
| Coconut meat, fresh............................. | 23 | 256 |
| Cod: | | |
| Cooked, broiled................................ | 110 | 407 |
| Dehydrated, lightly salted...................... | 8,100 | 160 |
| Coffee, instant, water-soluble solids: | | |
| Dry powder.................................... | 72 | 3,256 |
| Beverage...................................... | 1 | 36 |
| Coleslaw, made with French dressing (commercial)....... | 268 | 205 |
| Collards, cooked, boiled, drained, leaves, including stems, cooked in small amount of water .................. | 25 | 234 |
| Cookies: | | |
| Assorted, packaged, commercial.................... | 365 | 67 |
| Butter, thin, rich.............................. | 418 | 60 |
| Gingersnaps.................................... | 571 | 462 |
| Molasses....................................... | 386 | 138 |
| Oatmeal with raisins............................ | 162 | 370 |
| Sandwich type................................. | 483 | 38 |
| Vanilla wafer.................................. | 252 | 72 |
| Cookie dough, plain, chilled in roll, baked .............. | 548 | 48 |
| Corn, sweet: | | |
| Cooked, boiled, drained, white and yellow, kernels, cut off cob before cooking........................... | Trace | 165 |
| Canned: | | |
| Regular pack, cream style, white and yellow, solids and liquid..................................... | 236[2] | (97) |
| Special dietary pack (low-sodium), cream style, white and yellow, solids and liquid.................... | 2 | (97) |
| Frozen, kernels cut off cob, cooked, boiled, drained.... | 1 | 184 |
| Corn fritters.................................... | 477 | 133 |
| Corn grits, degermed, enriched, dry form.............. | 1 | 80 |
| Corn products used mainly as ready-to-eat breakfast cereals: | | |
| Corn flakes, added nutrients...................... | 1,005 | 120 |
| Corn, puffed, added nutrients...................... | 1,060 | ............ |
| Corn, rice, and wheat flakes, mixed, added nutrients... | 950 | ............ |
| Cornbread, baked from home recipes, southern style, made with degermed cornmeal, enriched.................. | 591 | 157 |
| Cornbread mix and cornbread baked from mix, cornbread, made with egg, milk............................ | 744 | 127 |
| Cornmeal, white or yellow, degermed, enriched, dry form. | 1 | 120 |
| Cornstarch...................................... | Trace | Trace |
| Cowpeas, including blackeye peas: | | |
| Immature seeds, canned, solids and liquid............ | 236[2] | 352 |
| Young pods, with seeds, cooked, boiled, drained....... | 3 | 196 |
| Crab, canned.................................... | 1,000 | 110 |
| Crackers: | | |
| Butter......................................... | 1,092 | 113 |
| Graham, plain.................................. | 670 | 384 |
| Saltines....................................... | (1,100) | (120) |
| Sandwich type, peanut-cheese..................... | 992 | 226 |
| Soda.......................................... | 1,100 | 120 |

TABLE 41—*Continued*

| Food and description | Sodium (Mg.) | Potassium (Mg.) |
|---|---|---|
| Cranberries, raw | 2 | 82 |
| Cranberry juice cocktail, bottled (approx. 33% cranberry juice) | 1 | 10 |
| Cranberry sauce, sweetened, canned, strained | 1 | 30 |
| Cream, fluid, light, coffee, or table, 20% fat | 43 | 122 |
| Cream substitutes, dried, containing: | | |
|   Cream, skim milk (calcium reduced), and lactose | 575 | . . . . . . . . . . |
| Cream puffs with custard filling | 83 | 121 |
| Cress, garden, raw | 14 | 606 |
| Croaker, Atlantic, cooked, baked | 120 | 323 |
| Cucumbers, raw, pared | 6 | 160 |
| Custard, baked | 79 | 146 |
| Dates, domestic, natural and dry | 1 | 648 |
| Doughnuts, cake type | 501 | 90 |
| Duck, domesticated, raw, flesh only | 74 | 285 |
| Eggs, chicken: | | |
|   Raw: | | |
|     Whole, fresh and frozen | 122 | 129 |
|     Whites, fresh and frozen | 146 | 139 |
|     Yolks, fresh | 52 | 98 |
| Eggplant, cooked, boiled, drained | 1 | 150 |
| Endive (curly endive and escarole), raw | 14 | 294 |
| Farina: | | |
|   Enriched: | | |
|     Regular: | | |
|       Dry form | 2 | 83 |
|       Cooked | 144 | 9 |
|     Quick-cooking, cooked | 165 | 10 |
|     Instant-cooking, cooked | 188 | 13 |
|   Unenriched, regular, dry form | 2 | 83 |
| Figs, canned, solids and liquid, syrup pack, light | 2 | 152 |
| Flatfishes (flounders, soles, and sand dabs), raw | 78 | 342 |
| Fruit cocktail, canned, solids and liquid, water pack, with or without artificial sweetener | 5 | 168 |
| Garlic, cloves, raw | 19 | 529 |
| Ginger root, fresh | 6 | 264 |
| Gizzard, chicken, all classes, cooked, simmered | 57 | 211 |
| Goose, domesticated, flesh only, cooked, roasted | 124 | 605 |
| Gooseberries, canned, solids and liquid, syrup pack, heavy | 1 | 98 |
| Grapefruit: | | |
|   Raw, pulp, pink, red, white, all varieties | 1 | 135 |
|   Canned, juice, sweetened | 1 | 162 |
| Grapefruit juice and orange juice blended, canned, sweetened | 1 | 184 |
| Grapes, raw, American type (slip skin) such as Concord, Delaware, Niagara, Catawba, and Scuppernong | 3 | 158 |
| Grapejuice, canned or bottled | 2 | 116 |
| Guavas, whole, raw, common | 4 | 289 |
| Haddock, cooked, fried | 177 | 348 |
| Hake, including Pacific hake, squirrel hake, and silver hake or whiting; raw | 74 | 363 |
| Halibut, Atlantic and Pacific, cooked, broiled | 134 | 525 |
| Ham croquette | 342 | 83 |
| Heart, beef, lean, cooked, braised | 104 | 232 |
| Herring: | | |
|   Raw, Pacific | 74 | 420 |
|   Smoked, hard | 6,231 | 157 |

TABLE 41—*Continued*

| Food and description | Sodium (Mg.) | Potassium (Mg.) |
|---|---|---|
| Honey, strained or extracted......................... | 5 | 51 |
| Horse-radish, prepared.............................. | 96 | 290 |
| Ice cream and frozen custard: | | |
| Regular, approximately 10% fat.................... | 63[8] | 181 |
| Ice cream cones................................... | 232 | 244 |
| Ice milk.......................................... | 68[8] | 195 |
| Jams and preserves................................ | 12 | 88 |
| Kale, cooked, boiled, drained, leaves including stems..... | 43 | 221 |
| Kingfish; southern, gulf, and northern (whiting); raw .... | 83 | 250 |
| Lake herring (cisco), raw........................... | 47 | 319 |
| Lamb, retail cuts.................................. | 70 | 290 |
| Lemon juice, canned or bottled, unsweetened........... | 1 | 141 |
| Lettuce, raw, crisphead varieties such as Iceberg, New York, and Great Lakes strains..................... | 9 | 175 |
| Lime juice, canned or bottled, unsweetened............ | 1 | 104 |
| Liver, beef, cooked, fried........................... | 184 | 380 |
| Lobster, northern, canned or cooked.................. | 210 | 180 |
| Loganberries, canned, solids and liquid, syrup pack, light | 1 | 111 |
| Macadamia nuts................................... | .......... | 264 |
| Macaroni, unenriched, dry form...................... | 2 | 197 |
| Macaroni and cheese, canned........................ | 304 | 58 |
| Margarine[9]....................................... | 987 | 23 |
| Marmalade, citrus ................................ | 14 | 33 |
| Milk, cow: | | |
| Fluid (pasteurized and raw): | | |
| Whole, 3.7% fat.............................. | 50 | 144 |
| Skim........................................ | 52 | 145 |
| Canned, evaporated (unsweetened) ................. | 118 | 303 |
| Dry, skim (non-fat solids), regular................. | 532 | 1,745 |
| Malted: | | |
| Dry powder.................................. | 440 | 720 |
| Beverage..................................... | 91 | 200 |
| Chocolate drink, fluid, commercial: | | |
| Made with skim milk.......................... | 46 | 142 |
| Made with whole (3.5% fat) milk................ | 47 | 146 |
| Molasses, cane: | | |
| First extraction or light.......................... | 15 | 917 |
| Third extraction or blackstrap..................... | 96 | 2,927 |
| Muffin mixes, corn, and muffins baked from mixes: | | |
| Muffins, made with egg, milk...................... | 479 | 110 |
| Muffins, made with egg, water..................... | 346 | 104 |
| Mushrooms: | | |
| Raw........................................... | 15 | 414 |
| Canned, solids and liquid......................... | 400 | 197 |
| Muskmelons, raw, cantaloupes, other netted varieties.... | 12 | 251 |
| Mussels, Atlantic and Pacific, raw, meat only........... | 289 | 315 |
| Mustard greens, cooked, boiled, drained............... | 18 | 220 |
| Mustard, prepared: | | |
| Brown......................................... | 1,307 | 130 |
| Yellow........................................ | 1,252 | 130 |
| Nectarines, raw................................... | 6 | 294 |
| New Zealand spinach, cooked, boiled, drained.......... | 92 | 463 |
| Noodles, egg noodles, enriched, cooked............... | 2 | 44 |

8. Value for product without added salt.

9. Values apply to salted margarine. Unsalted margarine contains less than 10 mg. per 100 grams of either sodium or potassium. Vitamin A value based on the minimum required to meet federal specifications for margarine with vitamin A added, namely 15,000 I.U. of vitamin A per pound.

TABLE 41—*Continued*

| Food and description | Sodium (Mg.) | Potassium (Mg.) |
|---|---|---|
| Oat products used mainly as hot breakfast cereals: | | |
| Oatmeal or rolled oats: | | |
| Dry form | 2 | 352 |
| Cooked | 218 | 61 |
| Oat products used mainly as ready-to-eat breakfast cereals: | | |
| Oats (with or without corn), puffed, added nutrients | 1,267 | .......... |
| Ocean perch, Atlantic (redfish): | | |
| Raw | 79 | 269 |
| Cooked, fried | 153 | 284 |
| Ocean perch, Pacific, raw | 63 | 390 |
| Oils, salad or cooking | 0 | 0 |
| Okra: | | |
| Raw | 3 | 249 |
| Cooked, boiled, drained | 2 | 174 |
| Olives, pickled; canned or bottled: | | |
| Green | 2,400 | 55 |
| Ripe, Ascolano (extra large, mammoth, giant jumbo) | 813 | 34 |
| Ripe, salt-cured, oil-coated, Greek style | 3,288 | .......... |
| Onions, mature (dry), raw | 10 | 157 |
| Onions, young green (bunching varieties), raw: | | |
| Bulb and entire top | 5 | 231 |
| Oranges, raw, peeled fruit, all commercial varieties | 1 | 200 |
| Orange juice: | | |
| Raw, all commercial varieties | 1 | 200 |
| Canned, unsweetened | 1 | 199 |
| Frozen concentrate, unsweetened, diluted with 3 parts water, by volume | 1 | 186 |
| Oysters: | | |
| Raw, meat only, Eastern | 73 | 121 |
| Cooked, fried | 206 | 203 |
| Frozen, solids and liquid | 380 | 210 |
| Oyster stew, commercial frozen, prepared with equal volume of milk | 366 | 176 |
| Pancake and waffle mixes and pancakes baked from mixes: | | |
| Plain and buttermilk, made with egg, milk | 564 | 154 |
| Parsnips, cooked, boiled, drained | 8 | 379 |
| Peaches: | | |
| Raw | 1 | 202 |
| Canned, solids and liquid, water pack, with or without artificial sweetener | 2 | 137 |
| Frozen, sliced, sweetened, not thawed | 2 | 124 |
| Peanuts: | | |
| Roasted, with skins | 5 | 701 |
| Roasted and salted | 418 | 674 |
| Peanut butters made with small amounts of added fat, salt | 607 | 670 |
| Pears: | | |
| Raw, including skin | 2 | 130 |
| Canned, solids and liquid, syrup pack, light | 1 | 85 |
| Peas, green, immature: | | |
| Cooked, boiled, drained | 1 | 196 |
| Canned, Alaska (Early or June peas): | | |
| Regular pack, solids and liquid | 236[2] | 96 |
| Special dietary pack (low-sodium), solids and liquid | 3 | 96 |
| Frozen, cooked, boiled, and drained | 115 | 135 |
| Peas, mature seeds, dry, whole, raw | 35 | 1,005 |

TABLE 41—*Continued*

| Food and description | Sodium (Mg.) | Potassium (Mg.) |
|---|---|---|
| Peas and carrots, frozen, cooked, boiled, drained......... | 84 | 157 |
| Pecans.................................................. | Trace | 603 |
| Peppers, hot, chili, mature, red, raw, pods excluding seeds | 25 | 564 |
| Peppers, sweet, garden varieties, immature, green, raw... | 13 | 213 |
| Perch, yellow, raw....................................... | 68 | 230 |
| Pickles, cucumber, dill.................................. | 1,428 | 200 |
| Pies: | | |
| Baked, piecrust made with unenriched flour: | | |
| Apple.............................................. | 301 | 80 |
| Cherry............................................. | 304 | 105 |
| Mince.............................................. | 448 | 178 |
| Pumpkin........................................... | 214 | 160 |
| Piecrust or plain pastry, made with, enriched flour, baked | 611 | 50 |
| Pike, walleye, raw...................................... | 51 | 319 |
| Pineapple: | | |
| Raw............................................... | 1 | 146 |
| Frozen chunks, sweetened, not thawed............... | 2 | 100 |
| Pizza, with cheese, from home recipe, baked: | | |
| With cheese topping................................ | 702 | 130 |
| With sausage topping............................... | 729 | 168 |
| Plate dinners, frozen, commercial, unheated: | | |
| Beef pot roast, whole oven-browned potatoes, peas, and corn.............................................. | 259 | 244 |
| Chicken, fried; mashed potatoes; mixed vegetables (carrots, peas, corn, beans)....................... | 344 | 112 |
| Meat loaf with tomato sauce, mashed potatoes, and peas | 393 | 115 |
| Turkey, sliced; mashed potatoes; peas............... | 400 | 176 |
| Plums: | | |
| Raw, Damson....................................... | 2 | 299 |
| Canned, solids and liquid, purple (Italian prunes), syrup pack, light........................................ | 1 | 145 |
| Popcorn, popped: | | |
| Plain.............................................. | (3) | ........... |
| Oil and salt added................................. | 1,940 | ........... |
| Pork, fresh: | | |
| Retail cuts, trimmed to retail level: | | |
| Loin............................................... | 65 | 390 |
| Pork, cured, light-cure, commercial, ham, medium-fat class, separable lean, cooked, roasted................ | 930 | 326 |
| Pork, cured, canned: | | |
| Ham, contents of can.............................. | (1,100) | (340) |
| Potatoes: | | |
| Cooked, boiled in skin............................. | 3[10] | 407 |
| Dehydrated mashed: | | |
| Flakes without milk: | | |
| Dry form....................................... | 89 | (1,600) |
| Prepared, water, milk, table fat added.......... | 231 | 286 |
| Pretzels................................................ | 1,680[11] | 130 |
| Prunes: | | |
| Dried, "softenized," cooked (fruit and liquid), with added sugar....................................... | 3 | 262 |
| Pudding mixes and puddings made from mixes: | | |
| With starch base: | | |
| Pudding made with milk, cooked................. | 129 | 136 |
| Pudding made with milk, without cooking.......... | 124 | 129 |

10. Applies to product without added salt. If salt is added, an estimated average value for sodium is 236 mg. per 100 grams.

11. Sodium content is variable. For example, very thin pretzel sticks contain about twice the average amount listed.

TABLE 41—*Continued*

| Food and description | Sodium (Mg.) | Potassium (Mg.) |
|---|---|---|
| Pumpkin, canned | 2 | 240 |
| Radishes, raw, common | 18 | 322 |
| Raisins, natural (unbleached): | | |
| Cooked, fruit and liquid, added sugar | 13 | 355 |
| Raspberries: | | |
| Canned, solids and liquid, water pack, with or without artificial sweetener, red | 1 | 114 |
| Frozen, red, sweetened, not thawed | 1 | 100 |
| Rennin products: | | |
| Tablet (salts, starch, rennin enzyme) | 22,300 | . . . . . . . . . . . . |
| Dessert mixes and desserts prepared from mixes: | | |
| Chocolate, dessert made with milk | 52 | 125 |
| Other flavors (vanilla, caramel, fruit flavorings): | | |
| Mix, dry form | 6 | . . . . . . . . . . . . |
| Dessert made with milk | 46 | 128 |
| Rhubarb, cooked, added sugar | 2 | 203 |
| Rice: | | |
| Brown: | | |
| Raw | 9 | 214 |
| Cooked | 282 | 70 |
| White (fully milled or polished): | | |
| Enriched: | | |
| Common commercial varieties, all types: | | |
| Raw | 5 | 92 |
| Cooked | 374 | 28 |
| Rice products used mainly as ready-to-eat breakfast cereals: | | |
| Rice flakes, added nutrients | 987 | 180 |
| Rice puffed; added nutrients, without salt | 2 | 100 |
| Rice, puffed or open-popped, presweetened, honey and added nutrients | 706 | . . . . . . . . . . . . |
| Rockfish, including black, canary, yellowtail, rasphead, and bocaccio, cooked, oven-steamed | 68 | 446 |
| Roe, cooked, baked or broiled, cod and shad[12] | 73 | 132 |
| Rolls and buns: | | |
| Commercial: | | |
| Ready-to-serve: | | |
| Danish pastry | 366 | 112 |
| Hard rolls, enriched | 625 | 97 |
| Plain (pan rolls), enriched | 506 | 95 |
| Sweet rolls | 389 | 124 |
| Rusk | 246 | 161 |
| Rutabagas, cooked, boiled, drained | 4 | 167 |
| Rye, flour, medium | (1) | 203 |
| Rye wafers, whole-grain | 882 | 600 |
| Salad dressings, commercial:[13] | | |
| Blue and Roquefort cheese: | | |
| Regular | 1,094 | 37 |
| Special dietary (low-calorie): | | |
| Low-fat (approx. 5 cal. per tsp.) | 1,108 | 34 |
| French: | | |
| Regular | 1,370 | 79 |
| Special dietary (low-calorie): | | |
| Low-fat (approx. 5 cal. per tsp.) | 787 | 79 |
| Mayonnaise | 597 | 34 |
| Thousand island: | | |
| Regular | 700 | 113 |

12. Prepared with butter or margarine, lemon juice or vinegar.

13. Values apply to products containing salt. For those without salt, sodium content is low, ranging from less than 10 mg. to 50 mg. per 100 grams; the amount usually is indicated on the label.

TABLE 41—*Continued*

| Food and description | Sodium (Mg.) | Potassium (Mg.) |
|---|---|---|
| Salad dressings, commercial:[12]—*Continued:* | | |
| Thousand island—*Continued:* | | |
| Special dietary (low-calorie, approx. 10 cal. per tsp.) | 700 | 113 |
| Salmon: | | |
| Coho (silver): | | |
| Raw. | 48[15] | 421 |
| Canned, solids and liquid. | 351[14] | 339 |
| Salt pork, raw. | 1,212 | 42 |
| Salt sticks, regular type. | 1,674 | 92 |
| Sandwich spread (with chopped pickle): | | |
| Regular. | 626 | 92 |
| Special dietary (low-calorie, approx. 5 cal. per tsp.). | 626 | 92 |
| Sardines, Atlantic, canned in oil, drained solids. | 823 | 590 |
| Sardines, Pacific, in tomato sauce, solids and liquid. | 400 | 320 |
| Sauerkraut, canned, solids and liquid. | 747[16] | 140 |
| Sausage, cold cuts, and luncheon meats: | | |
| Bologna, all samples. | 1,300 | 230 |
| Frankfurters, raw, all samples. | 1,100 | 220 |
| Luncheon meat, pork, cured ham or shoulder, chopped, spiced or unspiced, canned. | 1,234 | 222 |
| Pork sausage, links or bulk, cooked. | 958 | 269 |
| Scallops, bay and sea, cooked, steamed. | 265 | 476 |
| Soups, commercial, canned: | | |
| Beef broth, bouillon, and consomme, prepared with equal volume of water. | 326 | 54 |
| Chicken noodle, prepared with equal volume of water. | 408 | 23 |
| Tomato: | | |
| Prepared with equal volume of water. | 396 | 94 |
| Prepared with equal volume of milk. | 422 | 167 |
| Vegetable beef, prepared with equal volume of water. | 427 | 66 |
| Soy sauce. | 7,325 | 366 |
| Spaghetti, enriched, cooked, tender stage. | 1 | 61 |
| Spaghetti, in tomato sauce with cheese, canned. | 382 | 121 |
| Spinach: | | |
| Cooked, boiled, drained. | 50 | 324 |
| Canned: | | |
| Regular pack, drained solids. | 236[2] | 250 |
| Special dietary pack (low-sodium), solids and liquid. | 34 | 250 |
| Frozen, chopped, cooked, boiled, drained. | 52 | 333 |
| Squash, summer, all varieties, cooked, boiled, drained. | 1 | 141 |
| Squash, frozen: | | |
| Summer, yellow crookneck, cooked, boiled, drained. | 3 | 167 |
| Winter, heated. | 1 | 207 |
| Strawberries: | | |
| Raw. | 1 | 164 |
| Frozen, sweetened, not thawed, sliced. | 1 | 112 |
| Sturgeon, cooked, steamed. | 108 | 235 |
| Succotash (corn and Lima beans), frozen: | | |
| Cooked, boiled, drained. | 38 | 246 |
| Sugars, beet or cane, brown. | 30 | 344 |
| Sweet potatoes: | | |
| Cooked, all, baked in skin. | 12 | 300 |
| Canned, liquid pack, solids and liquid, regular pack in syrup. | 48 | (120) |
| Dehydrated flakes, prepared with water. | 45 | 140 |

14. For product canned without added salt, value is approximately the same as for raw salmon.

15. Sample dipped in brine contained 215 mg. sodium per 100 grams.

16. Values for sauerkraut and sauerkraut juice are based on salt content of 1.9 and 2.0 per cent, respectively, in the finished products. The amounts in some samples may vary significantly from this estimate.

TABLE 41—*Continued*

| Food and description | Sodium (Mg.) | Potassium (Mg.) |
|---|---|---|
| Tangerines, raw (Dancy variety) | 2 | 126 |
| Tapioca, dry | 3 | 18 |
| Tapioca desserts, tapioca cream pudding | 156 | 135 |
| Tartar sauce, regular | 707 | 78 |
| Tea, instant (water-soluble solids) carbohydrate added: | | |
| Dry powder | .......... | 4,530 |
| Beverage | .......... | 25 |
| Tomatoes, ripe: | | |
| Raw | 3 | 244 |
| Canned, solids and liquid, regular pack | 130 | 217 |
| Tomato catsup, bottled | 1,042[17] | 363 |
| Tomato juice: | | |
| Canned or bottled: | | |
| Regular pack | 200 | 227 |
| Special dietary pack (low-sodium) | 3 | 227 |
| Tomato juice cocktail, canned or bottled | 200 | 221 |
| Tomato puree, canned: | | |
| Regular pack | 399 | 426 |
| Special dietary pack (low-sodium) | 6 | 426 |
| Tongue, beef, medium-fat, cooked, braised | 61 | 164 |
| Tuna, canned: | | |
| In oil, solids and liquid | 800 | 301 |
| In water, solids and liquid | 41[18] | 279[18] |
| Turkey, all classes: | | |
| Light meat, cooked, roasted | 82 | 411 |
| Dark meat, cooked, roasted | 99 | 398 |
| Turkey potpie, commercial, frozen, unheated | 369 | 114 |
| Turnips, cooked, boiled, drained | 34 | 188 |
| Turnip greens, leaves, including stems: | | |
| Canned, solids and liquid | 236[2] | 243 |
| Frozen, cooked, boiled, drained | 17 | 149 |
| Veal, retail cuts, untrimmed | 80 | 500 |
| Vinegar, cider | 1 | 100 |
| Waffles, frozen, made with enriched flour | 644 | 158 |
| Walnuts: | | |
| Black | 3 | 460 |
| Persian or English | 2 | 450 |
| Watercress leaves including stems, raw | 52 | 282 |
| Watermelon, raw | 1 | 100 |
| Wheat flours: | | |
| Whole (from hard wheats) | 3 | 370 |
| Patent: | | |
| All-purpose or family flour, enriched | 2 | 95 |
| Self-rising flour, enriched (anhydrous monocalcium phosphate used as a baking acid)[19] | 1,079 | ....[20] |
| Wild rice, raw | 7 | 220 |
| Yeast: | | |
| Baker's, compressed | 16 | 610 |
| Brewer's, debittered | 121 | 1,894 |
| Yogurt, made from whole milk | 47 | 132 |
| Zweiback | 250 | 150 |

17. Applies to regular pack. For special dietary pack (low sodium), values range from 5 to 35 mg. per 100 grams.

18. One sample with salt added contained 875 mg. of sodium per 100 grams and 275 mg. of potassium.

19. The acid ingredient most commonly used in self-rising flour. When sodium acid pyrophosphate in combination with either anhydrous monocalcium phosphate or calcium carbonate is used, the value for calcium is approximately 120 mg. per 100 grams; for phosphorus, 540 mg.; for sodium, 1,360 mg.

20. 90 mg. of potassium per 100 grams contributed by flour. Small quantities of additional potassium may be provided by other ingredients.

# APPENDIX 7

## MINERAL ELEMENTS AND EXCESS OF ACIDITY OR ALKALINITY

### TABLE 42

MINERAL ELEMENTS* AND EXCESS OF ACIDITY OR ALKALINITY†
PER 100 GM. OF FOODS, EDIBLE PORTION

| FOOD | MINERALS | | | | | EXCESS‡ | |
| --- | --- | --- | --- | --- | --- | --- | --- |
| | Mag-nesium (Gm.) | Potas-sium (Gm.) | Sodium (Gm.) | Chlo-rine (Gm.) | Sul-phur (Gm.) | Acidity (Cc. of N Acid HCl) | Alkalinity (Cc. of N Alkali NaOH) |
| Almonds............ | 0.275 | 0.756 | 0.024 | 0.037 | 0.164 | 2.2 | 12.0–18.3 |
| *Apples:* | | | | | | | |
| fresh............. | 0.006 | 0.116 | 0.015 | 0.004 | 0.004 | .......... | 0.8–3.7 |
| dried............. | 0.029 | 0.557 | 0.072 | 0.019 | 0.019 | .......... | .......... |
| *Apricots:* | | | | | | | |
| fresh............. | 0.012 | 0.370 | 0.021 | 0.004 | 0.006 | .......... | 4.8–8.4 |
| dried............. | 0.062 | 1.924 | 0.109 | 0.021 | 0.031 | .......... | 31.3–41.9 |
| Asparagus.......... | 0.015 | 0.200 | 0.008 | 0.047 | 0.051 | 1.0 | 0.8 |
| Bananas............ | 0.024 | 0.412 | 0.023 | 0.163 | 0.013 | .......... | 4.4–7.9 |
| Barley, entire....... | 0.126 | 0.495 | 0.070 | 0.139 | 0.153 | 6.0–17.5 | .......... |
| *Beans:* | | | | | | | |
| dried............. | 0.165 | 1.284 | 0.189 | 0.007 | 0.224 | .......... | 18.0–23.9 |
| Lima, fresh........ | 0.067 | 0.606 | 0.089 | 0.009 | 0.068 | .......... | 14.0 |
| dried......... | 0.181 | 1.899 | 0.282 | 0.025 | 0.156 | .......... | 41.6 |
| string or green..... | 0.032 | 0.288 | 0.012 | 0.045 | 0.024 | .......... | 4.1–5.4 |
| Beef................ | 0.032 | 0.382 | 0.066 | 0.056 | 0.221 | 8.1–38.5 | .......... |
| Beets.............. | 0.027 | 0.235 | 0.053 | 0.040 | 0.017 | .......... | 8.9–11.4 |
| Beet greens.......... | 0.097 | 0.390 | ...... | ...... | 0.035 | .......... | .......... |
| Brains.............. | 0.016 | 0.269 | 0.160 | 0.155 | 0.130 | 17.7–20.7 | .......... |
| Bread, white........ | 0.034 | 0.110 | 0.517 | 0.602 | 0.083 | 1.5–7.1 | .......... |
| Broccoli............ | 0.024 | 0.352 | 0.030 | 0.076 | 0.126 | .......... | 3.6–4.9 |
| Brussels sprouts...... | 0.015 | 0.375 | ...... | ...... | 0.098 | .......... | 0.8–4.3 |
| Butter.............. | 0.002 | 0.019 | § | § | 0.009 | 0.4–4.3 | .......... |
| *Cabbage:*.......... | 0.016 | 0.217 | 0.038 | 0.034 | 0.074 | .......... | 1.4–8.2 |
| celery ........... | 0.011 | 0.400 | 0.028 | 0.023 | 0.013 | .......... | .......... |
| Cantaloupe.......... | 0.016 | 0.243 | 0.048 | 0.048 | 0.016 | .......... | 7.5 |
| Carrots............ | 0.020 | 0.219 | 0.050 | 0.035 | 0.019 | .......... | 4.4–10.8 |
| Cauliflower.......... | 0.023 | 0.292 | 0.048 | 0.038 | 0.074 | .......... | 1.4–5.3 |
| Celery............. | 0.025 | 0.320 | 0.101 | 0.225 | 0.021 | .......... | 2.5–11.1 |
| Cheese, hard........ | 0.031 | 0.116 | 0.900 | 0.972 | 0.214 | 0.3–11.8 | 3.6–5.1 |
| Cherries............ | 0.012 | 0.125 | 0.015 | 0.004 | 0.018 | .......... | 1.7–7.3 |
| Chestnuts.......... | 0.048 | 0.415 | 0.037 | 0.010 | 0.049 | .......... | 7.4–11.3 |
| Chicken............ | 0.047 | 0.402 | 0.054 | 0.034 | 0.303 | 9.6–25.4 | .......... |
| Chocolate.......... | 0.082 | 0.400 | 0.019 | 0.009 | 0.114 | 8.1 | 7.9 |
| Cocoa.............. | 0.192 | 0.534 | 0.060 | 0.050 | 0.197 | .......... | 0.7 |
| Coconut, fresh....... | 0.040 | 0.360 | 0.040 | 0.120 | 0.044 | .......... | 4.1–7.0 |
| Collards............ | 0.017 | | | | | | |
| *Corn:* | | | | | | | |
| field, mature....... | 0.142 | 0.300 | 0.110 | 0.041 | 0.124 | .......... | .......... |
| sweet | | | | | | | |
| fresh ........... | 0.047 | 0.278 | ...... | ...... | 0.037 | 1.8 | .......... |
| mature ........ | 0.121 | 0.415 | 0.148 | 0.050 | 0.146 | 6.0 | .......... |
| Cowpeas, dried....... | 0.265 | 1.305 | 0.036 | 0.019 | 0.250 | .......... | .......... |
| Crabs.............. | 0.117 | 0.271 | 0.366 | 0.570 | 0.255 | 39.5 | .......... |
| Cranberries.......... | 0.005 | 0.056 | 0.002 | 0.004 | 0.008 | .......... | 3.2‖ |
| Cream.............. | 0.006 | 0.112 | 0.031 | 0.067 | 0.033 | .......... | 0.4–3.2 |
| Cucumbers.......... | 0.020 | 0.170 | 0.026 | 0.028 | 0.011 | .......... | 3.2–31.5 |

---

* W. H. Peterson, J. T. Skinner, and F. M. Strong, Elements of food biochemistry (New York: Prentice-Hall, Inc., 1944), pp. 262–65.

† M. A. Bridges and M. R. Mattice, Food and beverage analyses (Philadelphia: Lea & Febiger, 1942), pp. 200–214.

‡ The ranges indicated come from reports of several authors, in which variety and method of preparation influence the results in part. For individual studies and sources of data see Bridges and Mattice, *op. cit.*

§ Variable.    ‖ Partly acid *in vivo.*

TABLE 42—*Continued*

| FOOD | MINERALS | | | | | EXCESS‡ | |
|---|---|---|---|---|---|---|---|
| | Magnesium (Gm.) | Potassium (Gm.) | Sodium (Gm.) | Chlorine (Gm.) | Sulphur (Gm.) | Acidity (Cc. of N Acid HCl) | Alkalinity (Cc. of N Alkali NaOH) |
| *Currants:* | | | | | | | |
| fresh | 0.031 | 0.208 | 0.015 | 0.010 | 0.021 | .......... | 0.7–8.8 |
| dried | 0.155 | 1.040 | 0.075 | 0.050 | 0.105 | .......... | 5.8–21.8 |
| Dates | 0.065 | 0.580 | 0.040 | 0.253 | 0.048 | .......... | 5.5–12.4 |
| Eel | 0.018 | 0.241 | 0.032 | 0.035 | 0.133 | 7.0–9.9 | .......... |
| Eggplant | 0.015 | 0.260 | 0.026 | 0.063 | 0.020 | | 4.5 |
| Eggs | 0.009 | 0.149 | 0.111 | 0.100 | 0.233 | 11.1–24.5 | .......... |
| Egg white | 0.011 | 0.149 | 0.175 | 0.131 | 0.211 | 4.8–8.3 | .......... |
| Egg yolk | 0.013 | 0.110 | 0.078 | 0.067 | 0.214 | 25.3–51.8 | .......... |
| *Figs:* | | | | | | | |
| fresh | 0.020 | 0.205 | 0.043 | 0.037 | 0.017 | .......... | |
| dried | 0.068 | 0.709 | 0.151 | 0.126 | 0.060 | | 10.0–100.9 |
| Fish (all kinds) | 0.024 | 0.375 | 0.064 | 0.137 | 0.199 | 8.5–20.1 | .......... |
| Flour, wheat, white... | 0.021 | 0.137 | 0.053 | 0.079 | 0.155 | 7.4–9.6 | .......... |
| Frog | 0.024 | 0.308 | 0.055 | 0.040 | 0.163 | 10.6–15.8 | .......... |
| Garlic | 0.008 | 0.130 | 0.009 | 0.004 | 0.318 | | |
| Goose | 0.031 | 0.406 | ..... | ..... | 0.326 | 7.7–24.5 | .......... |
| Gooseberries | 0.009 | 0.150 | 0.010 | 0.009 | 0.015 | | 2.1–7.6 |
| Grapefruit | 0.007 | 0.164 | 0.006 | 0.007 | 0.005 | .......... | 6.4 |
| Grapes | 0.004 | 0.267 | 0.011 | 0.002 | 0.009 | | 2.7–7.2 |
| Haddock | 0.017 | 0.334 | 0.099 | 0.241 | 0.225 | 8.5–19.7 | .......... |
| Heart | 0.035 | 0.329 | 0.102 | 0.204 | 0.151 | 27.6 | |
| Honey | 0.004 | 0.051 | 0.006 | 0.015 | 0.003 | 1.1 | 0.4–4.6 |
| Horse-radish | 0.028 | 0.550 | 0.094 | 0.013 | 0.234 | .......... | 2.7–5.8 |
| Kale | 0.055 | 0.486 | 0.050 | 0.120 | 0.160 | .......... | 4.0–17.0 |
| Kidney | 0.019 | 0.240 | 0.238 | 0.376 | 0.148 | 8.4–31.0 | .......... |
| Kohlrabi | 0.052 | 0.370 | 0.050 | 0.050 | 0.039 | .......... | 6.0 |
| Lamb (*see* Mutton) | | | | | | | |
| Leeks | 0.037 | 0.380 | 0.036 | 0.110 | 0.056 | | 5.5–11.3 |
| Lemons | 0.006 | 0.152 | 0.009 | 0.006 | 0.012 | | 5.5–9.9 |
| Lentils, dried | 0.082 | 0.662 | 0.754 | 0.062 | 0.123 | 5.2–17.8 | 0.4–2.0 |
| Lettuce | 0.015 | 0.256 | 0.028 | 0.085 | 0.014 | | 3.8–14.1 |
| Liver | 0.021 | 0.255 | 0.021 | 0.091 | 0.258 | 9.4–49.5 | .......... |
| Lobster | 0.022 | 0.258 | ..... | ..... | ..... | 38.4 | .......... |
| Macaroni, dry | 0.038 | 0.054 | 0.010 | 0.077 | 0.119 | 3.8–9.6 | .......... |
| *Milk:* | | | | | | | |
| cow | | | | | | | |
| fresh | 0.019 | 0.129 | 0.047 | 0.114 | 0.031 | .......... | 1.8–4.2 |
| evaporated | 0.038 | 0.258 | 0.094 | 0.228 | 0.067 | .......... | 4.6 |
| powder | 0.118 | 0.955 | 0.348 | 1.029 | 0.229 | .......... | 21.6 |
| goat | ..... | ..... | 0.026 | ..... | 0.163 | .......... | .......... |
| human | 0.005 | 0.055 | ..... | 0.058 | 0.142 | | |
| Mushrooms | 0.012 | 0.280 | 0.013 | 0.026 | 0.025 | | 1.8–4.0 |
| Mustard greens | 0.016 | 0.330 | 0.020 | 0.090 | 0.142 | | |
| Mutton | 0.033 | 0.260 | 0.070 | 0.069 | 0.187 | 4.5–22.5 | .......... |
| Oatmeal (rolled oats).. | 0.143 | 0.365 | 0.072 | 0.027 | 0.207 | 1.5–13.2 | .......... |
| Oats, entire | 0.150 | 0.450 | 0.168 | 0.089 | 0.187 | | |
| Onions | 0.016 | 0.200 | 0.020 | 0.053 | 0.065 | .......... | 0.2–8.4 |
| Orange juice | 0.014 | 0.200 | 0.006 | 0.008 | 0.005 | .......... | 4.5 |
| Oranges | 0.011 | 0.177 | 0.014 | 0.006 | 0.011 | .......... | 5.6–9.6 |
| Parsnips | 0.038 | 0.396 | 0.010 | 0.038 | 0.025 | | 6.6–11.9 |

TABLE 42—*Continued*

| FOOD | MINERALS | | | | | EXCESS‡ | |
|---|---|---|---|---|---|---|---|
| | Magnesium (Gm.) | Potassium (Gm.) | Sodium (Gm.) | Chlorine (Gm.) | Sulphur (Gm.) | Acidity (Cc. of N Acid HCl) | Alkalinity (Cc. of N Alkali NaOH) |
| *Peaches:* | | | | | | | |
| fresh | 0.015 | 0.174 | 0.012 | 0.006 | 0.005 | ......... | 3.8–6.1 |
| dried | 0.087 | 1.009 | 0.070 | 0.035 | 0.029 | ......... | 4.1–12.1 |
| Peanuts | 0.169 | 0.706 | 0.052 | 0.040 | 0.276 | 3.9–16.4 | ......... |
| Pears | 0.005 | 0.110 | 0.010 | 0.004 | 0.010 | ......... | 1.5–3.6 |
| *Peas:* | | | | | | | |
| green | 0.035 | 0.259 | 0.024 | 0.049 | 0.035 | 1.4–2.9 | 1.2–5.2 |
| mature | 0.121 | 0.943 | 0.072 | 0.034 | 0.178 | 0.5–3.4 | 1.2–10.3 |
| *Peppers:* | | | | | | | |
| green | 0.025 | 0.270 | 0.015 | 0.031 | 0.030 | ......... | ......... |
| red | 0.013 | 0.120 | 0.006 | 0.014 | 0.030 | ......... | ......... |
| Persimmons | 0.005 | 0.170 | 0.013 | 0.009 | 0.011 | ......... | ......... |
| Pike | 0.031 | 0.416 | 0.029 | 0.032 | 0.218 | 2.8–19.5 | ......... |
| Pineapple | 0.014 | 0.230 | 0.008 | 0.038 | 0.003 | ......... | 2.2–7.00 |
| Plums | 0.010 | 0.212 | 0.003 | 0.002 | 0.004 | ......... | 4.8‖ |
| Pork | 0.027 | 0.415 | 0.081 | 0.040 | 0.216 | 7.7–28.6 | ......... |
| Potatoes | 0.027 | 0.498 | 0.030 | 0.048 | 0.033 | ......... | 7.0–12.8 |
| Prunes, dried | 0.032 | 0.845 | 0.101 | 0.004 | 0.024 | ......... | 7.8–20.3‖ |
| Pumpkins | 0.021 | 0.198 | 0.011 | 0.025 | 0.016 | ......... | 0.3–7.8 |
| Rabbit | 0.029 | 0.415 | 0.047 | 0.051 | 0.184 | 14.8–22.4 | ......... |
| Radishes | 0.014 | 0.166 | 0.083 | 0.056 | 0.038 | ......... | 2.9–7.2 |
| Raisins | 0.017 | 0.796 | 0.120 | 0.068 | 0.043 | ......... | 23.7–27.0 |
| Raspberries | 0.018 | 0.141 | 0.007 | 0.010 | 0.012 | ......... | 4.1–6.1 |
| Rhubarb | 0.015 | 0.392 | 0.010 | 0.070 | 0.008 | ......... | 8.6–13.0 |
| *Rice:* | | | | | | | |
| entire | 0.141 | 0.334 | 0.068 | 0.066 | 0.121 | ......... | ......... |
| polished | 0.033 | 0.046 | 0.012 | 0.056 | 0.114 | 2.5–9.0 | ......... |
| Rutabagas | 0.015 | 0.210 | 0.052 | 0.031 | 0.069 | ......... | 8.5 |
| Rye, entire | 0.136 | 0.477 | 0.060 | 0.043 | 0.152 | 11.3 | ......... |
| Sardines, fresh | 0.035 | ...... | ...... | ...... | ...... | 11.4–26.5 | |
| *Shrimps:* | | | | | | | |
| dried | ...... | ...... | | | ...... | | |
| salted | 0.327 | 0.760 | § | § | 0.183 | 1.6 | |
| Soybeans, mature | 0.287 | 1.693 | 0.280 | 0.007 | 0.269 | ......... | |
| Spaghetti (*see* Macaroni) | | | | | | | |
| Spinach | 0.048 | 0.416 | 0.093 | 0.118 | 0.027 | ......... | 5.1–39.6 |
| Squash | 0.006 | 0.161 | 0.011 | 0.018 | 0.029 | | 2.8 |
| Strawberries | 0.019 | 0.205 | ...... | ...... | 0.013 | | 1.8–3.5 |
| Sugar beets | 0.041 | 0.440 | 0.130 | 0.180 | 0.021 | ......... | 3.3–9.4 |
| Sweet potatoes | 0.035 | 0.381 | 0.031 | 0.022 | 0.014 | ......... | 5.0–7.9 |
| Tomatoes | 0.016 | 0.277 | 0.013 | 0.048 | 0.017 | ......... | 5.6–13.7 |
| Turkey | 0.028 | 0.367 | 0.130 | 0.123 | 0.234 | 10.4–19.5 | ......... |
| Turnip greens | 0.079 | 0.300 | 0.260 | 0.390 | 0.051 | | 2.3 |
| Turnips | 0.019 | 0.193 | 0.104 | 0.054 | 0.048 | ......... | 2.7–10.2 |
| Veal | 0.030 | 0.380 | 0.086 | 0.073 | 0.199 | 9.8–28.5 | ......... |
| Venison | 0.029 | 0.336 | 0.070 | 0.041 | 0.211 | 23.8 | ......... |
| Walnuts | 0.132 | 0.606 | 0.013 | 0.030 | 0.120 | 7.9–9.2 | ......... |
| Watercress | 0.010 | 0.100 | 0.031 | 0.059 | 0.071 | | |
| Watermelon | 0.006 | 0.071 | 0.012 | 0.006 | 0.005 | ......... | 1.8–2.7 |
| *Wheat:* | | | | | | | |
| entire | 0.163 | 0.409 | 0.106 | 0.088 | 0.175 | 9.7–12.0 | |
| bran | 0.420 | 1.252 | 0.007 | 0.042 | 0.245 | | |
| Yams | 0.015 | 0.290 | 0.015 | 0.037 | 0.013 | ......... | |

# APPENDIX 8

## WEIGHT AND HEIGHT TABLES
### TABLE 43

### DESIRABLE WEIGHTS FOR MEN AND WOMEN, ACCORDING TO HEIGHT AND FRAME, AGES 25 AND OVER*

| HEIGHT (IN SHOES) | | WEIGHT IN INDOOR CLOTHING | | |
|---|---|---|---|---|
| | | Small Frame | Medium Frame | Large Frame |
| **MEN** | | | | |
| Feet | Inches | Pounds | Pounds | Pounds |
| 5 | 2....... | 112–120 | 118–129 | 126–141 |
| 5 | 3....... | 115–123 | 121–133 | 129–144 |
| 5 | 4....... | 118–126 | 124–136 | 132–148 |
| 5 | 5....... | 121–129 | 127–139 | 135–152 |
| 5 | 6....... | 124–133 | 130–143 | 138–156 |
| 5 | 7....... | 128–137 | 134–147 | 142–161 |
| 5 | 8....... | 132–141 | 138–152 | 147–166 |
| 5 | 9....... | 136–145 | 142–156 | 151–170 |
| 5 | 10....... | 140–150 | 146–160 | 155–174 |
| 5 | 11....... | 144–154 | 150–165 | 159–179 |
| 6 | 0....... | 148–158 | 154–170 | 164–184 |
| 6 | 1....... | 152–162 | 158–175 | 168–189 |
| 6 | 2....... | 156–167 | 162–180 | 173–194 |
| 6 | 3....... | 160–171 | 167–185 | 178–199 |
| 6 | 4....... | 164–175 | 172–190 | 182–204 |
| **WOMEN** | | | | |
| 4 | 10....... | 92– 98 | 96–107 | 104–119 |
| 4 | 11....... | 94–101 | 98–110 | 106–122 |
| 5 | 0....... | 96–104 | 101–113 | 109–125 |
| 5 | 1....... | 99–107 | 104–116 | 112–128 |
| 5 | 2....... | 102–110 | 107–119 | 115–131 |
| 5 | 3....... | 105–113 | 110–122 | 118–134 |
| 5 | 4....... | 108–116 | 113–126 | 121–138 |
| 5 | 5....... | 111–119 | 116–130 | 125–142 |
| 5 | 6....... | 114–123 | 120–135 | 129–146 |
| 5 | 7....... | 118–127 | 124–139 | 133–150 |
| 5 | 8....... | 122–131 | 128–143 | 137–154 |
| 5 | 9....... | 126–135 | 132–147 | 141–158 |
| 5 | 10....... | 130–140 | 136–151 | 145–163 |
| 5 | 11....... | 134–144 | 140–155 | 149–168 |
| 6 | 0....... | 138–148 | 144–159 | 153–173 |

* Derived from data of the 1959 Build and Blood Pressure Study, Society of Actuaries. Developed by the Metropolitan Life Insurance Company, Statistical Bureau.

# APPENDIX 9

## Energy Expenditure

Passmore and Durnin (1) have compiled more than five hundred values representing energy expenditures while carrying out personal necessities: sitting and walking at different speeds; during children's recreation; light indoor recreation of adults; domestic work; mental work; office work; during such "moderate" exercise as canoeing, horseback riding, cycling; during "heavy" exercise,

### TABLE 44

#### Daily Energy Expenditure of the Reference Man and Woman (2)
(Mean Annual Temperature 10° C.)

Calories

**Man, 65 Kg.**

A. 8 hr. *working activities:* mostly standing, over-all rate: 2.5 cal/min      1,200
B. 8 hr. *non-occupational activities*
     1 hr. washing, dressing, etc., at 3.0 cal/min..............    180
     1½ hr. walking at about 6 k.p.h. at 5.3 cal/min............    480
     4 hr. sitting activities at 1.54 cal/min...................    370
     1½ hr. active recreation and/or domestic work at 5.2 cal/min    470     1,500
C. 8 hr. *rest in bed* at basal metabolic rate...........................    500

      Total..................................................3,200

**Woman, 55 Kg.**

A. 8 hr. *working activities* in the home or in industry, mostly standing, over-all rate: 1.83 cal/min      880
B. 8 hr. *non-occupational activities*
     1 hr. washing, dressing, etc., at 2.5 cal/min..............    150
     1 hr. walking about 5 k.p.h. at 3.6 cal/min..............    220
     5 hr. sitting activities at 1.41 cal/min...................    420
     1 hr. active recreation and/or domestic work at 3.5 cal/min.    210     1,000
C. 8 hr. *rest in bed* at basal metabolic rate..............................    420

      Total ..................................................2,300

such as football, swimming, skiing, cross-country running, fishing; in various types of light and heavy industry, agriculture, lumber work, and the various activities of soldiers.

The unit used in expressing energy expenditure is in terms of the *total* energy expenditure in calories per minute rather than in *net* energy expenditure above basal calories. This unit has been recommended by the Committee on Calorie Requirements of the Food and Agriculture Organization in 1957 (2). Table 51 presents an example of how the energy expenditure may be distributed during the day.

## REFERENCES

1. PASSMORE, R., and DURNIN, J. V. G. A. Human energy expenditure, Physiol. Rev., **34**:801–40, 1955.
2. FOOD AND AGRICULTURE ORGANIZATION OF THE UNITED NATIONS. Calorie requirements. ("FAO Nutritional Studies," No. 15.) Rome, 1957.

# GLOSSARY OF DIETETIC TERMS REVISED, 1965

In 1931, members of The American Dietetic Association were actively working on the complexities of diets named after doctors, diseases, and many miscellaneous symptoms. The lack of consistent principles, nutritional inadequacies, and overlapping produced much confusion, controversy, and strain in the dietetic services. At that time, Grace Bulman, as chairman of a committee of the Diet Therapy Section, began collecting routine hospital diets used in sixty-five Class A hospitals in various parts of the country. With characteristic understatement, she reported: "These show a wide variation as to nomenclature and type of foods included" (1). Margery Ardrey, as chairman in the following year, carried on with some description of diets (2).

By 1939 the situation had reached the place where members felt the need for further revisions in nomenclature and descriptions of therapeutic diets that, among other things, would reflect the principle propounded earlier by Dr. Ruth Wheeler—that such diets should be regarded as modifications of the normal diet. At this time, Sister Jeanne d'Arc was appointed chairman of a committee to develop a glossary of dietetic terms. After two years of serious effort, a mimeographed list of terms was compiled and submitted to over two hundred members of the Association for review (3, 4). In the end, much order had been brought about by naming and describing diets in terms of dietetic principles rather than after doctors and diseases. Official use was made of this "Glossary of Dietetic Terms" in the first edition of the *Handbook of Diet Therapy* compiled for The American Dietetic Association in 1946 (5). Diets were named, defined, and described as set forth in this Glossary.

By 1948 rapid strides in diet therapy made members realize that corrections of inaccuracies, deletions, and additions were in order. Dr. Hazel Hauck as chairman and Dr. Helen Pilcher and Beatrice Finkelstein took the matter in hand, making extensive changes to bring the Glossary more closely in line with the newer findings in nutrition and with the wishes of the members. At this time the committee stated:

> In general the terms selected for inclusion in the Glossary of Dietetic Terms fall into the following categories: terms relating to the field of dietetics or the work of the dietitian; therapeutic diets; nutrients, or classes of nutrients required by man or thought to be useful in the human dietary; terms used in describing diets or foods, or relating to food composition; diseases associated with dietary deficiency or conditioned malnutrition; and some terms relating to digestion. The reader should consult a medical dictionary and appropriate texts for terms which are outside the scope of this glossary.

This revision was completed in 1950 and was used in naming and describing diets in the revised edition of the *Handbook of Diet Therapy* in 1952 (6). The complete Glossary appeared in this edition.

In 1956, members were again ready to reconsider the content of the Glossary. Under the chairmanship of Lorraine Weng, a committee of the Diet Therapy Section solicited recommendations from the state diet therapy sections regarding revisions in the *Handbook* which were incorporated in the third edition (7). In response to a question, "Do you use the Glossary of Dietetic Terms in naming and defining diets in your hospital manual?" approximately 70 per cent replied that they used it in some degree; 30 per cent that they did not.

The most recent revision of the Glossary was completed in 1965. Important contributors to this revision were: Elisabeth Yearick, Ph.D.; Annie Galbraith, Chairman, Diet Therapy Section, The American Dietetic Association; and Marion Seymour Noland, past-Chairman, Diet Therapy Section, The American Dietetic Association.

Since the purpose of the Glossary is to provide aid in the naming and the description of diets as well as in the use of other related terminology in diet manuals, recommendations from this committee have been included in the Glossary. In addition, recent findings relating to the chemical structure and function of certain nutrients have been incorporated from the National Academy of Science–National Research Council Publication No. 1164 (sixth revised edition). However, the guide lines established in 1950 have been retained.

## REFERENCES

1. WALLER, D. S. Report of Diet Therapy Section chairman, J. Am. Dietet. A., **7**:292, 1931.
2. Digest of committee reports, Diet Therapy Section. *In* American Dietetic Association Reports for 1931–32, J. Am. Dietet. A., Suppl. 8, p. 21, 1933.
3. Committee reports, Diet Therapy Section. *In* Annual Reports, 1939–40, and Proceedings New York meeting, J. Am. Dietet. A., **16**:1015, 1940.
4. Committee report, Diet Therapy Section. *In* Annual Reports, 1940–41, and Proceedings St. Louis meeting, J. Am. Dietet. A., **17**:999, 1941.
5. Glossary of dietetic terms. *In* TURNER, D. Handbook of diet therapy. Chicago: University of Chicago Press, 1946.
6. Revised glossary of dietetic terms. *In* TURNER, D. Handbook of diet therapy. 2d ed. Chicago: University of Chicago Press, 1952.
7. Revised glossary of dietetic terms. *In* TURNER, D. Handbook of diet therapy. 3d ed. Chicago: University of Chicago Press, 1959.

ACID, ARACHIDONIC—*See* Acids, Fatty, Essential.

ACID, ASCORBIC ($C_6H_8O_6$)—Vitamin C. A water-soluble vitamin destroyed by irreversible oxidation which is hastened by heat, light, and alkalinity. Occurs in metabolically active plant and animal tissues in two biologically active forms: ascorbic acid (reduced), and dehydroascorbic acid (oxidized). Essential for the formation of collagen of fibrous tissue, vascular endothelium, and matrices of bone and dentine; participates in biological oxidations and reductions. Certain clinical and biochemical manifestations occur well in advance of the deficiency disease, scurvy (1, 2).

ACID, DEHYDROASCORBIC ($C_6H_6O_6$)—The reversibly oxidized form of ascorbic acid; biologically active.

ACID, FOLIC—*See* Folacin.

ACID, FOLINIC ($C_{20}H_{24}N_7O_7$)—Citrovorum factor, formyl tetrahydrofolic acid; one of the functionally active forms of the folic acid group of vitamins. *See* Folacin.

ACID, LINOLEIC—*See* Acids, Fatty, Essential.

ACID, LINOLENIC—*See* Acids, Fatty, Essential.

ACID, NICOTINIC—*See* Niacin.

ACID, OXALIC ($C_2H_2O_4$)—A dicarboxylic acid which occurs as a result of metabolic processes in the body, and which is found in certain foods (especially cocoa, rhubarb, spinach, and certain other greens). Oxalic acid forms insoluble salts with calcium, magnesium, and iron.

ACID, PANTOTHENIC ($C_8H_{16}O_3NCOOH$)—A member of the B complex, thought to be essential for man; water-soluble, thermolabile. A constituent of coenzyme A which is essential for transacylations occurring in the energy cycle, in lipid synthesis and degradation, and in porphyrin synthesis. A deficiency has not been recognized in man on a natural diet; fatigue, gastrointestinal and neuromuscular disturbances have been observed after administration of an antagonist. It is distributed widely in plant and animal foods, synthesized by intestinal bacteria. Daily requirements appear to be provided by the average diet supplying 10–15 mg. (1, 4).

ACID, PARA-AMINOBENZOIC ($NH_2C_6H_4COOH$)—A component of the folacin molecule; a member of the B complex; originally considered to be a vitamin essential to humans.

ACID, PHYTIC ($C_6H_6 6H_2PO_4$)—Inositol hexaphosphoric acid; a phosphoric acid ester of inositol; occurs in nuts, legumes, and outer layers of cereal grains; the insoluble calcium-magnesium salt is called phytin. Because phytic acid forms insoluble salts with calcium, iron, and magnesium, it interferes with the intestinal absorption of these minerals.

ACID, PTEROYLGLUTAMIC—*See* Folacin.

ACID ASH RESIDUE—The preponderance in a food of inorganic (fixed) acid radicals, chiefly chloride, sulfate, and phosphate, which form acid ions (anions) in the body. The value is computed and expressed as the amount of 0.1N alkali which would be required for neutralization (5). See Table 42.

ACID-FORMING FOODS—Foods in which acid ash residue exceeds alkaline ash residue are meat, fish, poultry, eggs, cereals, and some nuts. Certain fruits, such as cranberries and some varieties of prunes and plums, although they have a predominantly alkaline residue, are acid-forming because the organic acids in them are not metabolized by the body. Pure starches, sugars, and fats, which produce carbonic acid during metabolism, are not included as "acid-forming" since carbonic acid is readily excreted by the lungs, without affecting alkaline reserve. *See* Acid Ash Residue.

ACIDOSIS—A condition caused by the abnormal accumulation of acids in the body or an excessive loss of base from the body; usually accompanied by a lowered alkali reserve. Acidosis may result from the accumulation of ketone bodies (diabetes), insufficient removal of acids (renal failure), inadequate removal of carbon dioxide (pulmonary), or excessive loss of alkaline intestinal secretions (diarrhea).

ACIDS, AMINO—Any one of a class of organic compounds containing the amino ($NH_2$) group and the carboxyl (COOH) group; the chief components of protein material.

ACIDS, AMINO, ESSENTIAL—Some twenty-two amino acids are known to be physiologically important. Of these, eight have been demonstrated to be dietary essentials for the adult human, since they are synthesized in inadequate quantity by the body. This group of "essential" amino acids includes isoleucine, leucine, lysine, methionine, phenylalanine, threonine, tryptophan, and valine. Dietary sources of a ninth amino acid, histidine, are probably necessary to maintain growth during childhood. The diet must include adequate sources of the essential amino acids and sufficient amounts of the other amino acids for maintenance in the adult and growth in children. Estimates of human requirements (6) appear in Table 45. Amino acids in foods (7) appear in Table 40.

ACIDS, FATTY—Any of a homologous series of open-chain monocarboxylic acids, containing only carbon, hydrogen, and oxygen. The saturated fatty acids ($C_nH_{2n}O_2$) of food fats are chiefly lauric ($C_{12}$), palmitic ($C_{16}$), and stearic ($C_{18}$). Mono-unsaturated fatty acids, such as oleic, have a single double bond ($C_nH_{2n-2}O_2$); polyunsaturated fatty acids, such as linoleic, have more than one double bond per molecule.

ACIDS, FATTY, ESSENTIAL—A group of unsaturated fatty acids, of which linoleic ($C_{17}H_{31}COOH$), and arachidonic ($C_{19}H_{31}COOH$) have been shown to be essential for growth and dermal integrity in human infants. Linolenic acid ($C_{17}H_{29}COOH$), formerly considered to be essential, does not prevent the dermatitis of fatty acid deficiency, nor is it as effective as linoleic in promoting growth. An intake of 1–3 per cent of total calories in the form of linoleic acid appears to meet the infant and probably adult needs. Excellent sources are corn, cottonseed, safflower, and soybean oils. The fatty acid content of additional foods appears in Table 36.

ADEQUATE—An amount sufficient to meet a specific requirement. The term "adequate diet" is often incorrectly used in reference to an individual diet which provides the dietary allowances of nutrients as recommended by the Food and Nutrition Board of the National Research Council. *See* Dietary Allowances, Recommended; Balanced Diet.

ALCOHOL—Ethanol. A term usually applied to ethyl alcohol ($C_2H_5OH$) which is distilled from the products of anaerobic fermentation of carbohydrate; yields about 7 calories per gram, of which more than 75 per cent is available to the body.

ALKALINE ASH RESIDUE—The preponderance in a food of the elements sodium, potassium, calcium, and magnesium, which form basic ions (cations) in the body. The value is computed and expressed as the amount of 0.1N acid which would be required for neutralization. *See* Table 42.

ALKALOSIS—A condition resulting from the abnormal accumulation of base or the excessive loss of acid from the body. Alkalosis may result from excessive administration of absorbable alkali, from prolonged vomiting of acid gastric juice, and from hyperventilation.

ALLERGEN—Any substance capable of inducing a condition of allergy or specific hypersensitiveness.

ALLERGY, FOOD—Hypersensitiveness to a substance (probably protein) in food which is ordinarily harmless in similar amounts for the majority of persons.

ANEMIA—A deficiency of hemoglobin in the blood, associated with either a decreased number of red blood cells, reduced corpuscular hemoglobin, or an abnormal type of hemoglobin. In the macrocytic anemias of folacin and $B_{12}$ deficiency, the red cells are large, immature, and few in number; in the microcytic hypochromic anemia of iron deficiency, the red cells are small and contain insufficient hemoglobin.

ANOREXIA—Lack or loss of appetite for food.

ANTIVITAMIN—Any substance that interferes with the synthesis or metabolism of a vitamin—for example, avidin, which combines with biotin and prevents its absorption; thiaminase in certain raw fish, which destroys thiamine; and sulfanilamide, which interferes with the synthesis of folic acid in the intestinal tract by competing with para-aminobenzoic acid for a place in the molecule.

APPETITE—A natural desire for food.

ARIBOFLAVINOSIS—A disease resulting from the deficiency of riboflavin; characterized by lesions of the tongue and at angles of the mouth, dermatitis, and ocular changes.

ARTERIOSCLEROSIS—A generic term which includes a variety of conditions which cause the artery walls to become thick and hard and lose elasticity. *See* Atherosclerosis.

ARTIFICIAL SWEETENERS—*See* Saccharin, Sulfamate, Sorbitol.

AS PURCHASED (A.P.)—Refers to food as offered for sale on the retail market. In tables which give nutritive value for food "as purchased," the nutrient content is stated in terms of the weight of the food before inedible portions usually discarded are removed; i.e., the nutritive value of refuse is not included. *See* Edible portion.

ASH—The total mineral matter residue after ignition of a food; always either neutral or alkaline, since acid in excess of that which can be neutralized is volatilized.

ATHEROSCLEROSIS—A kind of arteriosclerosis in which the inner layer of the artery wall is made thick and irregular by deposits of a fatty substance. These deposits (called atheromata) project above the surface of the inner layer of the artery, and thus decrease the diameter of the internal channel of the vessel. *See* Arteriosclerosis.

AVAILABLE—A nutrient is available to the body when it is in the form that can be absorbed from the digestive tract and then used for its intended function in the body.

AVIDIN—A glycoprotein in raw egg white which binds biotin and prevents its absorption from the intestinal tract. Avidin is rendered inactive by heating.

AVITAMINOSIS—A disease due to the dietary deficiency of a vitamin or vitamins or to failure of absorption or utilization of the vitamin.

BALANCE—In nutrition, the term balance refers to that condition in which the nutrients taken into the body are balanced by corresponding excretions. When the intake and output are the same, the condition is described as balance or equilibrium. When the intake exceeds the output, the balance is positive, and retention of the nutrient has occurred. A negative balance describes the state in which the intake is less than the output, and the body stores have been used. The balance study has been a useful tool for measuring protein and mineral metabolism, although the balance is greatly affected by other dietary components and by body stores.

BALANCED DIET—The term "balanced diet" has been loosely or incorrectly used to imply ideal proportions of all proteins, minerals, fats, and carbohydrates for "optimum" nutrition or that two or more food essentials are ideally proportioned to meet "optimum" nutritional needs. Since no one "diet" can be quantitatively "balanced" for "optimum" needs of all individuals, the term "balanced diet" should be used only in properly informative statements where its meaning is plainly evident and free of misleading implications.

BERIBERI—A deficiency disease due to lack of thiamine, and endemic in areas in which polished rice is the chief item of the diet; characterized by multiple peripheral neuritis, with paralysis, edema, or cardiac failure.

$\beta$-Carotene—*See* Carotene.

BIOLOGICAL VALUE—*See* Protein, Biological Value of.

BIOTIN ($C_{10}H_{16}O_3N_2S$)—Vitamin H, a vitamin of the water-soluble B complex. Occurs bound in nature in at least two active forms; participates in carbon dioxide fixation reactions associated with fatty acid synthesis and energy utilization. Deficiency states have been recognized in man only when the absorption of dietary biotin has been prevented by the ingestion of large amounts of avidin. Widely distributed in plant and animal foods, and synthesized by intestinal bacteria; daily requirements seem to be provided by an average diet supplying 150–300 $\mu$g.

BULK—*See* Carbohydrate, indigestible, which is the preferred term.

CALCIFEROL ($C_{28}H_{44}O$)—Vitamin $D_2$; a fat-soluble antirachitic factor, formed by the irradiation of ergosterol.

CALORIE (LARGE OR KILO-CALORIE)—The unit used to express food energy; the amount of heat required to raise the temperature of 1 kg. water 1° C.

CARBOHYDRATE, AVAILABLE—This term represents the portion of the carbohydrate of foods which is available to the human body for glycogen formation. It includes starch, dextrins, glycogen, maltose, sucrose, lactose, as well as the monosaccharides glucose, fructose, galactose, mannose, and pentoses.

CARBOHYDRATE, INDIGESTIBLE—Substances which make up the cell-wall structure of plants, consisting of varying amounts of cellulose, hemicellulose, lignin, pectin substances, gums, mucin, etc.; not hydrolyzed by enzymes of the human gastrointestinal tract.

CARBOHYDRATE, TOTAL, BY DIFFERENCE—Solids in foods other than protein, fat, and ash; includes both available and indigestible carbohydrates and some organic acids.

CAROTENE—Provitamin A. A group of yellow-red plant pigments which yield vitamin A upon oxidative scission. $\beta$-carotene ($C_{40}H_{56}$) is the most abundant form in green leafy and yellow vegetables. Because of inefficient conversion of carotene to vitamin A in the body, 2 I.U. of $\beta$-carotene are considered equivalent to 1 I.U. vitamin A in man; approximately two-thirds of the vitamin A activity of the average diet is provided by carotene.

CELLULOSE ($C_6H_{10}O_5$)$_n$—A polysaccharide made up of beta-glucose units; constituent of the cell walls of plants. *See* Carbohydrate, indigestible; Fiber, crude.

CELLULOSE, METHYL—A methyl ester of cellulose which swells in water to produce a colloidal solution; used as a thickening agent, an emulsifier, and as a non-caloric source of bulk.

CHOLESTEROL ($C_{27}H_{45}OH$)—A fat-like steroid alcohol found in animal tissues; may be synthesized in the body; excreted in the bile, but largely reabsorbed from the digestive tract in the presence of fat. Transported in serum attached to specialized proteins (lipoproteins). See Table 39 for food sources.

CHOLINE ($C_5H_{15}NO_2$)—A component of lecithin and acetylcholine; often considered a member of the B complex; necessary for fat transport in the body; acts as donor of labile methyl groups.

COOK MANAGER—One who by training and/or experience is qualified to assume the responsibility for food and beverage preparation of the food service in a hospital, nursing home, school food service, and other institutions.

Also supervises and instructs all personnel in food service, maintains and establishes standards of sanitation, safety, and housekeeping. May also be responsible for scheduling of work and hours for personnel; maintaining records including food costs, meal census, and personnel records; planning of menus and routine modified diets; and purchasing of food and supplies. The services of a qualified dietary consultant or a shared dietitian should be available.

CYANOCOBALAMIN—One form of vitamin $B_{12}$. *See* Vitamin $B_{12}$.

CYCLAMATES—The sodium or calcium salts of cyclohexylsulfamic acid; water-soluble, with a sweet taste (30 times that of sucrose). Used as non-caloric sweeteners.

DIET—Daily allowance of food and drink.

DIET, BALANCED—*See* Balanced Diet.

DIET, BLAND—A diet composed of mild-flavored foods. (See pp. 43–44 in text.)

DIET, CALORIC, HIGH—A diet* which has a prescribed caloric value above the total energy requirement.

DIET, CALORIC, LOW—A diet* which has a prescribed caloric value below the total energy requirement.

DIET, CHOLESTEROL, LOW—A diet* in which the intake of total cholesterol is restricted. The dietary prescription should include the permissible amounts of fat, and cholesterol. *See* Diet, Fat Modified, page 62 in text.

DIET, ELIMINATION—An allowance of foods which do not commonly produce sensitivity in human patients. Used for the diagnosis of food allergy.

DIET, FAT MODIFIED—A diet* prescribed to meet a specified level of fat in the diet, a percentage of fat calories, or specified amounts or ratios of fatty

---

* This diet is one planned to approximate the Recommended Dietary Allowances of the Food and Nutrition Board, National Research Council (1964), for healthy persons.

acids. When used for regulation of abnormal serum lipids or in treatment of patients with vascular disease, fat modification may be combined with cholesterol restriction. *See* Diet, Cholesterol, Low; Polyunsaturated: Saturated (P/S) Fatty Acid Ratio.

DIET, FIBER, HIGH—A normal diet,* including an additional 2–3 servings of foods high in indigestible carbohydrate and an unrestricted amount of connective tissue.

DIET, FIBER, LOW—A diet* which contains a minimum of indigestible carbohydrates and no tough connective tissue.

DIET, FULL HOSPITAL—A normal diet* for patients who do not require dietary modifications for therapeutic purposes; also known as House, Regular, or General diet.

DIET, GALACTOSE FREE—A diet which has been made almost free of galactose by the elimination of milk and milk products; or those containing complexed forms. Peas, Lima beans, and beets contain raffinose and stachyose which may release galactose. *See* text page ooo.

DIET, GENERAL—*See* Diet, full hospital.

DIET, GLIADIN-RESTRICTED—A diet without wheat, rye, oats, and barley. (See pp. 78–79 in text.)

DIET, "GLUTEN-FREE"—*See* Gliadin-restricted diet.

DIET, HOUSE—*See* Diet, full hospital.

DIET, KETOGENIC—A diet in which the ratio of fatty acid (ketogenic) value to glucose (antiketogenic) value equals 2 or more, i.e., is sufficiently high to produce ketosis. It provides small amounts of carbohydrate, approximately 1 gm. protein per kilogram of body weight, and sufficient fat to meet full caloric requirements.

DIET, LIQUID, CLEAR—This diet is most often used pre- and postoperatively. It supplies fluids but is of little importance nutritionally. Only fat-free broth, tea, and coffee with sugar but without milk or cream are allowed. Occasionally small amounts of ginger ale, clear fruit or vegetable juice, and gelatin may be added.

DIET, LIQUID, FULL—A diet* consisting of a variety of foods that are liquid or liquefy at body temperature.

DIET, MODIFIED—A diet based on the normal diet and designed to meet the requirements of a given situation. It may be modified in individual nutrients, caloric value, consistency, flavor, techniques of service or preparation, content of specific foods, or a combination of these factors. A diet is described as "high" in a specific nutrient when it provides substantially more of the nutrient than is ordinarily required; the converse is true of a diet which is "low" in a specific nutrient. A diet can be called "free" of a nutrient only if that nutrient has been completely eliminated from the diet. The adjectives "restricted" and "controlled" are applied to a diet in which the specific nutrient is provided in amounts less than usually consumed. See text for specific modifications.

DIET, PHENYLALANINE-RESTRICTED—A diet in which phenylalanine is limited to a prescribed amount (p. 71 in text) by the use of selected natural foods and a specially prepared commercial product (p. 73 in text).

DIET, PROTEIN MODIFICATIONS—A diet* prescribed to provide a specified level of protein, or protein fraction, or a specified ratio or amount of amino acids.

DIET, PURINE, LOW—A diet* in which the chief sources of purines, such as glandular organs, dried legumes, and meat extractives are eliminated. Other meat and fish may be restricted to 4 oz. weekly, thus reducing the daily intake of uric acid equivalent to approximately 35 mg. *See* Purines, pages 116–19.

DIET, REGULAR—*See* Diet, full hospital.

DIET, SALT, LOW—*See* Diet, sodium-restricted.

DIET, SODIUM-RESTRICTED—A diet in which the sodium content is limited to a prescribed level. (See pp. 104–15 in text.)

DIET, SOFT—A diet* modified in consistency, i.e., including liquid foods and those solid foods which contain a restricted amount of indigestible carbohydrate and connective tissue. (See pp. 39–46 in text.)

DIET, TEST—A meal or meals used as part of a diagnostic procedure (9). See *Annual Reports and Proceedings, American Dietetic Association*, (1945–46), p. 35.

DIET, THERAPEUTIC—*See* Diet, modified.

DIETARY ALLOWANCES, RECOMMENDED (R.D.A.)—The amounts of various nutrients recommended by the Food and Nutrition Board of the National Research Council as normally desirable objectives toward which to aim in planning practical dietaries in the United States; enough higher than the minimal requirements of average individuals to cover substantially all individual variations in the requirements of persons in normal health. Allowances are related to body size and are stated for the reference men and women at moderate physical activity; for pregnancy and lactation; and for children and adolescent boys and girls of various age groups. "Comparative Dietary Standards for Adults in Other Countries," appears in tabular form in Publication 1146, NAS-NRC. *Recommended Dietary Allowances*, 1964 (1).

DIETARY CONSULTANT (ALSO CONSULTANT DIETITIAN)—One who has followed a prescribed academic program resulting in a baccalaureate degree from an accredited College or University and has satisfactorily completed an approved dietetic internship or qualifying experience. Advises and assists public and private establishments, such as child care centers, hospitals, nursing homes, and schools in food service management and nutritional problems in group feeding. Plans, organizes, and conducts such activities as in-service training courses, conferences, and institutes for food service managers, food handlers, and other workers.

Develops and evaluates informational materials. Studies food service practices and facilities, and makes recommendations for improvement. Confers with architects and equipment personnel in planning for building or remodeling food service units.

DIETARY HISTORY—An informative description of an individual's food intake over a period of time. Should include socioeconomic factors affecting food habits. Usually serves as a basis for planning individualized dietary therapy and education. For use in research, specialized information may be included in detail.

DIETARY STATUS—Summation of information received in dietary history. *See* Dietary History.

DIETETIC INTERN—One who has followed a prescribed academic program resulting in a baccalaureate degree from an accredited College or University and is completing an approved dietetic internship. Learns to function as a professionally qualified dietitian while following the planned internship program. Gains professional and practical experience as requirement for positions in dietetics.

DIETETICS—The combined science and art of feeding individuals or groups under different economic or health conditions according to the principles of nutrition and management.

DIETITIAN—One who has followed a prescribed academic program resulting in a baccalaureate degree from an accredited College or University and has satisfactorily completed an approved dietetic internship or qualifying experience. Plans and directs food service programs in hospitals, schools, restaurants, and other public or private institutions. Plans menus and modified diets providing required food and nutrients to feed individuals and groups. Supervises workers engaged in preparation and serving of meals. Purchases or requisitions food, equipment, and supplies, and develops and analyzes food-cost control records. Inspects work areas and storage facilities to insure observance of sanitary standards. Counsels individuals and groups in application of principles of nutrition to selection of food. May prepare educational materials on nutritional value of foods and methods of preparation.

DIETITIAN, ADMINISTRATIVE—One who has followed a prescribed academic program resulting in a baccalaureate degree from an accredited College or University and has satisfactorily completed an approved dietetic internship or qualifying experience. Organizes, plans, and directs food-service programs, applying principles of nutrition and management to menu planning, food preparation, and service. Develops standards for selecting, purchasing, and inspecting food, equipment, and supplies. Develops standards of sanitation. Supervises selection and training of nonprofessional food-service personnel. Prepares reports of financial management, safety practices, and program efficiency. Evaluates physical layout and equipment, employee utilization, and work procedures, and coordinates dietary services with those of other departments to increase effectiveness of program.

DIETITIAN, DIRECTOR—One who has followed a prescribed academic program resulting in a baccalaureate degree from an accredited College or University and has satisfactorily completed an approved dietetic internship or qualifying experience. Administers, plans, and directs activities of department providing quantity food service. Establishes policies and procedures, and provides administrative direction for menu formulation, food preparation and service, purchasing, sanitation standards, safety practices, and personnel utilization. Selects professional dietetic staff, and directs departmental educational programs. Coordinates interdepartmental professional activities, and serves as consultant to management on matters pertaining to dietetics.

DIETITIAN, TEACHING—One who has followed a prescribed academic program resulting in a baccalaureate degree from an accredited College or University and has satisfactorily completed an approved dietetic internship or qualifying experience. Plans, organizes, and conducts educational programs in dietetics and nutrition, nursing, medical and dental students, and other personnel. Prepares manuals, visual aids, course outlines, and other material used in teaching. May provide dietary counseling for patients in hospital or public health center. May engage in research.

DIETITIAN, THERAPEUTIC—One who has followed a prescribed academic program resulting in a baccalaureate degree from an accredited College or University and has satisfactorily completed an approved dietetic internship or qualifying experience. Plans and directs preparation and service of modified diets prescribed by the physician. Consults medical, nursing, and social service staffs concerning problems affecting patients' food habits and needs. Formulates menus for therapeutic diets based upon indicated physiologic and ethnic needs of patients and integrates them with basic institutional menus. Establishes and maintains standards of palatability and appearance of patient meals. Counsels patients and their families on the requirements and importance of their modified diets, and on how to plan and prepare the food. May engage in research. May teach nutrition and diet therapy to dietetic, medical, dental, and nursing students.

DIGESTIBILITY, COEFFICIENT OF APPARENT—The percentage of an ingested nutrient which cannot be recovered in the feces; hence, the percentage of an ingested nutrient which is assumed to have been absorbed. The coefficients of digestibility of protein, fat, and carbohydrate in a mixed American diet have been estimated to be 92 per cent, 95 per cent, and 97 per cent, respectively.

DIGESTION—The process of converting food into substances which can be absorbed by the body.

EDIBLE PORTION (E.P.)—As used in food tables, this term refers to that part of a food which is most commonly eaten. Some parts, such as parings of potatoes, which are edible but not usually eaten, are excluded.

ENERGY, FOOD—Expressed in terms of calories per unit weight; represents the energy available after deductions have been made for losses in digestion and metabolism. Energy values stated in food composition tables have been computed on the basis of the specific fuel factors for the individual foods. The commonly used physiological fuel factors, when applied to the total daily intake of protein, fat, and carbohydrate from a typical American diet, provide a good estimate of the energy value of the diet. *See* Fuel factors, physiological and specific.

ENRICHED BREAD—May be made from enriched flour or by the addition of the required substances to the baker's formula or by the use of special high-vitamin yeast and iron. *See* Enriched flour.

ENRICHED FLOUR—White flour enhanced in thiamine, riboflavin, niacin, and iron value by changing the milling process to retain these constituents or by the addition of chemicals to white flour. The minimum levels specified in the standards of identity promulgated under the Food, Drug, and Cosmetic Act are: thiamine, 2.0 mg.; riboflavin, 1.2 mg.; niacin, 16 mg.; and iron, 13 mg. per pound. Certain levels of vitamin D and calcium are permitted as optional ingredients. States which require enrichment of white flour have generally been guided by federal legislation.

ENRICHMENT—A food may be labeled "enriched" if it contains added nutrients in kinds and amounts meeting standards established by the Food and Drug Administration; usually applied to addition to nutrients of cereal products.

EXCHANGES—*See* Food Exchanges.

ERGOSTEROL ($C_{28}H_{44}O$)—Provitamin $D_2$; a plant sterol found chiefly in yeast, which, upon irradiation, forms calciferol (vitamin $D_2$).

EXTRINSIC FACTOR—A term applied by Castle to the hemopoietic factor in foods. *See* Vitamin B₁₂.

FAT—A glyceryl ester of fatty acids, which on hydrolysis yields three molecules of fatty acids to one of glycerol. In food tables, figures for fat include, in addition to true fats, other ether-extractable substances (3).

FIBER—As used in reference to therapeutic diets, this term includes indigestible organic tissue, either plant or animal.

FIBER, CRUDE—Made up largely of cellulose, those hemicelluloses which are not readily soluble, and lignin; as usually determined, that portion of a food sample which resists solution when boiled in dilute acid and dilute alkali.

FOLACIN ($C_{19}H_{19}N_7O_6$)—Folic acid, pteroylglutamic acid; a vitamin of the B complex sparingly soluble in water; functionally active forms are formyl derivatives of reduced folic acid, among them, folinic acid. Essential to the transfer of single carbon units in amino acid metabolism and nucleoprotein syntheses. Deficiency occurs in sprue and other malabsorption syndromes, frequently in combination with deficiencies of vitamin B₁₂ or ascorbic acid; manifested by macrocytic megaloblastic anemia, glossitis, and gastrointestinal disturbances. Daily needs seem to be met by the average diet supplying 0.15–0.3 mg. of folic and folinic acid conjugates (0.05–0.1 mg. folacin); major sources (11) are liver, yeast, kidney, and green leafy vegetables; additional vitamin is synthesized by intestinal micro-organisms. Because folacin therapy promotes blood regeneration in pernicious anemia without correcting the neurological complications, sale without prescription of vitamin preparations recommending more than 0.1 mg. folic acid a day is prohibited.

FOOD EXCHANGES—Lists of foods grouped in terms of approximate equivalents in carbohydrate, protein, and fat content; as well as minerals and vitamins. Used for the purpose of planning diabetic, low-calorie, and other quantitative diets.

FOOD SERVICE SUPERVISOR—One who by education and/or successful completion of a planned in-service training program trains and supervises employees engaged in serving food in a hospital, nursing home, school or university food service department, and similar institutions. Supervises maintenance of established standards of cleanliness for food service areas, equipment, and dining areas. May assist in the direction of food and beverage production and in preparation of employee schedules. Instructs workers in methods of performing duties, assigns and coordinates work of employees to promote efficiency of operations. Maintains records such as food costs, meal census, and personnel records. Other duties may be performed as delegated by dietitian or food service director. In smaller institutions may be responsible for daily routine food service.

FORTIFICATION—The addition of a nutrient or nutrients to a food in amounts sufficient to make the total content larger than that contained in any natural (unprocessed) food of its class—for example, vitamin D milk, fortified margarine, fortified fruit juices. In general, no standards of identity have to be met when a food is labeled "fortified."

FORTIFIED MARGARINE—Most of the margarine on the market in the United States is fortified with 15,000 I.U. of vitamin A per pound.

FUEL FACTORS, PHYSIOLOGICAL (ATWATER)—The general energy values of protein, fat, and carbohydrate (4, 9, and 4 calories per gram, respectively) which are applicable to the total nutrient intake of the mixed American diet. These factors allow for incomplete oxidation of protein in the body, and for average losses in digestion. They are not applicable to specific foods which differ in their coefficients of digestibility.

FUEL FACTORS, SPECIFIC (ATWATER)—The energy values of protein, fat, and carbohydrate, expressed as calories per gram, determined for individual foods on the basis of the coefficients of digestibility which are specific for each food.

GALACTOSEMIA—The accumulation of the monosaccharide galactose in the blood, owing to a hereditary lack of an enzyme involved in the conversion of galactose to glucose; mental and growth retardation; liver enlargement and cataracts occur. See Diet, Galactose Free.

GLYCOGEN—A polysaccharide, also known as "animal starch," which yields glucose on hydrolysis; found in liver, muscle, and other tissues.

GOITER, SIMPLE—Enlargement of the thyroid gland, caused by an absolute or relative deficiency of iodine.

HEMICELLULOSE—A group of polysaccharides forming part of the cell wall of plants; indigestible, but may be broken down to a considerable extent by intestinal micro-organisms. It also absorbs water. See Fiber, crude.

HYDROGENATED FAT—Food fats commercially processed to harden fat by eliminating part of double bonds. Some of the natural cis double bonds change to the trans form.

INORGANIC ELEMENTS—See Ash; Minerals.

INOSITOL—$C_6H_6(OH)_6$ is an alcohol allied to the hexoses. It occurs in many foods, particularly bran of cereal grains. Inositol in combination with six phosphate molecules forms the compound phytic acid which hinders absorption of calcium and iron. See Acid, Phytic.

INSULIN—The hormone derived from the beta cells of the islands of Langerhans of the pancreas; essential for normal carbohydrate metabolism. Seven forms of insulin are now commercially available, each havings its own time effect ranging from rapid to very slow and prolonged. Products include Crystalline Insulin (regular), Semi-Lente, Globin Insulin with Zinc, Insulin Isophane (NPH), Lente Insulin, Protamine Zinc Insulin, and Ultra-Lente Insulin.

INTRINSIC FACTOR—A mucoprotein enzyme present in normal gastric juice; essential to the efficient intestinal absorption of dietary vitamin $B_{12}$; deficient in the gastric juice of the patient who has pernicious anemia.

IODINE VALUE (IODINE NUMBERS)—The number of grams of iodine absorbed by 100 grams of fat. One of several ways of expressing amounts of fatty acids in foods. A measure of total double bonds in a fat, but does not indicate particular fatty acids present. Ranges from about 10 for coconut oil to about 200 for safflower oil. See Polyunsaturated, Saturated Fatty Acid Ratio; Diet, Fat Modified.

KETOSIS—A condition in which there is an accumulation in the body of ketone compounds (beta-hydroxybutyric acid, acetoacetic acid, and acetone) as a result of incomplete oxidation of fatty acids; occurs when the amount of fat being oxidized is excessive, as with the use of ketogenic diets, in semi-starvation, and uncontrolled diabetes.

KWASHIORKOR—A nutritional deficiency syndrome observed in children subsisting on low-protein, cereal diets; owing chiefly to protein malnutrition, but complicated by deficiencies of other nutrients; characterized by edema, dermatitis, dyspigmentation of hair and skin, growth failure, and liver damage.

LIGNIN—A constituent of crude fiber, occurring in the cell wall of plants; resistant to hydrolysis by digestive enzymes, strong acids, and alkalis; not attacked to any extent by intestinal micro-organisms. *See* Carbohydrate, indigestible; Fiber, crude.

LIPIDS—Fat or fat-like substances, including fatty acids, soaps, triglycerides, sterols, waxes, and phosphatides.

MALNUTRITION—A condition of the body resulting from an inadequate or excessive supply, or impaired utilization of one or more of the essential food constituents.

MALNUTRITION, CONDITIONED—Deficiency or excess of one or more nutrients in the tissues, caused by factors other than diet alone; for example, deficiencies caused by factors which interfere with ingestion, digestion, absorption, or utilization of essential nutrients or by factors that increase their requirement, destruction, or excretion.

MALABSORPTION SYNDROME—A term used to grossly describe such conditions as the sprues; celiac disease, idiopathic steatorrhea which have in common the failure to absorb various nutrients as fats, calcium, and other minerals, as well as certain vitamins, notably the fat-soluble ones.

MARASMUS—Severe malnutrition characterized by extreme emaciation. Incidence is highest in young children who are not eating or utilizing sufficient amounts of food.

MENADIONE $(C_{11}H_8O_2)$—A synthetic compound, having greater vitamin K activity than the naturally occurring vitamin; used as a reference standard for biological assays of vitamin K. In large doses, synthetic vitamin K has produced toxic effects; consequently, a dose in excess of 5 mg. should be avoided.

METABOLISM—A general term to designate all chemical changes which occur to substances within the body after absorption. These changes include constructive (anabolic) and destructive (catabolic) processes.

MICRONUTRIENTS—Nutrients present in very small amounts in food; as applied to mineral elements, the term usually refers to those present in the body in amounts less than that of iron, as manganese, copper, iodine, cobalt, molybdenum, and zinc.

MINERALS—"Inorganic" elements. The following are known to be present in body tissue: calcium, cobalt, chlorine, fluorine, iodine, iron, magnesium, manganese, molybdenum, phosphorus, potassium, selenium, silicon, sodium, sulfur, zinc. It is generally accepted that a requirement exists for most of these. Mineral constituents, obtained from food, aid in the regulation of the acid-base balance of body fluids and of osmotic pressure, in addition to the specific functions of individual elements in the body. Some minerals are present in the body largely in organic combination, as iron in hemoglobin and iodine in thyroxin; others occur in the body in inorganic form, as calcium salts in bone, sodium and chlorine in sodium chloride. The terms "minerals" and "inorganic elements" do not imply that the element occurs in inorganic form in food or body tissue. *See* Ash.

NIACIN ($C_5H_4NCOOH$)—Anti-pellagra factor, nicotinic acid. A water-soluble, heat-stable vitamin of the B complex. Functionally active as the niacinamide coenzymes; essential to cell respiration, carbohydrate and protein metabolism, and lipid syntheses. Deficiency results in the skin lesions, gastrointestinal and cerebral manifestations which characterize pellagra. Dietary sources include preformed niacin and the precursor tryptophan; human requirements are expressed in terms of niacin equivalents and are related to caloric consumption (1, 2, 3).

NIACINAMIDE ($C_5H_4NCONH_2$)—Nicotinamide, the amide of niacin; principal form of the vitamin occurring in tissues; a component of the coenzymes nicotinamide-adenine-dinucleotide (NAD) and nicotinamide-adenine-dinucleotide phosphate (NADP), which are essential to cell respiration.

NIACIN EQUIVALENT—The Recommended Dietary Allowances for niacin are expressed by the Food and Nutrition Board of the National Research Council as niacin equivalents, on the assumption that 60 mg. tryptophan may be converted to 1 mg. niacin (1).

NICOTINAMIDE—*See* Niacinamide.

NUTRIENT—Any substance useful in nutrition; for example, proteins, fats, carbohydrates, minerals, vitamins, water. *See* Nutrition.

NUTRITION—The combination of processes by which the living organism receives and utilizes the materials necessary for the maintenance of its functions and for the growth and renewal of its components.

NUTRITION HISTORY—An informative and comprehensive description of laboratory, and clinical findings as well as dietary history of an individual. *See* Dietary History; Nutritional Status.

NUTRITION, NORMAL—A condition of the body resulting from the efficient utilization of sufficient amounts of the essential nutrients provided in the food intake.

NUTRITIONAL STATUS—The condition of the body resulting from the utilization of the essential nutrients available to the body. Nutritional status may be good, fair, or poor, depending not only on the intake of dietary essentials but also on the relative need and the body's ability to utilize them. *See* Nutriture.

NUTRITIONIST—One who has followed a prescribed academic program and received a Master's degree in public health nutrition from an accredited College or University. Organizes, plans, and conducts programs concerning nutrition to assist in promotion of health and control of disease. Instructs auxiliary medical personnel and allied professional workers on food values and utilization of foods by human body. Advises health and other agencies on nutritional phases of their food programs. Conducts in-service courses pertaining to nutrition in clinics and similar institutions. Interprets and evaluates food and nutrient information designed for public acceptance and use. Studies and analyzes scientific discoveries in nutrition for adaptation and application to various dietary problems. May be employed by voluntary or public health agency.

NUTRITIONIST-PUBLIC HEALTH—One who has followed a prescribed academic program and received a Master's degree in public health nutrition from an accredited College or University. In a public health agency, interprets and applies scientific knowledge of nutrition to planning, organizing, and carrying out or directing programs for the promotion of positive health, the prevention of chronic and debilitating diseases, and the treatment and rehabilitation of individuals. Consults with administrators, medical, and para-medical personnel on current scientific findings in food and nutrition and their application to agency programs. Conducts or participates in pre-service and in-service education of professional staff of own and related agencies. May design, conduct, or participate in dietary and nutrition studies, and other studies with a nutrition component. Prepares and evaluates technical and popular educational material. Cooperates with other agencies in the formulation and coordination of nutrition programs involving professional or lay groups. Should have post-graduate education in nutrition as it relates to public health and qualifying experience for the responsibilities entailed.

NUTRITIONIST-TEACHING—One who has followed a prescribed academic program and received a Master's degree in public health nutrition from an accredited College or University. Plans, organizes, and conducts education programs in nutrition for the preparation of professional workers as well as for the public. Develops curricula, course outlines, visual aids, pamphlets, and other materials used in teaching. The nutritionist in the college teaches the basic science and application of science of food and nutrition. Often engages in research. The nutritionist in the Extension Service advises agency administrators and county home economists and participates with the agent in training lay leaders. In business, the nutritionist gives technical advice and guidance in preparing and conducting consumer education programs. Should have post-graduate education in nutrition as it relates to public health, research, and teaching and qualifying experience.

NUTRITURE—Condition as to nourishment, either with respect to all nutrients (general nutriture) or to one nutrient at a time.

OXALIC ACID—*See* Acid, Oxalic.

PELLAGRA—A multiple deficiency disease caused by the lack of niacin or its equivalent, and associated with deficiencies of other B vitamins. Signs and symptoms involve the skin, gastrointestinal tract, and nervous system.

PHENYLKETONURIA—The excretion of phenylpyruvic acid and other phenyl compounds in the urine, resulting from the hereditary lack of an enzyme necessary for the conversion of the amino acid phenylalanine to tyrosine; phenylalanine accumulates in blood and tissues, and mental retardation occurs.

POLYUNSATURATED: SATURATED (P/S) FATTY ACID RATIO—One of several ways to express relative amounts of fatty acids in foods or diets. Usually refers to linoleic acid (polyunsaturated) and total saturated fatty acids. Mono-unsaturated fatty acids (chiefly oleic) are not considered in this ratio. *See*: Diet, Fat modified.

PROTEIN—Any one of a group of complex nitrogenous compounds (approximately 16 per cent nitrogen) which yields amino acids upon hydrolysis; widely distributed in plant and animal tissues; essential constituents of the cell protoplasm. Protein values as stated in food composition tables are generally computed from total nitrogen content and include, in addition to true protein, other compounds such as amino acids and purine bases.

PROTEIN, BIOLOGICAL VALUE OF—The percentage of absorbed nitrogen that is retained by the body. The numerical value obtained varies with the conditions of the experiment.

PROTEIN HYDROLYSATE—A mixture of amino acids and polypeptides prepared by the digestion of proteins by acids, alkalies, or proteolytic enzymes. Properly prepared hydrolysates may be used for either oral or parenteral administration. Some methods of hydrolysis lead to the destruction of certain essential amino acids.

PROVITAMIN—The precursor of a vitamin; for example, carotene, ergosterol.

PROXIMATE COMPOSITION—As applied to food, the term usually includes the percentages of protein, fat, total carbohydrate, ash, and water; calorie values may also be included.

PURINES—Purine bases; compounds which contain heterocyclic nitrogenous purine structure $(C_5H_4N_4)$; catabolized to uric acid; dietary purines are supplemented by endogenous synthesis. *See* Diet, Purine, Low (text, pp. 116-19).

PYRIDOXINE—*See* Vitamin $B_6$.

REFUSE—That portion of foods which is inedible (as bones, pits, shells) or usually discarded in preparation of food for the table (as potato parings and tough outer leaves of vegetables). In food values expressed on the "as purchased" basis, the nutrients in refuse have been disregarded.

REQUIREMENTS—Although the average minimal requirements for various nutrients cannot be stated with accuracy, certain "minimum daily requirements" for food-labeling purposes have been designated in regulations for enforcement of the Federal Food, Drug, and Cosmetic Act (Table 46). These should not be confused with the Recommended Dietary Allowances.

RESEARCH NUTRITIONIST (MAY BE DESIGNATED AS RESEARCH DIETITIAN)—One who has followed a prescribed academic program and received a Master's degree in public health nutrition from an accredited College or University. Originates or assists in planning, organizing, and conducting programs in nutritional research. Performs research in improvement of food as related to appearance, palatability, and nutritional value. Studies and analyzes recent scientific discoveries in nutrition for application in current research, for development of tools for future research, and for interpretation to the public (10).

RESIDUE, FECAL—The total solid of feces made up of undigested and unabsorbed food and metabolic and bacterial products. Some foods, such as milk, or fats which contain no fiber, may significantly increase fecal residue under abnormal conditions.

RIBOFLAVIN $(C_{17}H_{20}N_4O_6)$—A vitamin of the B complex; sparingly soluble in water, decomposed by exposure to light, heat-labile in alkaline solutions. Functions biologically as the coenzymes flavin mononucleotide (FMN), and flavin adenine dinucleotide (FAD), which are components of the flavoproteins, essential to protein and energy metabolism; participates in biological oxidations and reductions. The deficiency disease, ariboflavinosis, is frequently associated with deficiencies of other B vitamins. Human requirements are now considered to be more closely related to energy expenditure than to protein intake; recommended allowances have been computed on the basis of caloric intake (1, 2).

RICKETS—A condition, caused chiefly by deficiency of vitamin D in infancy and childhood, in which calcification of the growing bone does not occur normally; marked by softening and bending of the long bones, delayed closure of the fontanelles, and other deformities. The effects of hypovitaminosis D may be influenced by other factors affecting calcium absorption.

SACCHARIN—Ortho-benzosulfimide; usually marketed as the sodium or calcium salt of saccharin; 300 times as sweet as sucrose.

SALT, IODIZED—Table salt (sodium chloride) to which has been added 1 part per 10,000 of iodine as potassium iodide.

SATIETY VALUE—That quality of food contributing to satisfaction and resulting in a sustained sense of comfort or well-being.

SCURVY—A disease resulting from the relative or absolute deficiency of ascorbic acid; characterized by hemorrhage, anemia, delayed wound healing, and defective skeletal growth in children.

SORBITOL ($C_6H_{14}O_6$)—A hexahydric alcohol. Imparts a sweet taste; used in maintaining moisture and in inhibiting crystallization of certain commercial products. Contains 4 calories per gram.

STANDARD OF IDENTITY OF FOODS—The U.S. Food, Drug, and Cosmetic Act as Amended authorizes the U.S. Food and Drug Administration to establish food standards. Under this authority, the FDA has promulgated definitions and standards of identity, also standards of quality and fill of container, for approximately 200 foods. These standards apply to foods shipped in interstate commerce. Food standards have also been established by the Department of the Interior, Bureau of Commercial Fisheries, the Department of Agriculture, the Department of Defense, the Department of Commerce, the Federal Trade Commission, the Veterans Administration, and the General Services Administration.

SUPPLEMENT, NUTRITIONAL—A general term which usually refers to a concentrated source of nutrients, prescribed in addition to the daily diet to increase the nutrient intake. A supplement may be a food such as yeast or wheat germ, a concentrate such as cod liver oil, or a pharmaceutical preparation of vitamins or minerals.

SWEETENERS, NON-NUTRITIVE, ARTIFICIAL—Artificial sweetening ingredients are saccharin, sodium saccharin, sodium cyclamate, potassium cyclamate, calcium cyclamate, or any combination of these. *See* Saccharin; Cyclamates.

THIAMINE ($C_{12}H_{17}N_4OS$)—Antiberiberi factor, vitamin $B_1$; water-soluble, heat-labile in neutral or alkaline solution. Active form is thiamine pyrophosphate (TPP) or cocarboxylase, a constituent of the carboxylase and transketolase enzymes which function in carbohydrate metabolism. Thiamine deficiency results in polyneuritis (beriberi). Human requirements are related to carbohydrate utilization, recommended allowances are based upon caloric intake.

TOCOPHEROL—Vitamin E; a group of four phenolic compounds (designated $\alpha$, $\beta$, $\gamma$, and $\delta$) with vitamin E activity; fat-soluble, sensitive to oxidation and to ultraviolet light. As antioxidants, the tocopherols may retard oxidation of other fat-soluble vitamins and lipoperoxidation in adipose tissue associated with a high intake of polyunsaturated fatty acids; they may also be involved in cell respiration and in nucleoprotein synthesis. Evidence is accumulating that the tocopherols, long recognized as having vitamin activity for animals, may play an essential role in human nutrition. Richest sources are the vegetable oils, whole grains, and eggs; the average daily intake has been estimated at 24 mg. tocopherol (14 mg. $\alpha$ tocopherol). Human needs are related to the intake of polyunsaturated fatty acids and may vary between 10 and 30 mg. per day for adults (1, 12).

TRACE ELEMENTS—Minerals occurring in small amounts in food or body tissues; those which are known to be dietary essentials are also called "micronutrients."

TRIGLYCERIDES—Glyceryl esters of fatty acids. *See* Fat.

TRYPTOPHAN ($C_8H_6NCH_2CHNH_2COOH$)—An essential amino acid; a constituent of body proteins, a source of the vitamin niacin and of the vasoconstrictor serotonin. Animal protein contains approximately 1.4 per cent and vegetable protein 1 per cent tryptophan; an average daily diet may provide 500–1,000 mg. tryptophan. The dietary tryptophan available over and above the body's requirement (approximately 500 mg. for young men) may be converted to niacin in a proportion of 60 mg. tryptophan to 1 mg. niacin.

UNIT, INTERNATIONAL VITAMIN (I.U.)—A definite quantity of each International Standard of Reference, used for expressing the content of the respective vitamins in foods and other materials. Such units have been established for vitamins A, C, D, and thiamine but are used principally for vitamins A and D, since values for thiamine and vitamin C can now be conveniently expressed in weights. Originally established by a committee appointed by the Health Organization of the League of Nations, standardization of vitamin units is now under the supervision of subcommittees of the World Health Organization.

UNIT, INTERNATIONAL VITAMIN A—The activity of 0.300 μg. vitamin A alcohol (equivalent to 0.344 μg. vitamin A acetate, or to 0.550 μg. vitamin A palmitate), equal to 0.600 μg. of the provitamin β-carotene.

UNIT, INTERNATIONAL VITAMIN $B_1$—The vitamin $B_1$ activity of 3.0 μg. of the International Standard crystalline thiamine hydrochloride (vitamin $B_1$), therefore 1 mg. thiamine equals 333 I.U.

UNIT, INTERNATIONAL VITAMIN C—The vitamin C activity of 0.05 mg. of the International Standard crystalline ascorbic acid (vitamin C).

UNIT, INTERNATIONAL VITAMIN D—The vitamin D activity of the International Standard solution of irradiated ergosterol in oil, containing 0.025 μg. of calciferol.

UNIT, U.S.P. (UNITED STATES PHARMACOPEIA)—Equal to the corresponding International Units.

VIOSTEROL—A general name for preparations of irradiated ergosterol in oil, in which the active agent is calciferol (vitamin $D_2$).

VITAMIN—An organic substance occurring in minute quantities in plant and animal tissues; must be either supplied in the diet of animals or synthesized from essential dietary or metabolic precursors; essential for specific metabolic functions or reactions to proceed normally.

VITAMIN A ($C_{20}H_{29}OH$)—A fat-soluble vitamin occurring in several biologically active forms; sensitive to oxidation and exposure to light; an unsaturated alcohol which may be found as an aldehyde or an ester; synthesized in animal tissue from plant precursors (carotenes). Functions in the development of normal skin and bone and in the maintenance of scotopic vision; essential for regeneration of visual purple, participates in synthesis of mucopolysaccharides. Deficiency may be manifested by night-blindness, keratinization of epithelial tissue, and xerophthalmia. Excessive doses of the vitamin produce toxic effects (1, 2).

VITAMIN A VALUE—The combined potency of a food or diet, represented by its content of vitamin A, carotene, and other plant precursors (1, 3).

VITAMIN B₁—*See* Thiamine.

VITAMIN B₂—An obsolete term for riboflavin.

VITAMIN B₆—A collective term which includes three water-soluble, heat-stable pyridine derivatives: pyridoxine ($C_8H_{11}O_3N$) in plant products, pyridoxal ($C_8H_9O_3N$) and pyridoxamine ($C_8H_{12}O_2N_2$) in animal products; all exhibit activity in humans, functioning as the phosphorylated derivatives. Principally concerned with the metabolism of amino acids, as a coenzyme in transaminations, deaminations, and decarboxylations, and in the metabolism of tryptophan; also involved in carbohydrate and fat metabolism. Symptoms attributed to a vitamin B₆ deficiency in humans include convulsions in infants receiving a synthetic diet, lesions of the skin and mucous membranes of adults receiving an antagonist. Widely distributed in plant and animal foods, excellent sources include yeast, wheat germ, liver, kidney, and muscle meats. Although there is evidence that vitamin B₆ requirements increase with protein intake, the needs seem to parallel those of thiamine; a tentative adult allowance of 1.5–2.0 mg. per day is readily provided by ordinary mixed diets.

VITAMIN B₁₂—Animal protein factor, anti-anemic principle, extrinsic factor; a group of cobalt-containing compounds (cobalamins) with hemopoietic activity, of which cyanocobalamin ($C_{69}H_{90}N_{14}O_{14}PCo$) is the prototype; soluble in water, relatively stable to heat; occurs bound.to protein in animal tissues. Functions in nucleic acid and protein syntheses; facilitates reduction reactions; necessary for activity of folic acid coenzymes. Deficiency occurs in the absence of the gastric intrinsic factor (pernicious anemia, post-gastrectomy syndrome), in the malabsorption syndromes, and as a consequence of a strict vegetarian diet; manifested by a macrocytic megaloblastic anemia, spinal cord degeneration, and gastro-intestinal changes. Daily needs are met by the average diet supplying 3–5 µg. vitamin B₁₂; major sources are liver, kidney, and muscle meats (13).

VITAMIN B COMPLEX—As originally used, this term referred to the water-soluble vitamins occurring in yeast, liver, meats, and whole-grain cereals, but some of the newer B complex vitamins, for example, folic acid and Vitamin B₁₂, do not correspond to this distribution; includes a number of compounds which have been identified, isolated, and synthesized, viz., thiamine, riboflavin, nicotinic acid, vitamin B₆, pantothenic acid, biotin, folic acid, inositol, and choline; vitamin B₁₂, the structure of which has been determined; and others which have been only partially demonstrated or identified.

VITAMIN C—*See* Ascorbic Acid.

VITAMIN D—A group of fat-soluble factors which have antirachitic activity; structurally related to the sterols. Vitamins D₂ and D₃ are derived from their respective provitamins ergosterol and 7-dehydrocholesterol by ultraviolet irradiation. Vitamin D increases the availability, retention, and utilization of calcium and phosphorus for proper mineralization of the skeleton. Deficiency of vitamin D is a major cause of rickets in the infant, and one of the causes of osteomalacia in the adult. The requirements of infants are generally met through the use of vitamin D milk; the needs of adults are probably supplied by the average diet and casual exposure to sunshine. Excessive doses of the vitamin produce toxic effects (1, 2).

VITAMIN D₂—*See* Calciferol.

VITAMIN D₃ ($C_{27}H_{44}O$)—A fat-soluble antirachitic factor, obtained by ultra-violet-ray activation of 7-dehydrocholesterol; occurs in fish-liver oils and in irradiated foods of animal origin; termed "natural" vitamin D.

VITAMIN D MILK—May be produced by three different methods: (1) "fortified" milk, which is now more generally distributed than the other types, is that to which a vitamin D concentrate has been added; (2) "metabolized" milk is produced by feeding the cows irradiated yeast; and (3) "irradiated" milk has been exposed directly to ultraviolet rays. The standard amount used for fortification is 400 I.U. vitamin D per quart of fresh or reconstituted milk.

VITAMIN E—*See* Tocopherol.

VITAMIN INHIBITORS—*See* Antivitamins.

VITAMIN K—"Koagulationsvitamin." A group of fat-soluble, light-sensitive vitamins possessing a common naphthoquinone structure; natural forms include vitamin K₁ ($C_{31}H_{46}O_2$) occurring in green leaves, and vitamin K₂ ($C_{41}H_{56}O_2$) produced by intestinal bacteria; synthetic forms, such as menadione, are available as water-soluble esters. Vitamin K is required for the maintenance of normal prothrombin time; it may be involved in cell respiration and associated phosphorylations. Deficiency, which is characterized by hemorrhagic tendencies, may result from reduced synthesis by intestinal bacteria or poor intestinal absorption; prophylaxis is achieved with 1–2 mg. vitamin K, administered orally.

VITAMINS, FAT-SOLUBLE—Vitamins A, D, E, and K, which are extractable from foods with fat solvents.

VITAMINS, WATER-SOLUBLE—Members of the B complex and vitamin C which can be extracted from foods with water as the solvent.

WATER, ENDOGENOUS—Water which is provided by metabolic processes.

WATER, EXOGENOUS—Water ingested as such or as a component of food. In food composition tables, "water" includes volatile substances in addition to free water.

WATER, REQUIREMENT—Determined by body heat production, amounts of dissolved materials to be excreted by the kidney and its concentrating capacity, and losses due to sweating. Water and salt requirements are intimately related. Under ordinary environmental conditions, the daily requirement of a 70-kg. man on a 3,200-calorie diet is about 2,300–3,100 ml., much of which is contained in foods as eaten.

## TABLE 45

### TENTATIVE MINIMUM REQUIREMENTS OF AMINO ACIDS BY YOUNG ADULTS

| AMINO ACID | MINIMUM REQUIREMENTS* (GM. PER DAY) | |
|---|---|---|
| | Women | Men |
| Isoleucine........... | 0.45 | 0.70 |
| Leucine............. | 0.62 | 1.10 |
| Lysine............. | 0.50 | 0.80 |
| Methionine⎱ Cystine ⎰ ········ | {0.55 | {1.10 |
| Phenylalanine........ | 0.22⎱ | {1.10 |
| Tyrosine........... | 0.90⎰ | |
| Threonine........... | 0.31 | 0.50 |
| Tryptophan......... | 0.16 | 0.25 |
| Valine............. | 0.65 | 0.80 |

\* Values for women are from R. M. Leverton in *Protein and Amino Acid Nutrition*, ed. A. A. Albanese. New York: Academic Press, 1959, p. 504. Values for men are from W. C. Rose, Fed. Proc., **8**:546, 1949.

## TABLE 46

### MINIMUM DAILY REQUIREMENTS OF CERTAIN VITAMINS AND MINERALS*

Established by the Food and Drug Administration for Labeling of Special Purpose Foods. If a food or food supplement is represented to be for special dietary use by man by reason of its vitamin or mineral properties, the label must bear a statement of the proportion of the minimum daily requirement for such vitamins or minerals supplied by the food or food supplement when consumed in specified quantity during the period of 1 day. For the purpose of regulation, the minimum daily requirements are stated as follows:

| | Infants under 1 Year | Children 1-5 | Children 6-11 | Children 12 yrs. and Over | Adults | Pregnancy or Lactation |
|---|---|---|---|---|---|---|
| Calcium, gm.............. | ....... | 0.75 | 0.75 | 0.75 | 0.75 | 1.5 |
| Phosphorus, gm.......... | ....... | 0.75 | 0.75 | 0.75 | 0.75 | 1.5 |
| Iron, mg................ | ....... | 7.5 | 10.0 | 10.0 | 10.0 | 15.0 |
| Iodine, mg.............. | ....... | 0.1 | 0.1 | 0.1 | 0.1 | 0.1 |
| Vitamin A, U.S.P. units... | 1,500 | 3,000 | 3,000 | 4,000 | 4,000 | ....... |
| Thiamine, mg........... | 0.25 | 0.5 | 0.75 | 1.0 | 1.0 | ....... |
| Riboflavin, mg.......... | 0.5 | ....... | ....... | 2.0 | 2.0 | ....... |
| Niacin, mg............. | 5.0 | 5.0 | 7.5 | 7.5 | 10.0 | ....... |
| Ascorbic acid, mg........ | 10.0 | 20.0 | 20.0 | 30.0 | 30.0 | ....... |
| Vitamin D, U.S.P. units... | 400 | 400 | 400 | 400 | 400 | ....... |

\* Food and Drug Administration, U.S. Department of Health, Education, and Welfare: Title 21, Code of Federal Regulations and 21 CFR, 1959 Supplement, and amended as in Federal Register, June 1, 1957.

## REFERENCE LIST FOR GLOSSARY

1. NATIONAL ACADEMY OF SCIENCES, NATIONAL RESEARCH COUNCIL. Recommended Dietary Allowances. 6th revised ed. Washington, D.C.: National Academy of Sciences, National Research Council Publication 1146, 1964.
2. U.S. FOOD AND DRUG ADMINISTRATION. Minimum Daily Requirements of Certain Vitamins and Minerals. U.S. Department of Health, Education, and Welfare, Food and Drug Administration, Federal Register, 22:3841, 1957. Also in Code of Federal Regulations, Title 21, and 21 CFR Supplement 1959. (See Table 46.)
3. WATT, B. D., and MERRILL, A. L. Composition of Foods—Raw, Processed, Prepared. U.S. Department of Agriculture Handbook No. 8, revised 1963.
4. ZOOK, E. G., MACARTHUR, M. J., and TOEPFER, E. W. Pantothenic Acid in Foods. U.S. Department of Agriculture Handbook No. 97, 1956.
5. MATTICE, M. R. Bridges' Food and Beverage Analyses. Philadelphia: Lea and Febiger, 1950, pp. 201–15.
6. LEVERTON, R. M. Amino Acid Requirements of Youg Adults. In Protein and Amino Acid Nutrition, ed. A. A. ALBANESE. New York: Academic Press, 1959, p. 504.
7. ORR, M. L., and WATT, B. K. Amino Acid Content of Foods. U.S. Department of Agriculture, Home Economics Research Report No. 4, 1957. (See Table 40.)
8. Nutritive Value of Foods, U.S. Department of Agriculture, Home and Garden Bulletin No. 72, Washington, D.C., revised September, 1964.
9. Annual Reports and Proceedings, American Dietetic Association, 1945–46, p. 35.
10. Occupational Analysis Branch, U.S. Employment Service, Dictionary of Occupational Titles, Second Ed., Suppl. I. (Washington: U.S. Department of Labor, Bureau of Employment Security, Division of Placement Methods, March, 1955.)
11. TOEPFER, E. W., ZOOK, E. G., ORR, M. L., and RICHARDSON, L. R. Folic Acid Content of Foods. U.S. Department of Agriculture Handbook No. 29, 1951.
12. HARRIS, P. L., QUAIFE, M. L., and SWANSON, W. J. Vitamin E content of foods. J. Nutr., 40:367, 1950.
13. LICHTENSTEIN, H., BELOIAN, A., and MURPHY, E. W. Vitamin $B_{12}$—Microbiological assay methods and distribution in selected foods. U.S. Department of Agriculture, Home Economics Research Report No. 13, 1961.

# INDEX